Cyberprotest

CU00746912

Since the Seattle anti-globalization protests in 1999 the adoption of new information and communications technologies (ICTs) by social movement activists has offered the prospect of a serious challenge to traditional forms of political participation. With its transnational, many-to-many communication facility, the internet offers revolutionary potential for social movements to speak directly to the citizens of the world, circumventing the 'official' messages of political organizations and traditional media. Furthermore, electronic mail, mailing lists, websites, electronic forums and other online applications provide powerful tools for coordinating activity among geographically dispersed individuals, and for shaping collective identity.

This book critically assesses how ICTs are finding their way into the world of social movements, considering overarching issues and providing examples of cyberprotest movements from across the globe. It will be valuable reading for students and academics in politics, media and communication, public administration, sociology and ICT. It will also be of great interest to policy makers and social activists.

Wim van de Donk is Professor of Public Administration at Tilburg University, The Netherlands and member of the Scientific Council for Government Policy in The Hague. **Brian D. Loader** is Director of the Community Informatics Research and Applications Unit based at the University of Teesside, UK. He is also Editor of the international journal *Information, Communication & Society*. **Paul G. Nixon** is a Senior Lecturer in Political Science at the Haagse Hogeschool, The Hague, The Netherlands. **Dieter Rucht** is Professor of Sociology at the Social Science Research Center, Berlin, Germany.

Cyberprotest

New media, citizens and social
movements

**Edited by Wim van de Donk,
Brian D. Loader, Paul G. Nixon,
Dieter Rucht**

Foreword by Peter Dahlgren

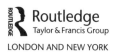

Routledge
Taylor & Francis Group

LONDON AND NEW YORK

First published 2004
by Routledge
11 New Fetter Lane, London EC4P 4EE

Simultaneously published in the USA and Canada
by Routledge
29 West 35th Street, New York, NY 10001

Routledge is an imprint of the Taylor & Francis Group

© 2004 selection and editorial matter, Wim van de Donk,
Brian D. Loader, Paul G. Nixon, Dieter Rucht; individual
chapters, the contributors

Typeset in Sabon by BC Typesetting Ltd, Bristol
Printed and bound in Great Britain by
MPG Books Ltd, Bodmin, Cornwall

British Library Cataloguing in Publication Data
A catalogue record for this book is available from the British Library

Library of Congress Cataloging in Publication Data
A catalog record for this book has been requested

ISBN 0–415–29784–2 (hbk)
ISBN 0–415–29785–0 (pbk)

Contents

Contributors

W. Lance Bennett is Professor of Political Science and Ruddick C. Lawrence Professor of Communication at the University of Washington, USA. He directs the Center for Communication and Civic Engagement (www.engagedcitizen.org) and has begun a project on global citizenship and communication technology (www.globalcitizenproject.org). lbennett@u.washington.edu

Kerry Brown is a Senior Lecturer in the School of Management at Queensland University of Technology, Brisbane, Australia. ka.brown@qut.edu.au

Gustavo Cardoso is an Assistant Professor of Information and Communication Sciences at the Department of Information Sciences and Technologies at ISCTE Lisbon, Portugal. He lectures in the degrees of Sociology in the MCs of Communication, Culture and Information Technologies and Digital Libraries, and in the Post-Degree on Journalism. He also works as a researcher at the Communication Studies Research Team of ISCTE and, during the past five years, he has been conducting research related to the Information Society national policies and working as an adviser for 'Information Society and Telecommunications' at the Portuguese Presidency of the Republic. gustavo.cardoso@iscte.pt

Rita Cheta is a PhD candidate in Sociology and Communications Studies at ISCTE, Lisbon, Portugal. She is a junior research-member at CIES and is a researcher of the Communication Studies Research Team at ISCTE. Her previous research related to Portuguese mass media representations of crime, social contexts of ICT uses in Portugal and the underlying identity transformation processes. rita.cheta@totalise.co.uk

Arthur Edwards is senior lecturer at the Department of Public Administration, Erasmus University, Rotterdam. His research fields are: ICTs and democracy, local democracy, and the public sphere. His most recent research concerns comparative research on interactive policy making in Dutch municipalities and also on new forms of local democracy in European countries. edwards@fsw.eur.nl

Brigitte le Grignou is Professor of Political Science at the Paris Dauphine University, France. Her research focuses on political communication, particularly in relation to the use of television as a political communication media, on social movements and audience studies. b.legrignou@free.fr

Brian D. Loader is Director of the Community Informatics Research and Applications Unit (www.cira.org.uk) based at the University of Teesside, UK. He is also General Editor of the international journal *Information, Communication & Society* (www.infosoc.co.uk) and has edited a number of books including *The Governance of Cyberspace* (Routledge, 1997), *Cyberspace Divide* (Routledge, 1998), (with Barry Hague) *Digital Democracy* (Routledge, 1999), (with Doug Thomas) *Cybercrime* (Routledge, 2000), (with Leigh Keeble) *Community Informatics* (Routledge, 2001), (with Bill Dutton) *The Digital Academe* (Routledge, 2002), and (with David Bell, Nicholas Pleace, and Doug Schuler) *Key Concepts in Cyberculture* (Routledge, 2004). He has also published articles and reports on technological change and social and political restructuring. b.d.loader@tees.ac.uk

Pedro Pereira Neto is conducting research in the field of the impact of ICTs on the Mass Media and of Social and Economic Inclusion and ICTs. He is an affiliate researcher at CAV_ISCTE (Center for Audiovisual Technologies at ISCTE). His recent research projects and publications concern: digital libraries and citizens' use of the internet, and social movements and new media. pedropneto@netcabo.pt

Joyce Y.M. Nip is Assistant Professor in the Department of Journalism at Hong Kong Baptist University. joycenip@hkbu.edu.hk

Paul G. Nixon is a Senior Lecturer in Political Science at the Haagse Hogeschool, Den Haag, The Netherlands. He is a visiting Professor of European Politics at Mitthögskolan, Sweden. He has contributed chapters to many edited collections on the use of ICTs, particularly in the fields of political parties, electronic democracy and social welfare. He is at present editing a book, *Political Parties and the Internet*, for Routledge (with Steve Ward and Rachel Gibson). He has also published in the fields of culture and literature, including editing a collection entitled *Representations of Education in Literature* (Edwin Mellen Press, 2000). p.nixon@sost.hhs.nl

Charles Patou is a PhD student in Political Science at the Paris Dauphine University, France. His research focuses on political communication, social movements and social movement expertise. charles.patou@dauphine.fr

Barbara Pini is a Postdoctoral Researcher in the School of Management at Queensland University of Technology, Brisbane, Australia. b.pini@qut.edu.au

Josephine Previte is Associate Lecturer at University of Queensland Business School, Ipswich, Australia. j.previte@business.uq.edu.au

Jacob Rosenkrands is a journalist and commentator for the weekly magazine *Mandag Morgen*, based in Copenhagen, Denmark, which offers selective news coverage and analysis for those working at a senior level in business, politics and the third sector in Denmark. He covers topics centred around business affairs, politics, political campaigning, protest, and social movements, and has a particular interest in issues relating to the renewal of democracy. jacobr@jacobr.dk

Dieter Rucht is Professor of Sociology at the Social Science Research Center, Berlin, Germany. His research interests include modernization processes in a comparative perspective, social movements and political protest. Among his recent books are: (together with Ruud Koopmans and Friedhelm Neidhardt, eds) *Acts of Dissent*, Boulder, CO: Rowman and Littlefield, 1999; (together with Donatella della Porta and Hanspeter Kriesi, eds) *Social Movements in a Globalizing World*, Basingstoke: Macmillan, 1999; (together with Myra Marx Ferree, William Gamson, and Jürgen Gerhards) *Shaping Abortion Discourse: Democracy and the Public Sphere in Germany and the United States*, Cambridge: Cambridge University Press 2002; (together with Lee Ann Banaszak and Karen Beckwith, eds) *Women's Movements Facing the Reconfigured State*. Cambridge: Cambridge University Press, 2003. rucht@medea.wz-berlin.de

Peter Van Aelst is a member of the Communication Department and a researcher in the 'Media, Movements and Politics' group of the University of Antwerp (Belgium). His research focuses on social movements and political campaigns, with special interest in the role of the (new) media. vanaelst@uia.ua.ac.be

Wim van de Donk is Professor of Public Administration at Tilburg University, and a member of the Scientific Council for Government Policy in The Hague. He has published widely on the meaning of informatization for the democratic arena, e.g. books published in the IOS Press series on 'informatization developments in the public sector', notably *Orwell in Athens* (IOS, 1995) and *Public Administration in an Information Age* (IOS, 1998), and (together with Steve Coleman and John Taylor) *Parliaments in an Information Age* (Oxford University Press, 2000). wim.b.h.j.vddonk@uvt.nl

Stefaan Walgrave is Professor of Political Science and Co-ordinator of the Media Movements and Politics Group (M2P) at the University of Antwerp, Belgium. His current research focuses on social movements, civil society, extreme right parties and media and politics. walgrave@uia.ua.ac.be

Steve Wright is a Research Fellow at the University of Monash, Australia. His PhD concerned workers' responses to industrial restructuring in Italy during the 1960s and 1970s, and is to be published by Pluto Press in Britain. Workplace politics in Italy and Australia remain among his research interests, along with the place of information technologies in social movements, and the question of online access for disadvantaged groups, such as people with disabilities. steven.wright@sims.monash.edu.au

Foreword

Peter Dahlgren

Since the early 1990s the signs of democracy's dilemmas have internationally become increasingly apparent. Political systems modelled on the Western liberal model show signs of stagnation; the margins of governmental manoeuvrability are narrowing. Institutions central to democratic life, in particular political parties, seem less responsive in the face of the major changes of late modernity. The sovereignty of the nation-state itself is being downsized in the face of neo-liberal globalization, as well as – in the European context – the EU. In the latter case democracy is being challenged to develop at the supranational regional level. In Central and Eastern Europe, the new democratic institutions struggle to take root. In Asia, Latin America and Africa, many societies are still in the process of trying to make the transition from authoritarian to democratic regimes.

Among citizens in the West, the arena of official politics has witnessed a decline in support and participation. Voter turnouts are decreasing, party loyalty is in decline, especially among the young. One can see signs of contempt for the political class, with a climate of cynicism emerging in some places. The extensive disenchantment with formal politics and the crisis of citizenship are themes addressed by many today. Economic insecurity, unemployment, low wages, declining social services, growing class cleavages, ecological dilemmas, and a sense of powerlessness among many citizens are all part of the picture. One can speak of a retreat from public culture, with an ever-increasing emphasis on private consumption and life style.

However, we also have evidence of alternative developments, a more optimistic renewal of democracy, largely outside the parliamentarian context, that can be said to represent forms of alternative or 'new politics', 'life politics', life-style politics', or 'sub-politics'. There are a variety of labels, and many variations in the way these alternatives manifest themselves. There are many kinds of social movements, special interest organizations, activist groups, single-issue coalitions, and civic networks. These all suggest that if we look beyond the formal political arena, we can see clear signs that many people have decidedly not retreated from the arena of common concerns and abandoned political engagement. Rather, they have refocused their political attention in other arenas, developed other political targets, and developed other modes of political engagement.

This type of political activity tends to be more *ad hoc*, less dependent on traditional organizations and on elites mobilizing standing cadres of supporters. Some activists are even in the process of redefining just what constitutes politics, guided more by personal values than traditional ideologies; often the focus is on single issues rather than across the board social change. The boundaries between politics, cultural values, identity processes and collective self-reliance become fluid; politics becomes not only an instrumental activity for achieving concrete goals, but even at times an expressive and performative activity, entwined with the development of the self.

Various forms of extra-parliamentarian political activity have of course long been a part of the history of democratic societies. We can note an array of collective action in the informal political domain, including the new social movements of the 1970s and 1980s, the protest movements of the 1960s, as well as class-based struggles and women's movements dating back to the nineteenth century. Yet it is safe to say that such political phenomena took an impressive step forward somewhere in the mid-1990s; in a few years, with some historical hindsight, we may well speak of the start of a new wave of social movements and alternative politics.

Just about concurrent with the growing crisis of democracy in the 1990s we witnessed the emergence of the internet and other digital information and communication technologies (ICTs). It did not take long before many observers began to link the two phenomena: not least, there was considerable armchair theorizing about how the internet might help promote democratic involvement among citizens, or even how it might 'save' democracy. The internet has truly constituted an impressive – even if globally a highly uneven – revolution in communication, and has had an impact on just about all spheres of society and culture. It certainly seemed reasonable to expect that even the dynamics of democracy would experience an impact.

Yet, after a few years of somewhat unfulfilled anticipation, the conventional wisdom has it that the internet, while certainly of political significance, is not about to engender major alterations in the overall way that democratic systems function. Even the results of ambitious experimentation where so-called e-democracy is inserted into the dynamics of the formal system have been modest. A view of 'business as usual' has emerged – at least as far as the formal political system is concerned. However, at the margins of the system, in the domain of informal politics, we see something different emerging. Though the picture is still rather sketchy, we have indications that the new ICTs are playing a much more significant role in the extra-parliamentarian context, in fact even enabling forms of participation that would not have been possible without them.

Theories of democracy have generally treated the communicative interaction among citizens as vital. Talk among citizens is seen as basic to their political participation, to the functioning of the public sphere. This view resides at the centre of most formulations of neo-republicanism, radical or 'strong' democracy, and certainly of what is called deliberative democracy. Today, a good deal of civic discussion takes place on the internet, not only in explicit public forums and within varieties of online journalism, but also within the vast networking of activist organizations and social movements. Though the internet is threatened by both government control and commercialization via market forces, it still offers an incomparable communicative civic space. We observe the emergence of new, fluid publics, citizen networks and affinity groups via the horizontal civic communication that it facilitates.

Not least, we see how the internet helps promote what are called alternative or counter public spheres that can offer a new, empowering sense of what it means to be a citizen. In the context of social movements and activist networks, this is taken one step further via mobilization and the various forms of political practices that they embody. We would do well, however, to avoid idealizing these developments. For one thing, the activists one finds on the net are not all necessarily democratic in character: there are also racists, neo-nazis, and other unsavoury types. Also, given the fluid character of many of these net-based movements, and the ease of joining and withdrawing, it is really difficult to estimate what portion of the citizenry is actually involved. Yet contemporary social movements and their use of ICTs constitute a major element in the landscape of late modern democracy.

It is against the backdrop of this turbulent period in the history of democracy, with an emergent wave of social movements, together with the spread of new ICTs, that this outstanding and ground-breaking anthology makes its intervention. It makes an important contribution precisely by weaving together two trajectories of research: on the one hand, on the current wave of social movements, citizen engagement and mobilization, and on the other, on studies of the new ICTs and their relevance for democracy. Building largely on a series of empirical case studies – and even including, laudably, cases beyond the English-speaking world – this collection moves beyond generalizations and speculation by addressing concretely the implications that ICTs have for various forms of contemporary social movements. The studies highlight the specific attributes of ICTs, in particular the internet, by elucidating the ensemble of attributes and the forms of communication, social relations, and organizational practices that they help foster. Attention is paid to patterns of communication both within the social movement organizations and between them and the external social environment.

Even if many movements today operate in transnational contexts, the impact of national, regional and local political cultures can still be of relevance. Thus, even global movements articulate in complex ways with dominant national political cultures. There have been over the years a number of notable analyses of the strategies that social movements develop *vis à vis* the dominant mass media. Yet, thus far, there has been little work done on how the newer means of communication that movements have at their disposal are used to negotiate their relations with their surroundings. Moreover, our understanding of how the media logic of the digital age enables and modifies the structures and organizational dynamics of these movements is limited. Not least, we need to know more about what impact the ICTs have on the democratic character of the movements, how the use of ICTs affects recruitment and membership of new members, as well as the relationship between online and offline activities for the participants.

Also, we still know little about the impact of media on a related set of concerns that is salient to contemporary social movement research; these concerns derive from versions of late modern social theory. I have in mind such culturalist themes as meaning, identity, subjectivity, and reflexivity – topics that are prominent especially in the European literature. One of the characteristics of late modern society is the emergence of the self as a reflexive project, an ongoing process of the shaping and reshaping of identity, in response to heterogeneous social forces, cultural currents and personal contexts encountered by individuals. These themes have been addressed in regard to ICTs from a variety of angles in some quarters of media and communication studies, as well as in a sector of cultural studies focused on cybercultures. However, their link to ICTs has not been much explored in the social movement literature.

There a number of other topics that weave through these chapters and will continue to be on our research agendas, but I will just mention one more, that of information and knowledge. The new ICTs in general can be seen to be contributing to new ways of knowing, new strategies for gathering, storing, retrieving and utilizing information. The multimedia, digital quality of the ICTs modifies traditional communication forms. To take but one example: hyperlinks on the world wide web erode the strict linearity of traditional text culture. Placed in the context of social movements and the new modes of political engagement, these developments remind us of the old adage that information is power. An essential element in the external strategies of the social movements, as well as in the empowering of their members, has to do with the many ways in which knowledge and expertise can be redistributed, relayed horizontally, even on a global basis. For example, lessons and experiences can be shared with like-minded allies all over the world. Also, the tactical use of information for organizing and coordinating actions, both large and small, provides these movements with an efficacy they could never have had before. Moreover, in the new media environment, traditional hierarchies based on differential knowledge and information access are challenged. Counter-expertise and counter- information, not least in the form of alternative interpretation of current events and access to important data banks, modifies to an important degree traditional imbalances of power between elites and protesters.

The social movement literature as such has been well established for some years; there are a number of traditional analytic approaches that together convey an overall picture of a social terrain characterized by considerable heterogeneity. Thus the book is rightly cautious about drawing too many over-arching conclusions from these case studies. Yet, what it does is provide us with valuable contours of the current state of research – offering us a range of approaches, models, theories and methodologies – as well as pointing explicitly and implicitly toward directions for future research. Contemporary alternative, informal politics involves a variety of organizational forms, strategies, tactics, goals. The net and other ICTs unquestionably play a key role in this emerging realm of political intervention and manifestation. Yet, as this collection reminds us, we should avoid becoming obsessed with just the communication technology itself. Instead we need to include in our analytic horizons the complex ways in which ICTs interplay with the dynamics of the social movements, as well as with mainstream political structures and contemporary cultural trends that frame these movements.

Social movements and ICTs, separately and together, constitute fast-moving and fast-changing analytic targets, and a challenge for research. We who strive to study these areas can feel very grateful to the editors and authors of this volume for providing us with both resources and inspiration.

Peter Dahlgren
Lund University, Sweden

Preface

As a means of facilitating the creation of cross-national, 'dis-organized' networks for collective action on the basis of negotiated common concerns, the internet might almost have been purpose-built for social movements (SMs). A growing body of literature during the last decades of the twentieth century attests to the significant impact SMs have had upon the restructuring of the political landscape. Recently some attention has turned to the potential synergy between the transforming qualities of emerging information and communications technologies (ICTs) and the social movement-driven new cultural politics (Castells 1997, 2001; Webster 2001). What has particularly stimulated this interest is the perceived ascendancy of this cyber-cultural politics against a backdrop of the declining salience of traditional political organization and discourse. The *cyber* organizing of global protests and campaigns is making a strong contrast to declining party membership and falling electoral turnouts in many countries. Drawing upon a series of case studies from various countries, this book provides a critical analysis of the politics of *cyberprotest* by exploring the way the internet and related applications of modern ICTs are actually changing the internal and external organization of SMs.

The introduction of new ICTs into the political domain has been studied extensively in the past decade. Often these studies have tended to explore how such new applications might fuel new possibilities for traditional political institutions (politicians, parliaments, political parties) rather than their possible consequences for SMs. Many of these publications have also contributed to all kinds of digital idealism, which often simply (and even naively) project technological possibilities into social 'realities'. In contrast, in a recent anthology of the social and political implications of new media (1740–1915), Gitelman and Pingree have suggested that initially, 'the place of these new media tends to be ill-defined and that their ultimate meanings and functions are shaped over time by that society's existing habits of media use (which of course, derive from experience with other, established media), by shared desires for new uses, and by the slow process of adaptation between the two' (Gitelman and Pingree 2003: xii). Although their book focuses on media (such as *zograscopes, optical telegraphs* and the *physiognotrace*) that failed to survive for very long, their analysis of 'dead media' is highly interesting for those who explore the meaning of digital ICTs for SMs. Some of the lessons they learned from these historical case studies seem to be highly relevant indeed for the case studies on the meaning of digital ICTs in the domain of SMs that are presented in this book. Their analysis shows how the success of new media is shaped by the 'surviving systems' (concrete historical and institutional contexts) by which they are developed, introduced and socially diffused. The acceptance of such an approach in this collection enables the authors to place the adoption and shaping of ICTs by SMs into everyday life experiences of activists rather than as some kind of completely new phenomena unconnected to past academic analyses of SMs. It thereby attempts to foreground *continuity* as well as *innovation* in discussions of cyberprotest.

Most of the contributions originate from a working-group that was formed within the larger framework of the European Union's COST Action (A14) on government and democracy in the Information Age. This action facilitated the formation of a European and even global network of researchers to undertake an exploration of frontline perspectives on the ways ICTs are changing the internal and external functioning of SMs. It has been further complemented by scholars from around the world whose chapters have been previously published in the journal *Information, Communication & Society* (www.infosoc. co.uk). Although this network has been a virtual network most of the time, using the internet to discuss and exchange papers and chapters, some persons in very real places and organizations have crucially contributed to the production of this book.

The editors would consequently like to thank the scientific officers of the COST Action, Mr Vesa-Mathi Lahti and Mrs Bjørg Ofstad, both of Directorate General on Research; also the chair of the management committee, Prof. Dr Jens Hoff from Copenhagen University for his enthusiasm and diligence throughout the life of the programme. We are indebted for her support to our commissioning editor, Edwina Welham, and wish her enjoyment in her retirement. Special thanks go to Catherine Lincoln, Leigh Keeble and Wilma Bosmans for helpful feedback, excellent organization and helping us to get the manuscript into a publishable format. Finally, we would like to thank our partners

Kim Loader, Evelin Riefer-Rucht, Caroline van de Donk-Evers and
Margaret Nixon for their unerring forbearance and encouragement,
and our younger helpers William and Christopher Loader, Ann and
Maud van de Donk and Patrick Nixon (his dad dedicates his contribution to this book to him), the bringers of joy and playful interludes!

Wim van de Donk, Tilburg, the Netherlands
Brian Loader, Swainby, UK
Paul Nixon, Den Haag, The Netherlands
Dieter Rucht, Berlin
December 2003

1 Introduction

Social movements and ICTs

Wim van de Donk, Brian D. Loader, Paul G. Nixon and Dieter Rucht

Internal and external communication of social movements was and is heavily based on direct interaction among physically present people. However, for at least two hundred years, direct interaction has been complemented by various media such as leaflets, brochures and newsletters to reach large numbers of people both within and outside the movements. Moreover, newspapers and, in later periods, radio and television covered major movement activities. By the late 1960s, probably for the first time in history, some movements conducted protest actions in the knowledge that, literally, 'The Whole World is Watching' (Gitlin 1980). Internal as well as external communication of social movements was facilitated – but certainly not revolutionized – by telephones, copy machines and fax machines. With the most recent information and communication technologies, hereafter called ICTs[1] (particularly portable computers, now morphing with mobile phones to give easy access information), and their links via the world wide web (internet), citizen groups and social movements, like many other organizations and institutions, are likely to reach a new level in the ways in which they mobilize, build coalitions, inform, lobby, communicate, and campaign (Hajnal 2002). Contemporary forms of protest seem to combine 'old-fashioned' technologies such as 'banners' with high-tech mobile tools of communication. Moreover, not only the use of ICTs *within* movements, but also the use of ICTs by some actors in the relevant environment of these movements (e.g. governmental organizations, political parties, citizens, corporations and media organizations) seems to present some threats as well as opportunities for social movements.

This volume seeks to contribute to the scholarly investigation of the use of ICTs by social movements. More specifically it seeks to critically explore, analyse and assess the implications of the use of ICTs (such as the internet) for citizen mobilization and the formation, activities, legitimacy and effectiveness of old, new and 'newest' social movements. The various contributions in this volume present a series of case studies into the use of email, newsgroups, mailing lists, forums, websites, streaming, and 'hacktivism' in the field of citizen groups and social movements. The volume tries to explore to what extent and in which forms social movements and, more specifically, social movement organizations (SMOs) use ICTs. It tries to give an insight into how this use affects the structure and operation of SMOs, including their relationships with members and adherents. Some of the chapters investigate how ICTs change the way SMOs communicate with each other; some others study how SMOs mobilize and intervene in public debates and political conflicts.

By investigating these questions, this volume seeks to contribute to the larger research agenda in the field of ICTs and democracy. This inevitably means that it is an explorative volume. ICTs not only are a relatively recent phenomenon but also have changed so rapidly in the past two decades that we can hardly build on solid ground. Although some research has been done in the field (e.g. van de Donk and Tops 1992; van de Donk *et al.* 1995; Hajnal 2002; Gibson *et al.* 2003), the rapid development of new applications of – especially – digital communication technologies constantly challenges the research agenda.

This lack of systematic knowledge probably applies more to the use of ICTs by mostly informal citizen groups and network-based social movements than to well-established organizations in the realms of business, science, and state administrations. In recent anthologies on ICTs and democracy (e.g. Gibson *et al.* 2003; Hoff *et al.* 2000; Hague and Loader 1999), the more traditional players such as political parties are thoroughly examined. Yet one will look in vain for detailed questions, let alone significant research results, on how other important players in the democratic game, interest groups and social movements, are using ICTs. It appears that the research community has particularly neglected the role of ICTs in the extra-institutional sphere of 'politics' in which loosely structured groups and social movements play a prominent role (but see, for example, Myers 1998; Naughton 2001) This is all the more remarkable in light of the much-debated 'extra-institutional' characteristics and capacities of ICTs (especially the internet) that, allegedly, offer a substantial potential for increased citizen participation. According to leading authors in the field of informatization, ICTs, and more specifically the internet are a challenge to traditional forms of (political) organization in general and to traditional – and mainly representative – democratic practices in particular (e.g. Bekkers 1998; Frissen 1999).

Compared to the clearly identifiable and well-established actors such as major political parties and interest groups, the use of ICTs by social movements is difficult to study because of the very nature of social movements. As stated time and again in and beyond this volume, these tend to be fuzzy and fluid phenomena often without clear boundaries. Although they may include formal organizations as components, on the whole they are not an organization. A social movement typically lacks membership forms, statutes, chairpersons, and the like. It may expand or shrink considerably over relatively short periods of time, and exhibit phases of visibility and latency. Also, unlike political parties, social movements may have significant overlaps with other movements. Moreover, a social movement may quickly change its forms, strategy, tactics, and even some of its goals. In sum, a social movement is a 'moving target', difficult to observe.

While some scholars have stressed the informal, fragmented or even disorganized character of social movements (Gerlach and Hine 1970), others have pointed to the key role of SMOs as the backbone of movements, regardless of their size or thematic focus. Other observers have argued that the degree of organization of social movements is a function of time, usually assuming an early stage in which a social movement is highly informal and later stages in which it becomes more and more institutionalized, eventually developing into a full-blown bureaucratic organization which has lost its character as a (true) movement (Alberoni 1984; Calhoun 1995). Whether there exists such a 'natural life cycle' or – in terms attributed to Robert Michels – an 'iron law of oligarchy' is heavily disputed. However, in defining social movements, most observers would agree that they need some structure and are to some extent 'organized'.[2] This structure, however, is not an organization but a network, or even a *network of networks*, that both rests on and maintains a sense of collective identity. In addition to this structural feature, most recent definitions converge in stressing that social movements, unlike most thematically narrow and short-lived political campaigns, seek to change a given social (and political) order instead of only trying to modify an existing law or replace a political leader. In striving for social change, movements typically, though not exclusively, use 'unconventional' means. Based on these three constitutional elements – aiming for social change, identity-based network structure, and means of protest (Rucht 1994) – it is a matter of the preferred analytical perspective whether the emphasis is more on the interactive nature of a social movement as a series of contentious challenges to authorities (Tilly 1986: 392), the symbolic construction and maintenance of a collective identity (Melucci 1989: 34), or the ensemble of interconnected SMOs striving for similar goals (Zald and McCarthy 1980: 3).

Whatever the preferred definition of a social movement, it is clear that social movements cannot exist without sustained interactions both internally and with their external reference groups. This points to the centrality of communication and, given both the network structure of social movements and their limited financial resources, to the attractiveness of using ICTs.

Whereas the more traditional social movements, e.g. those of peasants and workers, were essentially based on closely-knit and relatively homogeneous milieux bound to particular territories and social locations, this seems to be less true for the more recent social movements, including the so-called new (or even 'newest') social movements. Some of the latter, e.g. the environmental movements, the women's movement, and the Global Justice movements, have a relatively heterogeneous constituency that is only loosely coupled but easily stretches beyond national borders. Moreover, these new movements tend to embrace concepts such as diversity, decentralization, informality and grassroots democracy rather than unity, centralization, formality and strong leadership (Gundelach 1984). Therefore, we would speculate that new social movements are particularly keen to adopt ICTs because these fit their ideological and organizational needs.

It is, indeed, interesting to see how the new social movements (such as the environmental movements) are using the internet for coordinating successfully at the international level, a level that is, to a large extent, characterized by an unsettled mix of institutional indolence and emptiness as far as the formal institutions are concerned (see Reinicke 1998; Hudock 1999). It is also interesting to see how SMOs such as Greenpeace or Friends of the Earth frequently use the internet and related applications to be effective in the public arena (e.g. in mobilizing the 'electorate'). They sometimes almost seem to be more effective than regular political parties in shaping public opinion. As far as the younger generation of citizens is concerned, such SMOs are especially attractive, and the internet is a prime tool to foster this strength. Of course, political parties have also discovered ICTs and the internet (e.g. Frantzich 1989; Bogumil and Lange 1991; van de Donk and Tops 1992; Depla and Tops 1995; Nixon and Johansson 1999;

Smith 2000; Löfgren 2000; Gibson *et al.* 2003), as have with some delay, the trade unions in various countries (see: www.labournet.org). Strikingly, political parties using the internet seem to rediscover some of the movement-like qualities and characteristics they have often lost since they have transformed themselves from the social movements they, to a certain extent, once were, into the tightly organized, centralized and professional organizations they – most of the time – have become. In the machine age, they were much more decentralized at the level of constituencies, wrote petitions and mobilized masses based on their anchorage in specific social milieux. Now, they are smoothly managed political enterprises that more often suppress than encourage dialogue and open debates because such openness might endanger their image and thus their power in the political arena – an arena increasingly defined and constrained by the needs of modern media.

Whether or not such a defensive attitude will last remains to be seen, but it is interesting to see that political parties of the Information Age are in many cases using digital means in an attempt to democratize their party organizations, create discussion groups, and involve 'ordinary' or *ad hoc* members in the drafting of political agendas, voting on selected issues and so on (see also Nixon and Johansson 1999; Löfgren 2000). The scope and effects of such attempts are still unclear, however, and it is especially difficult to predict how the use of ICTs will relate to other factors that transform the political parties as we know them. But is it unthinkable that political parties will be using ICTs to redesign themselves into a more 'social movement'-like type of organization, or that social movements are using them to compete with political parties? ICTs might perhaps not profoundly change the very 'logic' of collective action, but they seem to change, in any case, the structure of some players and probably also affect the kind and speed of political communication and mobilization.

While political parties may also undergo changes partly due to the use of ICTs, we might expect these technologies to be of greater value and have deeper impacts for citizen initiatives and (new) social movements. Thus, in this volume, we focus on the use of ICTs by citizen groups and SMOs, and how that use is shaping, and shaped by, the way these actors operate. Some evidence that they are doing quite well, thanks to the internet, can be found at the international level: the 'battle of Seattle' in December 1999 was – at least for the time being – won by a multifaceted and partly electronically organized coalition of social movements, some of them already of a predominantly virtual character themselves (Smith 2000). After 'Seattle', a series of events in which 'new media strategies' and 'cyber activism' played a dominant role have attracted yet more attention. However, as Bennett shows in Chapter 6, cyber activism is not so new. Yet more and more, the internet seems to be being developed as a new 'strategic platform' that helps a variety of movements to mobilize and to organize protest (Warkentin 2001). De Wilde *et al.* (2003) suggest a *Wahlverwandschaft* (an elective affinity) between the nongovernmental organizations (NGOs) and social movements on the one hand and the internet on the other, and show how these have influenced each other: 'The internet is not used as a mere supplement to traditional media, it also offers new, innovative opportunities for mobilizing and organizing individuals. The new technologies, however, do not determine these innovations. The internet provokes innovation, but this innovation has to be organized and disseminated. NGOs are specially innovative in this field: not only has the internet helped these organizations, NGOs were also very important for the further development of the internet' (De Wilde *et al.* 2003: 48). Many chapters in this volume confirm these general contentions about the role of the internet.

Before we will be able to explore that role, we want, in this introductory chapter, to discuss how some of the existing conceptual approaches in the field of social movement theory can support our endeavour, thus developing a more systematic research agenda, and establishing a link between two realms that so far are mainly 'disconnected': theoretical approaches to the study of social movements and the actual use of ICTs by SMOs. Moreover, we seek to avoid an excessively exclusive (or even 'deterministic') focus on technology in studying its 'impacts' on social and political practices. It is important to underline that these 'impacts' must be considered as 'outcomes' that emerge from a complex interplay between existing institutions and practices on the one hand and (the characteristics of) new technologies on the other hand (see van de Donk and Snellen 1998).

Later in this chapter we will briefly present those approaches to social movements that are potentially relevant for aspects of internal and external communication, and thus also relevant for the study of the use of ICTs by social movements. Secondly, we will single out some dimensions relevant to the empirical case studies that are presented in this book and offer some hypotheses on the use of ICTs by SMOs. Lastly, we will give a brief outline of the chapters that follow.

Social movements theories: the role of communication and mobilization

Social movements vary greatly in ideology, aims, size, social background, organizational structure and activities. Even when looking at the same movement, different analysts highlight different aspects, often following their specific scientific paradigms and research interests. Several scholars have provided overviews on what they perceive to be the most influential or distinct social movements theories. Not surprisingly, these categorizations also exhibit some variation. Dalton (1994), for example, partly drawing on the work of others, has typified five approaches: the classic (collective behaviour) perspective, the resource-mobilization perspective, the perspective of the political opportunity structure, the ideologically structured perspective, and the discourse or social constructionist perspective. A similar typology can be found in Hellmann (1998), who distinguished between 'movement paradigms' focusing on structural strain, collective identity, framing, resource mobilization, and political opportunity structures. Others, drawing mainly on the literature in the 1970 and 1980s, have juxtaposed the resource mobilization approach originating from the US, and the new social movements approach developed by European scholars, but also stressed the links of these approaches to more specific concepts referring to relative deprivation, political opportunities and process theories (Neidhardt and Rucht 1991; Rucht and Neidhardt 2002). Looking further back in history, one may additionally identify a mass psychology approach, which flourished at the turn of the twentieth century. Broadening the perspective, one can also point to a rational choice approach that reduces social movement to nothing more than an aggregate of individual decisions to participate in joint action. Things become even more complicated when taking into account that each of these approaches, which can be seen as having a distinct label, is, indeed, internally differentiated. For example, with regard to the 'collective behaviour' approach, one can distinguish between a structural and a symbolic interactionist school. In sum, things are less simple than most typologies suggest.

In the context of this book, it is not our intention to discuss these typologies, let alone to present a further one, nor do we want to present one or several of these approaches in much detail. Instead, we refer to various approaches only to the extent that they focus on aspects that are relevant to our concern, that is the internal and external communication of social movements, and the way they present themselves to the public and mobilize their constituency.

Communication as a tool of resource mobilization

Whereas some social psychologists considered social movements as a result of 'contagion' among more or less irrational people lacking clear goals and the will or capacity to organize and act strategically, proponents of the resource mobilization perspective took the opposite stance. It was the involvement of many middle-class people, including intellectuals and professionals, in the movements of the 1960s (e.g. the civil rights movement) that led analysts to take a more positive and realistic view on social movements in general. Schwarz, for example, claimed that 'participants in social movements are at least as rational as those who study them' (Schwarz, cited in Buechler 2000: 34). Rational, instrumentally oriented action requires organization, and therefore the role of social movement organizations (SMOs) was put at the centre of interest and investigation (McCarthy and Zald 1977). According to this view, SMOs can be paralleled to economic activities in a competitive field with relatively scarce resources. In consequence, resource mobilization theorists also suggested categories such as 'social movement industries' and 'social movement entrepreneurs'. Unlike in earlier theories, the rise and fall of movement activity was considered to be a function not of structural strain (Smelser 1962), objective (Karl Marx) or relative deprivation (Gurr 1970), or the existence of charismatic leaders (Max Weber), but of the SMOs' ability to collect and use resources such as money, activists' time, commitment, and knowledge. When overviewing the course of social movements in the US over a long time span, resource mobilization theorists argued that there is a general trend towards organization-building and professionalization – a trend that they found quite logical and, as engaged citizens, would hardly oppose. Other social movement scholars such as Piven and Cloward (1977) confirmed such a trend but, on normative and political grounds, heavily criticized it as a way for movement leaders to pursue their personal interests, to de-power and pacify the rank and file, and to integrate the movement into the established system.

Within the resource mobilization approach resources were usually measured as the amount of money and numbers of staff, volunteers and members, but the actual process in which these resources were gathered or mobilized was either neglected or studied in a mainly descriptive fashion by focusing, for example, on particular techniques such as canvassing or direct mailing. From a resource mobilization perspective, however, these techniques are potentially powerful tools to build organizations, to collect and disseminate information, and to mobilize for action. Moreover, resource mobilization theorists have pointed to the existence of different movement structures, distinguishing, for example, between more centralized and more federated structures, again without paying much attention to what such structures imply in terms of different ways and means of communication and their consequences. While the more conventional means of communication were relatively expensive and tended to foster just a few centres of communication (and often related to this, of power and decision-making), ICTs do not necessarily exhibit an inherent tendency to be concentrated and controlled in the hands of a few movement entrepreneurs. To be sure, ICTs can be effectively used to build and maintain powerful and centralized organizations, but empirical evidence also suggests that ICTs can be effective tools to establish and run decentralized networks that allow those who are technically linked to air their views, and, if needed, to mobilize a virtual or physical community of activists.

One of the criticisms levelled against the resource mobilization approach is that it reduces multidimensional processes to mere organizational matters, thereby devoting (too) little attention to the ideological and cultural aspects of the functioning of social movements (Buechler 1993, 2000). Additionally, it considers communication only as an instrument to mobilize resources without considering that both an instrumental attitude in general and the use of particular techniques of mobilization are not neutral approaches but have consequences for the internal structure of an SMO and its relationships with adherents, allies, and bystanders. Moreover, resource mobilization theories have focused mainly on the micro- and meso-levels, largely ignoring the connection with the macro-level and thus the structural setting in which social movements act.

Communication as structured interaction with external reference groups

Perspectives that are labelled 'political opportunity' and 'political process' approaches share with resource mobilization theory the assumption that social movements are essentially rational and instrumentally oriented actors. In contrast to the resource mobilization theory, which focuses on the relations within and between SMOs, the two other approaches put much emphasis to the way social movements interact with external reference groups (e.g. allies, opponents, state authorities, mass media, bystanders) in a given setting. The two approaches differ somewhat in their focus. While political opportunity (structure) perspectives, as represented for example by Tarrow (1998), Kitschelt (1986) and Kriesi *et al.* (1995), consider relatively inert structural features (e.g. regime structures, access to the decision-making system) as crucial explanatory factors for the levels and/or forms of social movement mobilization, the political process perspective pays more attention to (a) the interactive dynamics between movements and their reference groups, and (b) the changing (political) opportunities which, in part, can also be influenced by social movements (Tilly 1978; McAdam 1982; Rucht 1996; Gamson and Meyer 1996). Various dimensions and factors usually located at the macro- and meso-levels are considered to be of critical importance to the functioning of social movements. This is especially apparent in international comparative research that was partly responsible for the development of these approaches. Why was the peace movement strong in Germany and The Netherlands, but not in France? Why do French movements tend to be more radical than those in Scandinavian countries? The explanations could be found not in the capability to organize the available resources, but rather in the structure and combination of opportunities that were connected to the political system in particular or, more generally, to the 'societal context structure' (Rucht 1996). Within these approaches, the focus is on the most important political divisions/contradictions (can a social movement break free of the dominant divisions between left and right, and how does an electoral system contribute to that?), the formal institutions (e.g. the level of vertical centralization, horizontal concentration, the representativeness of the electoral system, and the role of direct democracy), and the dominant strategy towards social movements that is employed by the formal political institutions (facilitating, assimilative, cooperative; or repressive, confrontational, polarizing).

In spite of these approaches' emphasis on interaction, relatively little attention has been paid to the content, means and channels of communication of the groups involved. Interaction is essentially conceived as a power game in which the actors choose certain arenas, strategies and tactics, forge alliances, challenge and probably threaten opponents, seize or miss opportunities, etc. The concrete communication and mobilization processes that underlie these interactions, however, are largely neglected. Collective actors are mainly studied as 'entities' appearing on a public stage and addressing themselves to other actors, whereas their internal communication, their forms of organization, and all the activities preceding or following the (joint) action at the public stage, remain essentially a black box. Moreover, the fact that much of the communication between social movements and their reference group is indirect in so far as the actors observe and talk to each other via the mass media, is, at best, acknowledged but hardly studied in its implications. Hence it would be important to analyse and interpret the latent and explicit messages to the audience. Also, political opportunity and process theories have not reflected on the implications of different ways to keep an SMO or a whole movement together. It may well be that movements which are primarily built on direct communication of people knowing each other tend to operate differently, even in public arenas, to movements whose adherents are structurally isolated from each other, and therefore have to be bound together mainly by media such as newsletters, journals, or mass actions.

From the political opportunity and political process perspective, the use of ICTs is likely to have consequences for the ways in which social movements interact with their environment. For example, ICTs could improve a movement's capacity to act in a coordinated and coherent way, to react more quickly to an external challenge, and to become less dependent on the established mass media in conveying their messages to a broad audience. More generally, we would expect that action and reaction follow each other in ever shorter cycles, and the speed of diffusion of new ideas, tactics and arguments will increase considerably. Also, the availability of ICTs could facilitate mobilization across large territories, as illustrated by recent campaigns such as the protests against the World Trade Organization in Seattle in December 1999. In addition, the availability of ICTs could make certain kinds of actions, e.g. collections of signatures, more likely than, say, those where participants have to physically meet each other, e.g. a street blockade.

Ideology, identity and persuasion aspects of communication

Using an analogy inspired by the language of ICTs, one could say that all approaches mentioned so far concentrate on the 'hardware' of social movements and their environment. In contrast, other approaches deal with the 'software' of internal and external social movement communication, pointing to the relevance of content, and the non-instrumental, expressive side of social movements. According to this view, social movements cannot be understood without considering their ideological beliefs, their need to create a collective identity, and their attempts to persuade and mobilize their followers to frame the problems they deem relevant and to appeal to their wider environment. According to this perspective, aims and content matter. Dalton, for example, argues that the choice of specific goals and actions is mainly dependent on the core values and ideological principles of a movement rather than an intelligent anticipation of its opportunity structure, although – more in line with opportunity structure theories – he also finds that movements that are financially supported by their government are less inclined to use radical means, and are focused on influencing policy rather than mobilizing public opinion. In his empirical research of the structure and recent history of European environmental movements, he concludes that 'Any systemic differences between nations are outweighed by the variation across groups within nations' (Dalton 1994: 209). His 'data support Lipsky's dictum that protest is the politics of the powerless, organizations with abundant resources were more likely to work through conventional channels' (Dalton 1994: 202).

Other approaches concentrating on the content of social movement messages were inspired by social constructionist theories. They study social movements from the perspective of so-called 'frames': organizing ideas (catchwords, images) that describe or represent a problem that, from the viewpoint of the scientific observer, is not inherently given but a social construction. A variant of this perspective is known as the discursive approach. It studies behavioural practices in relation to competition about 'frames' and 'discourses'. For example: is the problem of congested roads an environmental problem or an obstacle to the desire for, or economic need of, mobility? How are the perceptions of a certain 'problem' managed? (Important authors in this tradition are Snow and Benford 1992; Klandermans 1989; Gamson 1998.) 'Frames' are clues for identifying and interpreting a problem, its dimensions, causes, and probably potential remedies. For example, civil nuclear power can be interpreted according to a 'progress' frame, a view that dominated until the 1960s, or a subsequent 'devil's bargain' frame, according to which nuclear power has advantages but also inherent risks (Gamson and Modigliani 1989). Frames can be specific but may also overarch a set of interrelated issues. Snow and Benford (1992) argue that 'master frames' are crucial as they can provide an entire social movement with a sense of direction: master frames 'provide the interpretive medium through which collective actors associated with different movements within a cycle assign blame for the problem they are attempting to ameliorate' (1992: 139). Because of their generic nature, master frames may colour and constrain the punctuations, attributions and articulations 'of any number of movement organizations' (1992: 138). For this reason, the concept provides a potential bridge between the largely micro-level focus of the frames that relate to everyday experiences and the macro-level of a movement's ideology and its links to broader cultural values such as equality, solidarity, and injustice (Buechler 2000: 42; see also Pellow 1999; Capek 1993; Perrolle 1993).

When considering the role and impacts of frames, we can hardly assume that ICTs are just a technical expansion of existing means of communication. Compare, for example, the oral word in a conversation, the written word on, say, a flyer or in a newspaper, and the word transmitted by electronic means. In the first case, the word is usually ephemeral and irreversibly lost after the encounter. Nevertheless, it may have a deep impact once we feel that the speaker is honest and authentic. Conversely, mimics and tone may tell us that the speaker is unsure or may even lie. In the second case, we can assume that the word is not spontaneously chosen but well-reflected, probably being the result of a long process of deliberation. In the case of an electronic message, we tend to give more weight to speed than to accuracy. Moreover, if messages come from unknown persons, we can assume in many cases that they did not pass the filter of professional journalistic criteria such as providing a correct, balanced account and checking the credibility of sources. Thus we may read electronic information from an unknown sender with more suspicion than the same information in a well-established newspaper.

Important in this approach is what Gamson refers to as 'robust collective-action frames': these connect everyday experiences, media discourse and more or less clear core values (equality, justice). The role of media (who has access, who determines images?) and information-ecologies (who owns, produces, controls relevant data?) is likely to be a relevant dimension that might be influenced by new media or ICT development. What does it mean that the internet will facilitate citizen action groups and SMOs to have their own unmediated broadcasting channels?

In Table 1.1, we try to condense some aspects of the discussion above by listing the key dimensions that are stressed by three different approaches dealing with social movement communication and mobilization.

In this volume we have used these 'key dimensions' to guide our exploration into the use of ICTs by SMOs. Each of these dimensions suggests some specific research questions. Now we will see how these dimensions may help us to formulate these questions by looking

Table 1.1 Initial key elements of approaches to social movements

Approach	Some key dimensions
Resource mobilization	• Organizational structure and linkages/ mobilization of members and other resources; • Professionalization/Institutionalization.
Political opportunity structure and political process	• Structural conditions and reference groups in the movement's environment, interaction shaped by both structural and contingent factors.
Ideology, identity, persuasion	• Core values, collective identity, management of frames and perceptions.

more specifically into the use of ICTs in the domain of the environmental movement organizations.

Social movements using ICTs: preliminary observations and questions for research

The domain of environmental movements

Even when considering one single but broad movement such as the environmental movement in a given country, one is struck by the plethora of ideological tendencies, issue areas, networks and organizations, and forms of action. We would speculate that the quality of these features has an effect on the extent to which and the way in which ICTs are used. Some of them do relate more or less explicitly to the SMOs that are mentioned below. Let us examine some of these questions before moving to specific empirical examples of various environmental SMOs' websites.

Ideology

In terms of their basic ideology, several observers have distinguished between three major strands: an apolitical conservationism, a political but mainly pragmatic environmentalism, and a more radical and fundamentalist political ecology (Rucht 1989, Diani 1995). We would speculate that over the past decade or so pragmatic environmentalist groups have become more prone to the use of ICTs than the two other tendencies because they are used to thinking in terms of an instrumental rationality and are more open to any kind of organizational and technical innovation concerning their own operations.

Issues

Although the environmental movement, broadly speaking, can be identified with all sustained efforts of non-state collective actors to protect the natural environment, in practice the movement is differentiated, if not fragmented, into a broad variety of issue domains which, in turn, can be subdivided into more specific thematic concerns and campaigns. Some groups are fighting against the civil use of nuclear power, others try to protect the rainforests, still others oppose the pollution of the oceans. In each of these areas, there exist more specialized networks or groups, e.g. fighting against the construction of a nuclear reprocessing plant, specializing in the rainforest in Brazil, or campaigning against the transport of hazardous waste across the oceans. At this point, we have little reason to assume why actors in certain issue areas, by the very content of these areas, are more prone to use ICTs than actors in other issue areas. However, we would hypothesize that the use of ICTs is particularly widespread and sophisticated in areas where transnational, let alone global, problems are tackled. A telling example is the concern about global warming and climate change. Here we find much cross-national cooperation based on an extensive use of ICTs. For example, Climate Action Network (CAN), with its few and relatively small offices, is heavily dependent on the use of the internet since it disseminates information to and, occasionally, mobilizes groups from all parts of the globe.

Networks and organizations

Also in structural terms we find a great variety of forms within the environmental movements, ranging from small and informal local groups to regular membership organizations on a national level, to decentralized or centralized supranational organizations, to worldwide but loosely coupled networks. We expect that two of these structures are more inclined to use ICTs than others. First, we assume that large and powerful organizations, e.g. the Sierra Club in the USA, are very quick in recognizing and exploiting the advantages of ICTs to facilitate internal communication, to keep their (physically distant) members informed, to present themselves to outsiders via homepages, and to communicate with other groups. This process is enhanced by the fact that the big players have the financial means to buy the necessary hardware and to hire specialists creating websites and running the systems. Second, we also assume that organizations and networks spanning larger territories, even when they are relatively poor in resources, are prone to adopt ICTs simply because these technologies are more effective and cheaper than distributing letters, papers, brochures, and calls for action by regular mail. Hence we should not be surprised that groups such as Greenpeace International, Friends of the Earth International and the World Wide Fund for Nature are among those who were early adopters of ICTs and continue to use them extensively.

Strategies and forms of activities

If one locates strategies on a spectrum marked by a pole of extreme radicalism on the one hand and extreme pragmatism/conformity on the other, we hypothesize that on both ends ICTs are less frequently used compared to the middle ground. Radical groups are usually quite segregated from their moderate environments and focus more on dense and personal communication within small circles for which ICTs are of limited value, although the changing natures of ICTs such as the use of mobile telephony may cause pause for thought here. Moreover, radical groups must also fear surveillance by control agencies that may tap or reconstruct electronic communication. For different reasons, the very moderate and pragmatic groups also appear to be less eager to use ICTs (apart from office technologies) because, in relative terms, they have good access to established interest groups, the mass media and political decision-makers, often by relying on formal meetings or informal contacts.

It is obvious that characteristics in these dimensions can be combined in many ways. Sometimes they may reinforce each other in favour of or against the use of ICTs; at other times they may work in opposite directions and neutralize each other. For example, we can assume that an organization such as Greenpeace is very keen on the use of ICTs for several reasons mentioned above: it deals with a number of environmental problems that transcend national borders, it is composed of sections in many countries, it links a great number of adherents in a large number of territories, it is a centralized organization with considerable financial resources, and it acts, though at times breaking the law, in a disciplined and strictly non-violent way.

As noted earlier, the actual use of ICTs by various social movements has undergone limited investigation to date. From casual observations and remarks in the literature we know that ICTs are generally making their way within social movements and other political groups, though to different degrees and at different paces (Bieber 1999). Recent transnational social movement campaigns, e.g. mobilizations against meetings of the World Trade Organization, the International Monetary Fund and the World Bank, indicate that these protests are heavily dependent on the internet. But also national or sub-national conflicts, e.g. the struggle of the Zapatista movement in Mexico or the movement against the Narmada dam system in India, are widely discussed and supported in the internet. According to an analysis based on the websites and a questionnaire of all political groups to be found in 1996 in Germany (excluding student organizations), more than 30 per cent of the groups could be attributed to social movements, followed by parties and their sub-units, employers' organizations, trade unions and other groups (Prümm 1996). The current recent research of Rucht and Roose (2001) on environmental organizations in Germany suggests that probably two-thirds of the nationwide players investigated in 1997/98 offered websites on the internet.

A 'quick scan' of websites of various environmental organizations – e.g. Greenpeace, Friends of the Earth, World Wide Fund for Nature, the Institute for Global Communications EcoNet, the Sierra Club and Earth First! – can ascertain the ways in which these groups take advantage of some of the possibilities offered by the ICTs. It seems, at first sight, to confirm the widely held belief that technology is currently a facilitator of social movement activities. Writing letters, mobilization and donations are all, of course, possible in the physical world, but have been made easier and more accessible by means of technology. With the activities of many of these SMOs largely comparable, the diversity in movements is clearly expressed in mission statements and site layout, accentuating different aspects of social movement activity. Notable is the absence of the use of the internet's interactive possibilities. Although all of the sites mentioned here have email addresses, only a few provide online discussion forums, and communication is still largely a one-way street, the SMO providing the visitor with information. The absence of links to like-minded movements is also remarkable. Although movements like Greenpeace and the World Wide Fund for Nature (WWF) refer to their numerous national sites, hardly any of the SMOs mentioned above refer the visitor to one of the others. However, as hints on various sites prove, collaborative initiatives do exist, though not as part of the individual websites. Instead, a separate website is created, devoted to a single issue or event, a trend started by the already legendary site devoted to the WTO Summit in Seattle.

ICTs and social movements: preliminary observations

- Our discussion of various theoretical perspectives on social movements has shown that these approaches address different levels of attention to internal and/or external communication processes. They also highlight different aspects of these processes. In addition, these approaches suggest that some movements, and some groups within movements, are more inclined than others to introduce and use some applications of ICTs. Inspired by a scan of the way ICTs are used by environmental SMOs, we are able to list a number of hypotheses and preliminary observations, which are addressed in the empirical chapters that follow this introductory chapter. Our tentative exploration suggests that ICTs are increasingly used by various kinds of SMOs, to remarkably different degrees and purposes, and with varying levels of sophistication. Characteristics of different applications of ICTs as well as different characteristics of SMOs will have to be taken into account. The heterogeneous nature of SMOs will be reflected in different patterns and implications of the introduction and use of ICTs. We assume that the internet is used particularly by two kinds of movement structures: (a) informal networks with a large geographical reach, and (b) big, powerful and more centralized social movement organizations. Moreover, the internet appears to play an especially crucial role in issue-focused, transnational campaigns (such as the recent protests against the World Trade Organization, the International Monetary Fund and the World Bank).
- The internet may facilitate the traditional forms of protest such as rallies, demonstrations, and collection of signatures, but it will hardly replace these forms.[3] So far, we remain sceptical. The very ease of virtual mobilization may well devalue it as a political resource that attracts public attention and respect. In addition, virtual mobilization may be devalued by the activists themselves because it lacks the attraction of the group experience and the 'fun' and 'adventure factor' accompanying some forms of protest.
- What the internet certainly does is to allow for immediate mobilization across the globe, as practised for example by Earth Action, an environmental group that alerts its worldwide constituency to urgent matters calling for immediate targeting of the political leaders in each territory.

- The internet may also serve as a tool to provide information that tends to be suppressed by the more established media. This was the rationale for creating Indymedia (see www.indymedia.org), a leftist-oriented loose network of groups that now exists in dozens of countries. More generally, citizen groups and SMOs using ICTs become less dependent on coverage by the established mass media to convey their messages to a large audience. In addition, ICTs themselves may become both a means of mobilization and a target to hit, for example when tens of thousands of emails or faxes are sent to a target in order to block its systems of communication or when politically motivated hackers enter and probably modify the communication system of target institutions.

- It is likely that the use of the internet affects the *internal structure* of social movement organizations, above all the density and direction of their links. In the long run, ICTs may help to intensify communication among all parts of an organization (including the rank and file), thereby challenging to some extent the top-down flow of communication domination so far. Whereas the impact of ICTs on the internal structure of SMOs is still an open matter, there is ample evidence that ICTs are conducive to forging (temporary) alliances and coalitions, both vertical and horizontal, across different movements. It appears that the emergence of global justice (or global solidarity) movements (often called anti-globalization movements) that closely link a number of issues such as human rights, social rights, poverty and environmental issues has been greatly facilitated by the use of ICTs. In addition, specialized structures that are supporting the flow of communication, e.g. Institute for Global Communication (IGC) and the abovementioned Indymedia network, have emerged. While some of these structures aim to be politically neutral, others take an ideological stance to support a broader 'movement family' regarding their matters of communication. Whether the internet enhances the chances of 'democratic' and 'egalitarian' communication among movements still remains to be seen. While several writers have expressed great hopes, others remain sceptical and try to demystify the internet (Münker and Roesler 1997, 2000).

- Because not only social movements but also their opponents profit from ICTs' advantages, we do not assume that the existing constellation of powers is fundamentally changed as long as all actors use ICTs to similar degrees.

An overview of explorative case studies presented in this volume

The chapters in this volume present a series of explorative case studies of a variety of social movement organizations. In most of them, the internal and/or external impacts and patterns of use of the internet and related applications (databases, email, multimedia applications) are explored and subjected to tentative evaluation. The cases and analysis seek to contribute to the development of a research agenda. The first group of chapters examine the changing levels and domains of political action.

In his chapter on media strategies employed by three kinds of progressive protest movements – the New Left of the 1960s, the New Social Movements of the 1970s and 1980s, and the most recent global solidarity movements, Rucht (Chapter 2) shows that these strategies emerge in a complex interplay between the 'logic' of movement organizations and the dominant characteristics of the (mass) media. Although ICTs can be expected to represent some new characteristics (greater openness of new media, which are more amenable to be 'controlled', at least partly, by SMOs), it is clear that their importance should not be overstated. Moreover, traditional or mainstream mass media remain important (they still have to be seen as crucial actors in mobilization and agenda-setting), and the fragmented nature of new media severely limits the possibilities for a social movement strategy that tries to create its own and independent media (or public forums of communication) that promise to reach an external audience.

In Chapter 3, Rosenkrands shows how another change is facilitated by the internet. In his analysis of the new anti-corporate movement, he demonstrates how a new field of political action is entered by 'culture-jammers', '(h)activists', 'ad-busters' and, last but not least, ordinary consumers and citizens. Rosenkrands examines how the new anti-corporate movement is attempting to hold big business democratically accountable: the *raison d'être* of a movement that has turned the market into a political battleground. This chapter explores the role played by the internet in the targeting of corporations. A number of popular anti-corporate websites are analysed and the following questions answered: Which kinds of goals are pursued? Which types of organizations and groups run anti-corporate websites? Who are targeted? How are the special functionalities and features of the internet utilized? Which types of organizational strategies do the websites reflect? How are websites linked to other websites?

In Chapter 4, Wright presents an overview of the way ICTs are (re)shaping patterns of information and communication in the domain of contemporary anti-capitalist movements. His analysis confirms some of the findings presented by Rucht in Chapter 2. He claims that it is far too early for a well balanced and informed account of how the use of ICTs is influencing traditional patterns of information and communication in the field of social protest. More than facilitating all kinds of new 'revolutionary' patterns, ICTs (e.g. the internet, internal and external forms of communication) tend to be integrated (e.g. adapted) into existing patterns and practices. However, some of these traditional routines of 'knowledge management' in social movement organizations are challenged by the use of the internet. The internet itself seems to become a platform that facilitates all kinds of 'subterranean' information and communication channels that affect traditional participatory structures and cultures. Problems of excess volume and chaotically organized information seem to challenge not only the way analysis and action are integrated in decision-making processes, but also the existing configuration of power in the internal and external environment of SMOs.

The next set of chapters focuses on the way ICTs contribute to new strategies and stratagems that are developed by the social movement organizations of the information age.

Van Aelst and Walgrave, in Chapter 5, show how virtual networks seem to have contributed decisively to the formation of a truly transnational anti-globalization movement. Although they demonstrate that ICTs (the internet) help to organize political action at a global level, by lowering costs for and promoting a more universal access to political participation, they also provide evidence that the new forms of computer-mediated political communication associated with ICTs are still clearly different from the more permanent and stable patterns that breed stable SMOs. Although virtual forms of mobilization and organization have clearly contributed to the development of common ideas, counter-expertise, discourses and frames, these were most of the time very much summit-related. The linking of websites in itself is not enough to overcome the geographical and ideological distances that characterized these anti-globalization movements. Indeed, the internet seems to contribute to all kinds of vertical and horizontal forms of coalition formation, but also furthers the segmented, polycentric nature of these movements.

Bennett, in Chapter 6, shows that many observers doubt the capacity of digital media to change the political game. The rise of a transnational activism that is aimed beyond states and directly at corporations, trade and development regimes offers a fruitful area for understanding how communication practices can help create a new form of politics. The internet is implicated in the new global activism far beyond merely reducing the costs of communication, or transcending the geographical and temporal barriers associated with other communication media. Various uses of the internet and digital media facilitate the loosely structured networks, the weak identity ties, and the patterns of issue and demonstration organizing that define a new global protest politics. Analysis of various cases shows how digital network configurations can facilitate permanent campaigns, the growth of broad networks despite relatively weak social identity and ideology ties, transformation of individual member organizations and networks, and the capacity to communicate messages from desktops to television screens. The same qualities that make these communication-based politics durable also make them vulnerable to problems of control, decision-making and collective identity.

Cardoso and Neto in Chapter 7 address the pro-East Timor movement in Portugal in 1999, and the role the ICTs and the traditional mass media played in its emergence and orientation. The authors aim to identify the usage of these media by the agents directly implicated and, on the other hand, to ascertain changes prompted by such usage on the underlying organizational structure and communication fluxes. Through the intertwining of the constructive insights of different analytical approaches in the social movements field, the authors shed light not only on the societal context in which the protest evolved and the resources it mobilized but also on how the cultural identity framing it was promoted. It is argued that the pro-East Timor movement qualifies as a networked social movement, that is, a movement focused on cultural values, acting from the local in an attempt to influence the global, using the ICTs as a fundamental tool.

Le Grignou and Patou in Chapter 8 present a case study on ATTAC. It seeks to provide an analysis of how the internet is shaping new relations in this movement, especially regarding the use of knowledge and information. It raises issues such as the mobilization of expertise in a new movement context, the role of epistimic community, the formation of a counter-expertise, and democracy within the movement organization. It critiques many of the 'promises' of the internet literature, which the authors see as not being met in this case.

The final set of chapters deal with issues around the notions of citizenship, identity and virtual movements. Edwards in Chapter 9 examines the Dutch women's movement online. He shows how the internet is being used to reshape the organizational infrastructure of the movement, focusing on how this affects its ability to influence the political agenda. His analysis of new forms of virtual organization rejects the dominant hypothesis in this field that ICTs contribute to disintermediation. The use of the internet tends to reinforce existing power relationships rather than contributing to radical shifts in existing power configurations. However, there is some evidence of the use of ICTs facilitating internal democratization and interactive forms of policy-making within the movement.

Cheta in Chapter 10 examines the relationships between disability social movements (DSMs) and new technologies, which the author argues are crucial to understanding the problems of DSM identity politics, its framing and transformation as it accompanies the evolution of DSMs. She provides a case study analysis of the Portuguese Accessibility Special Interest Group (GUIA), an excellent example of a communicative means of protest, and seeks to portray how GUIA contributed to redefining/challenging outdated frames on disability and new technologies. The chapter identifies the framing processes that underline GUIA's actions and analyses how GUIA has launched a new ethos and new *modus operandi* with repercussions at the national, European and international levels during its short life. The chapter illustrates some of the most striking GUIA initiatives, such as the popularity achieved with the first electronic petition to improve internet accessibility launched in Portugal and Europe, and online protests for multiple accessibility to ICT. The author seeks to present a dual strategy that affirms the ICT accessibility principle as a core value of framing identity, and the mobilization and management of ICT as means of protest, and thus recharacterizes GUIA within the DSMs.

Nip in Chapter 11 examines the impact of internet facilities (bulletin boards, mail, etc.) on offline social movement mobilization within a women's group in Hong Kong (the Queer Sisters). It puts a particular emphasis on the notion of identity-building and thus gives a different perspective on some of the issues raised in Chapter 10. This case study uses content analysis, online survey, interviews and observation in order to offer a picture of the movement and the way in which it uses ICTs. It shows the realization of the creation of counter culture(s) and the role of a virtual community. Although her results show that whilst ICTs may have the potential to help achieve this, the evidence leads her to conclude that it is not sufficient in itself in terms of the creation of an identity-building process.

In the final chapter, Pini, Brown and Previte present a case study that examines how Australian women in the domain of agriculture construct and reconstruct new ICTs for political activism. The case study draws on interviews, content analysis and observation, and questions whether cyberspace is developing as a new (public) space for political engagement. The research conducted suggests that the internet has helped to form new opportunities for mobilization in geographically dispersed and male-dominated 'territories' such as that in the study. At the same time, the study has identified how the women have used ICTs to set their own agenda by promoting topics in mainstream debates while acknowledging the problems in engaging less active, marginal actors. The authors demonstrate the importance of 'private' space to supporting women in their political discussions and development of ideas and argue that in this case study, this issue has not been addressed in relation to online communications within the group (while acknowledged in terms of offline meetings). Thus, the authors argue that consideration needs to be given to how new configurations in computer-mediated communication lead to new patterns and possibilities and foster new coalitions of ideas/identities/frames that challenge existing ones in the 'real' world.

Concluding remarks

As the internet and new media become ever more ubiquitous in our world, such technologies begin to look less like revolutionary phenomena and more a familiar aspect of everyday life. As a consequence the earlier heroic rhetoric from cyber utopians is displaced by more considered analyses of the role and influence of ICTs within our political institutions and practices. It is our hope that the contributions to this book go a considerable way in exploring how social movements are shaping the new media in ways that are both innovative and consistent with past traditions.

Notes

1 Although the term 'ICT' is broader and includes relatively conventional technologies (e.g. telephone), we use this acronym here only with reference to digital technologies based on microchips, in particular computers.
2 This is recognized in the following definition: 'Social movements are a strategically and/or thematically connected series of events, produced in interaction with adversaries and carried out by a coherent network of organizations and participants who use largely unconventional means in

attaining political goals' (Duyvendak 1995). For a similar definition, see Diani (1992: 4).

3 Only in a few and relatively marginal cases do ICTs indeed replace traditional means of mobilization. One example is the use of 'telephone trees' in order to mobilize a given group of activists. This task can be more easily performed by email.

Part I

Changing the levels and domains of political action

2 The quadruple 'A'

Media strategies of protest movements since the 1960s

Dieter Rucht

In contemporary societies, mass media are extremely important for almost all political actors (Zaller 1992). This is particularly true for social movements and protest groups. As a rule, they are outsiders *vis-à-vis* the institutionalized political game, having few means to get their voices heard and their activities seen. Joachim Raschke, a German political scientist, aptly – although not literally – highlighted the importance of media coverage when he said 'A movement that does not make it into the media is non-existent' (Raschke 1985: 343), underlining the fact that groups and events that are not reported by the media are known only to the immediate participants and bystanders, and not by the broader public.

Most, but not all, social movements and protest groups strive to get media attention and, if possible, positive media coverage, which in turn may be crucial to influencing people's hearts and minds and, eventually, policy decisions. Some groups are very successful in dealing with the media; others attain media resonance only to a small extent, or in rare moments, while still others fail completely. If they fail, however, this does not necessarily mean that their cause is definitely lost. They may try to develop their own means of communication to spread their word, to reframe their goals and demands, to change their forms of action and/or to reorient their media strategies so that they become more attractive to the media, or parts of it. In other words, movements have different ways of dealing with the media.

The media, in turn, have different ways in dealing with social movements. They can ignore them or react to them only under particular circumstances; they can proactively contact movement activists and eagerly seek information; they may comment positively or negatively on movements' goals and activities, or side issues such as the activists' outlook or personal background, thereby following a more general tendency 'to downplay the big social economic, or political picture in favour of the human trials and triumphs that sit at the surface of events' (Bennett 1996: 39). Because of the variety of these options and because of the fact that neither social movements nor the media represent a coherent entity, we can expect complex patterns of relationships. Moreover, any variation is increased by the extent to which both social movements and the mass media undergo structural changes over time.

One of the most crucial changes is the introduction and growing role of the ICTs and, in particular, the internet. While many activists and observers assume that the internet tends to revolutionize the media strategies of social movements (e.g. Frederick 1993), this chapter takes a more sceptical view. Only when comparing over time can we see the extent of any changes. Therefore, a longitudinal view is taken by focusing on the media strategies of social movements in recent decades. It will be shown that social movements in the past sought to rely on both their own media and the established mass media, though to strikingly different degrees depending on the circumstances. The internet, in spite of its advantages, will not make other media unimportant. It mainly serves as a highly efficient tool to gather and spread information for those who not only have the technical facilities but also know what they are looking for. The internet will not replace the physical encounters of social movement groups. Nor will it devalue the traditional mass media, which, as pre-selectors of credible information and as 'serious' political commentators, remain crucial to the broader populace to which most movements seek to appeal.

As this topic of social movements' changing media strategies is very broad, it will be narrowed in three respects. First, I will focus on 'progressive' movements because these are more explicit in their media work than their counterparts from the Right. Also, their relationship with the mass media is more complex and varied compared to right-wing movements. Secondly, to avoid over-complexity, only the period from the rise of the New Left in the 1960s to the present time will be covered. This length of perspective is sufficient to identify both continuities and discontinuities in the movements' media strategies. Thirdly, the main field of empirical reference is Western Europe and, occasionally, the US, simply because this is the field on which most material is available and which allows for a feasible scope of generalization.

In the first section of this chapter, some theoretical considerations on the interactions between social movements and mass media are presented. Secondly, reference will be made to the empirical cases with special emphasis on three types, or generations, of 'progressive' social movements: the New Left and student movements of the 1960s, the new social movements of the following two decades, and the recent transnational movements challenging neo-liberal globalization. In the third section, some conclusions will be drawn with regard to both empirical observations and theoretical considerations.

Theoretical framework

Social movements and mass media share an engagement in undertaking struggles to attract attention. However, because of the different functions and aims of social movements on the one hand and mass media on the other, these struggles take very different forms. Only by taking into account their respective characters and underlying conditions can we hope to obtain a better understanding of how social movements and mass media interact.

Social movements and their audience

Social movements, by definition, strive for change in society. The ways such changes are sought may differ considerably. Some movements, or groups within a given movement, try to persuade people mainly through personal contacts, hoping that the growing number of people supporting the cause ultimately will make a difference. Other movements, or groups in the same movement, consider the opportunities to change people's minds and hearts to be slim unless structural changes take place. In the social movement literature, scholars have suggested an analytical distinction between movements 'changing individual and member behaviour versus [those] changing society' (Zald and Ash 1966: 331). Moreover, drawing on earlier work of Scipio Sighele dating from 1894, a distinction between inward- and outward-oriented movements has been proposed (Lang and Lang 1961: 498). The two concepts are not identical but overlap. They are a useful reminder that not all movements are necessarily seeking wide public attention.

Some movements are primarily concerned with reaching their immediate target audience. They prefer forms of *qualitative* mobilization (Rucht 1988). Relying primarily on face-to-face interaction, they seek a profound impact on a limited number of people instead of a more superficial impact on large groups or the 'masses'. A typical example was the creation of consciousness-raising groups in the new women's movements during the 1970s and 1980s.

For many other social movement groups, public attention and support is the key means to impress and influence policy-makers who otherwise might ignore the challengers' aims and claims. These groups tend towards forms of *quantitative* mobilization, attempting to reach as many people as possible. In this case, the modern mass media become crucial because millions of people cannot be targeted by face-to-face interaction. Even when personal change is a primary goal, the mass media may become a central reference point in so far as a relatively small impact on many people, in its aggregate effect, may dwarf an intensive impact on just a few individuals. An example of such an attempt at quantitative mobilization is a campaign for environmentally friendly consumer behaviour.

Given the reach of modern mass media, and the dependency of power-holders on public opinion and voting behaviour, it is clear that mass media play a crucial role for most social movements. We can hypothesize that reactions of the mass media are a precondition for the ultimate success or failure of these movements. Therefore, from the local to the global levels, movements struggle for public visibility as granted (or refused) by the mass media. When outward-oriented movements fail to get visibility, they tend to shrink, to fall apart, to take a sectarian course, or to radicalize. While the latter guarantees attention, it does not often trigger much applause.

Protest groups' struggles for visibility may have a different relevance and may take different forms. From an analytical perspective, we can discern two basic situations. The first is the more or less spontaneous collective expression of emotion such as rage. Almost by definition, this occurs without much strategic consideration. When people are deeply angry, they often do not care about the reactions of others, including the media. However, there may also be situations in which the actors deliberately show their anger so that others get a sense of the intensity of the protesters' feelings. While in the first case media attention is not a goal but a side-effect, in the second case media attention may be welcomed, though the action was not designed to get coverage.

A different situation exists when protest groups seek large visibility and accordingly choose, and carefully design, their activities. In this case, the media become a crucial reference point. This implies a careful understanding of the needs and rules of the mass media. Some groups, particularly those who are provocative and radical, primarily seek attention but cannot hope to receive positive resonance. Others try to get positive coverage so that their goals and demands are perceived as legitimate and their actions as appropriate. Reaching and influencing the broad populace via the media may be the ultimate target. However, we can also imagine situations when influencing masses of people is, ultimately, only a tool to impact on the power-holders who, in democratic societies, cannot or dare not ignore voters' opinions.

In order to gain media coverage, though not necessarily in a positive fashion, social movements have a variety of strategies at hand. In terms of their public activities, they can try to mobilize masses of people (usually in rallies, collections of signatures, etc.) to stage disruptive or even violent actions, to carry out innovative protests, or to find prominent and/or politically relevant allies. The more one, or several, of these strategies materialize, the greater the chances of getting media coverage. This is probably what Ralph Turner had in mind when stating with regard to disruptive protests: 'A combination of threat and appeal serves to gain attention and to create a sense of urgency necessary to overcome the resistance of acknowledging protest' (Turner 1969: 821).

While certain kinds of activities are likely to be ignored and others are likely to be covered, protest groups can influence this process not only by shaping and framing their public action but also by using other means. For example, they can try to establish continuous relationships with certain media and/or certain journalists; they can privilege some journalists by providing background information; they can facilitate the journalists' jobs by preparing well-crafted press releases and/or offering contacts to particular spokespeople, specialists, etc. The effect of such strategies, however, is usually limited, because, unlike senior political leaders, protest groups seldom possess information that journalists desperately seek. Hence the protest action itself remains the key activity to get media coverage.

Mass media and their audience

The mass media are engaged in a different struggle for attention. They seek to attract as many people as possible to buy newspapers, listen to the radio, watch television, or browse the world wide web. When they reach masses of people, the media's mission is fulfilled, provided that the large audience can also be converted into economic survival and success. Whether the audience likes or dislikes the messages is of no, or perhaps only secondary, importance. In this regard, the media clearly differ from social movements, which, in most cases, not only seek attention but also support and commitment. Unlike movements, the media are not, or only in rare instances, engaged in a partisan struggle. Thus they usually lack a distinct opponent. Instead, their basic frame of reference is that of delivering a service within the framework of economic competition.

In their constant and daily struggle to attract an audience, the media have relatively clear measures of success (e.g. circulation of newspapers, number of people listening to a radio station or watching a television channel). This leads to a direct and tough competition, which, in many instances, follows the logics of a zero-sum game. Again, this differs to some extent from social movements, that tend to form – at least within certain ideological lines – broad alliances, and do not compete, or compete only indirectly,[1] with other groups of the same network.

Given the media's context and their particular kind of struggle for visibility, they follow some basic functional principles. An overriding feature of most mass media is their extreme selectivity. For the most part, the media are confronted with an oversupply of inputs delivered by a variety of sources. In order to filter out what shall and shall not be reported, the media generally follow some guidelines and rules that, according to communication theories, can be summarized under the heading of 'news values' (Schulz 1976; Staab 1990). Compared to the news values, other criteria of selection, such as the ideological leaning of the particular medium or the personal preference of the gatekeeper who selects what to cover, are of secondary importance. While there is no coherent and universally acknowledged list of news values, most researchers in this area would agree that conflict, spectacle, newness, prominence, physical closeness to the medium and its audience, and severe and direct consequences of events on people's lives should be included in such a list. Another feature of the media is their high degree of internal division of labour and, related to this, level of professionalization. This usually implies a particular training of the journalists, the acknowledgment and practice of certain rules, and a set of professional ethics that, among other things, requires the journalist to separate information from opinion, not to present merely one view on conflictual topics, to verify certain 'facts', and so on. The definition of the basic role of a journalist is that of a fair and largely non-partisan 'reporter' of events (Kaplan 2002), though it is evident that certain kinds of journalists notoriously deviate from this role. This prescriptive requirement as well as the extent to which it is actually met clearly differ from the situation of a social movement. Most social movement activists are fighting for a particular cause, whatever their professional background may be. Even those who devote, unpaid or paid, most of their time to a social movement cannot rely on a standard set of rules and professional ethics. While   other people agitating is the basic requirement for social movement activists, this would be considered an evil among most journalists. These different roles partly explain why the relationship between social movements and the media is not an easy one (Gitlin 1980; van Zoonen 1992; Gamson and Wolfsfeld 1993; Neidhardt 1994; Gamson 1998; Neveu 1999).

The interplay between movements and mass media

As discussed above, social movements and mass media have several features in common: they are engaged in a struggle for attention; they want to maximize their outreach; they are confronted, though to different degrees, with competitors. Nevertheless, they not only follow a different functional logic but also have a strikingly asymmetric relationship when dealing with each other. This becomes clear when we consider the structural positions of the movements offering conflict, spectacle, surprise, threat, etc. on the one hand and the media (potentially) granting coverage, importance, sympathy, etc. on the other hand. In a nutshell, this asymmetry stems from the fact that most movements need the media, but the media seldom need the movements.[2]

The reason why social movements need the mass media has been explained above. To recap, without the media a movement remains unknown to a large audience. Therefore, its impact would remain limited to its immediate environment. Thus, the media are extremely attractive to social movements. Consequently, many movements are ready to make concessions in order to meet the media's criteria and requirements. For instance, even groups praising equality and spontaneity may nominate 'speakers' or schedule their activity according to the production time of the media in order to get coverage.

The mass media, on the contrary, can easily survive and even flourish without social movements. As noted above, particularly those media with many resources and reaching a large audience do not lack input but rather agonize as to what to select from a daily avalanche of offers. However, under certain conditions, protest groups may become attractive to the media so that, particularly in the case of radical groups, an 'adversary symbiosis' emerges (Gitlin 1980: 29). The mass media, particularly when existing in a competitive context, want to appear interesting, innovative, fast, and – to some extent – fair and balanced (Tuchman 1972). This gives protest groups some leverage that otherwise would have little value to the media.

Protest groups, even if small and not overly professional, can be of interest to journalists because they tend to be more innovative and more surprising than most other actors. Movement activities often involve drama and spectacle, passion and emotion, conflict and threat – aspects in which the mass media are generally interested (Molotch and Lester 1974; Gitlin 1980; Wolfsfeld 1984; Kielbowicz and Scherer 1986). Moreover, differences of opinions on many issues within established groups are often minor or subtle allowing journalists to actively search for dissenting views. To some extent, this promise of spectacle can compensate for the otherwise weak position of most protest groups, particularly in terms of their lack of resources and professional knowledge in dealing with the media. In some cases, these features may even become an asset in so far as the challengers are sympathetically framed as 'Davids versus Goliaths'. Nevertheless, there is no guarantee of getting media coverage merely on the basis of being a protest group. Too many issues are of potential interest for the media, and usually too many groups compete within a given issue domain to secure media attention for each actor involved. Thus those groups that take the principles of the media system into account are likely to get advantages relative to other groups who do not care about these principles.

The quadruple 'A': four social movement reactions to a lack of media resonance

As mass media are extremely selective in both what they cover and which aspects they focus on (Hilgartner and Bosk 1988), protest groups, particularly if minor and/or radical, often feel ignored or grossly distorted. Various studies found that as a result of the media's selectivity, only a few per cent of protest events that occur are actually reported by at least one national newspaper (Hocke 1999; Fillieule 1999; McCarthy *et al.* 1996). Moreover, time and again movements complain that media do not portray them adequately, specifically when it comes to their reasons for protest. Simplified, one can identify four reactions to such frustrating experiences, which can be symbolized by a quadruple 'A': abstention, attack, adaptation, and alternatives.

Abstention is born out of resignation based on negative experiences with the established media. In analogy to abstention from voting, it implies the withdrawal from attempts to influence the mass media and the retreat to inward-directed group communication. This is an option that, in an empirical study, was found among both radical pro-life and pro-choice groups in Germany. Some of the interviewed groups, based on their negative experiences with the mainstream media, simply gave up all efforts to have an impact on these media. One group representative bitterly stated: 'The right-to-life movement finds no open doors with the media. The newspapers take practically no press releases from the right-to-life groups' (Ferree *et al.* 2002: 168).

Attack, the second reaction, consists of an explicit critique of, and sometimes even violent action against, the mass media. Activists who feel ignored or grossly misrepresented by certain media may write a letter of complaint to the editor, start a collection of signatures against unfair treatment or neglect, or contact a more or less established rival medium that they hope will do a better job. For example, the US AIDS movement, particularly Act Up, blamed the media for portraying AIDS as a 'gay' disease, even suggesting that this was contributing to death rates caused by AIDS.

Adaptation, the third type of reaction, means the acceptance/ exploitation of the mass media's rules and criteria to influence coverage positively. Predominantly, the more 'established' movement groups tend to apply this strategy. In its most advanced form, it may include hiring a professional journalist or even creating a separate public relations unit that knows how to play the game with the established media. A typical example of this is Greenpeace, which has an undisputed reputation for its professional media work.

The fourth type of reaction – the search for *alternatives* – is the attempt by social movements to create their own and independent media (or public forums of communication) in order to compensate for a lack of interest, or bias, on the part of the established media. One example is the US magazine *Lies of Our Times* that existed in the early 1990s. It was set up to correct mainstream reports on issues and activities of left and liberal groups. Another example is the creation of a regular daily newspaper such as the French *Libération*.

Two of these four reactions – abstention and alternatives – result in inward-directed activities of social movements, whereas the remaining two – attack and adaptation – are outward-directed in so far as these target the mass media. Another underlying dimension is the amount of resources required for these reactions. Adaptation and alternatives are viable options only when considerable resources are invested more or less continuously, while no, or relatively few, resources are required for abstention and attack, respectively. Thus, the four reactions could be represented in a diagram organized along the two dimensions of the basic orientation (inward/outward) and the resource demand (high/low).

The question is, under which circumstances social movements tend to which, or which combination, of the four non-mutually exclusive options. This question can be studied best when looking at various kinds of movements in different contexts and time periods.

Changes over time

What has been said so far is a generalization, ignoring not only differences within social movements and the media but also structural and technical changes over time. For example, the European labour movements from the late nineteenth century to the first half of the twentieth century were perceived as a threat to the established system and particularly to the educated elites who controlled the mass media. As these movements had little hope of gaining both extensive and fair coverage, they created their own mass media to reach their adherents in an effective way, preferably on a daily basis. Other groups, including the main opponents of the labour movements, followed a similar strategy. As a result, the mass media were differentiated or 'pillarized' along ideological lines, with each camp basically serving its own clientele by reflecting and reinforcing a particular worldview. For a number of reasons, this partisan structure faded away, while at the same time less ideologically driven mass media made ground, targeting a broader audience than ever before. Today, the traditional partisan press (in German dubbed *Gesinnungspresse*) has largely disappeared. The major newspapers are no longer inherently part of a particular political camp. Though they may still roughly follow a certain political line and, for the most part, can be situated along the left–right axis in many countries (Voltmer 2000), they rather see themselves as, or indeed are, 'pluralistic', often presenting different views on important matters within the same medium.

Other important structural changes are the rise of new media such as radio and television, the increasing numbers and growing role of privately run stations, their dependency on paid advertisements, and the ever tough competition within and across different kinds of media.

It is clear that such changes affect social movements in their attempts to reach a large audience. To the extent that the major mass media become more diversified, more open to various kinds of political actors, and offer different views on divisive matters even within the same paper or channel, social movements no longer need mainly rely on their own media. Instead, they can realistically hope that their existence will not be ignored and their cause and activities not completely distorted, particularly when different media are competing with each other and, in their political leaning, occupy different positions on the political spectrum. However, some changes also weaken the position of social movements. For example, dependency on paid advertisement from big corporations can sometimes engender pressure on journalists not to report in a favourable way on groups that challenge these corporations.

Another factor that is likely to make the job of social movements more cumbersome concerns broader societal transformations. As long as most social movements in the past were confined to certain social classes, which stood in stark contrast or even opposition to each other, every movement was basically referring to its 'natural' base without struggling to reach other social strata. Today, with the decline of class cleavages and the proliferation of issues that are not related to particular social classes (e.g. environmental protection, homosexuality, genetic engineering), social movements tend to address a broader and more diverse audience but also have to invest more in discursive struggles. Related to this, social movements can hardly count on 'natural allies' within the established media. Rather, they have to work hard to get attention at all.

Media and progressive movements since the 1960s

In the following, an attempt will be made to illustrate how different social movements relate to the media. I will focus on progressive movements since the 1960s, drawing mostly, though not exclusively, on examples from Western Europe.

New Left and student movements in the 1960s

Movement-controlled media

The New Left emerged probably most distinctively in Great Britain and France during the 1950s and early 1960s, later spreading to other European countries and the USA which, however, also had their own intellectual and organizational roots. As a basically intellectual movement, the early New Left was centred around discussion groups and existing, or newly created, political journals. In Great Britain, *The New Reasoner* and *Universities and Left Review* were first published in 1957 and, in 1959, merged to become the *New Left Review*. The journal, with a circulation of 9,000 copies in 1960, was a crucial focus of intellectual debates and social bonds. It considered itself as part of a broader intellectual and political movement that deliberately refused to be part of, or become, a political party. 'Clubs, discussion centres will be places beyond the reach of the interference of the bureaucracy where the initiative remains in the hand of the rank and file.'[3] By the end of 1960, around 40 New Left clubs, partly overlapping with local chapters of the Campaign for Nuclear Disarmament, existed in England, particularly in cities with universities.

In France, two independent journals, *Socialisme ou Barbarie* and *Arguments* played a similar role, serving as catalysts for the emergence of the French New Left. *Socialisme ou Barbarie* was already established in 1949, and gradually developed into a New Left journal (existing until 1966). *Arguments* was created in 1956 and ended six years later. It was modelled according to the Italian journal *Ragionamenti* (which means reasons, arguments) from which it also borrowed its name.[4] Similarly to the situation in England, these journals triggered the creation of circles of readers.[5] In Paris, the first circles emerged in 1959 and subsequently spread to other French cities.

In Germany, the name and the structure of the French *Arguments* – with the combination of journal and press, volunteering writers, and discussion groups – was adopted with the creation of *Das Argument*. The first issue was published in 1959. The journal continues to exist today, though not in its original form. Another important journal was *Neue Kritik* (1960 through 1970). It was an organ of the Socialist German Students' Alliance (SDS, Sozialistischer Deutscher Studentenbund), the most influential group of the student movement in the 1960s, but had a wider readership than just the members of the SDS.

In the USA, though there were traditional left organs such as *Dissent*, no New Left journals of nationwide significance existed.[6] Unlike their European counterparts, the new generation of US activists engaged less in reading Marxist literature and in intense theoretical debates about the correct ideological line (Diggins 1992). Whereas the European New Left had to define its position in a political space that was densely populated by various significant leftist parties, groups, movements and prominent intellectual figures, the space in the US was more open. In a later period, the US also provided a fertile ground for the flourishing of the underground press (Peck 1985). Because traditional leftist parties and groups had a low profile, the

New Left could easily agree on a number of general principles such as participatory democracy and the key role of intellectuals (instead of the working class) as an agent of change. Also, it could largely agree on a single document such as the Port Huron Statement that was essentially drafted by one person, the SDS activist Tom Hayden, in 1962 (Students for a Democratic Society (SDS) was based in the USA). The more pragmatic attitude of the US New Left is also exemplified by C. Wright Mills, an 'academic outlaw' (Jamison and Eyerman 1994: 36) who, though in close contact with leading European leftists, never considered himself to be a communist or Marxist.

Critique of the established press

The New Left journals were limited in two ways. First, unlike daily newspapers, they did not cover the news of the day but were organs of more general intellectual and political debates. Second, probably with the exception of Italy, they reached only a very small audience, thus appearing virtually non-existent to the wider populace.[7] For the large majority of the population, tabloid papers and, since the 1960s, television were the main sources of information about political and societal matters beyond the readers' immediate environment. These sources were basically oriented towards the *status quo*.[8] From the perspective of New Left activists, they were part and parcel of the ruling system, contributing to the maintenance of a 'false consciousness' about the nature of power relations in capitalist societies. To the New Left, this became particularly obvious in the way their aims and activities were portrayed by the mainstream media and especially the tabloid press. Consider, for example, the comments of a British local paper on an anti-apartheid demonstration of students protesting against a visiting South African Rugby Union team in 1969:

> We are becoming all too familiar with those 'again it' – the lean, savage-looking, longhaired student type who appears to be 'anti-everything'. They are those who are all too ready to carry their protest into the realm of violence. To them protest is not enough. They have to provoke. This is the kind of protest the British people are heartily sick of. They are sick of the young who join in without knowing what the protest is all about.[9]

Time and again, the protesters of the 1960s found that their arguments were ignored or distorted. Tabloids not only misrepresented realities and promoted prejudice in quite a number of cases (Gitlin 1980), but also occasionally bluntly lied (Sack 1984: 188). No wonder that the media became a target of the New Left. In West Germany in 1967, the Socialist Students Alliance (SDS) passed a 'resolution to fight manipulation and to democratise the public sphere', strongly criticizing the mass media:

> Press, radio, television and film create an illusionary world in which the 'secret seducers' of private capitalism and political dominance functionally integrate the desires of humans and cause psychic misery and the destruction of reasoned political judgement.
>
> (Oy 2001: 125)

In the wake of this resolution, a number of publications, protest actions and initiatives[10] were launched. Strong critique was not only one-way. Segments of the press, in turn, contributed to a climate of hostility against the protesters so that 'ordinary people' felt encouraged to take action. One victim of this aggression spurred by the media was Rudi Dutschke, a famous spokesperson of the German SDS, who was shot down by a young right-wing-oriented worker in Berlin on 11 April 1968. This assault was preceded by an intense campaign to discredit the student movement, spearheaded by the conservative Springer press, which, among other things, owned the largest tabloid in Europe and controlled 70 per cent of the West Berlin newspaper market. Clearly, the movement saw a causal chain between the shooting of Dutschke and how the media had portrayed the movement and its leaders ('long-haired apes') in the previous months. It regarded the Springer press, along with the state authorities, as being responsible for the shooting.[11] The movement's answer was to attack this kind of media both verbally and physically. During Easter 1968, students tried to stop the distribution of Springer newspapers in Berlin by blocking the doors of the printing factory – an act that escalated into violent clashes with the police and massive destruction of property (Hilwig 1998). Also in a few other cities students launched activities against the Springer press, which, for example in Frankfurt, also turned into violent clashes (Kraushaar 1998: 305–309).

The 'Anti-Springer' or 'Expropriate Springer' campaign was soon echoed in Italy. On 1 June 1968, student activists, without success, tried to storm the Turin-based headquarters of *La Stampa*, a newspaper that earlier had characterized the students as left fascist (Gilcher-Holtey 2001: 103). One of their slogans was 'La Stampa = Springer', thereby directly relating to the events in Germany (Hilwig

1998). Although the press in most European countries was not covering the student activities in a uniform and exclusively discriminatory
fashion,[12] the students felt that the differences were essentially a
matter of degree. Overall, the students thought that they had little if
any influence in shaping the way their demands and activities were
presented to the wider audience. In consequence, they tried to develop
a concept of counter-institutions and, more particularly, of counter-
publics (*Gegenöffentlichkeit*).

The creation of counter-publics

The idea of creating counter-institutions materialized only to a small
extent. Examples were the proclamation of a 'Free University' (in
Berkeley), a 'Critical University' (Berlin) and an 'anti-university'
(London) as an alternative to the existing campuses. These would be
places of intense intellectual and political exchange without the hierarchical and formal structures and the competitive pressure of the
established universities. These attempts, however, were mainly of symbolic significance. The critical universities never went beyond a series
of seminars and discussions that the students organized autonomously.
Other and partly more enduring examples of counter-institutions were
communes, anti-authoritarian kindergartens (*Kinderläden*) and, in a
later period, alternative schools, health centres and the like. 'The creation of counter-publics' was promoted in the late 1960s, hence parallel
to the 'march through the institutions' that could be considered as an
alternative political strategy. The message and material substance of
counter-publics remained largely confined to the range of intellectual
journals mentioned above and a number of political clubs, congresses,
and spectacular acts of protest. During the late 1960s and early 1970s,
the infrastructural basis of this counter-public remained small in terms
of resources, number of journal copies, etc. To the wider public,
the existence of some sort of counter-public became known mainly
through the mainstream media, particularly when students staged
spectacular events. In Berlin, such activities included the Anti-Vietnam
Congress in February 1968 (Fraser 1988: 177–180). In Berkeley, there
was an attempt to transform a parking lot owned by the university
into a 'People's Park' (Gitlin 1988: 354–361; Morgan 1991: 185–
186). Another tactic was to turn an established procedure, for example
a trial in court, into some sort of a political theatre by behaving in
unconventional ways or trying to switch roles so that the situation
became absurd. It appears that the radical students deliberately

designed some of their provocative and shocking activities to attract media attention, hoping to create a kind of counter-public with the unintended help of the established public. These tactics were often useful to get attention but, had counterproductive effects in other respects.

In summary, the New Left emphasized different strategies over time. In its nascent period, internal communication centred around intellectual magazines and discussion clubs. Communication with the outside world was very limited. Yet this reliance on their own channels of communication was not exactly the 'alternative' media strategy typified above. It did not result so much from negative experiences with the established media as from the desire to engage in a collective learning process. In a second period, when the movement became more visible in the public sphere due to its growing size and its provocative actions, the movement learnt that it received wide coverage but could not use the mainstream media for its own purposes. To a large extent, these media were hostile to the ideas and activities of the movement. Therefore, the movement shifted towards the 'attack strategy' by analysing, criticizing, and – occasionally – directly attacking these 'bourgeois media' without putting much effort into expanding movement-controlled media. Beyond a range of other factors, this strategy of attack contributed to widening the gap between the movement and its broader social environment.

New social movements in the 1970s and 1980s

In several ways, the new social movements (NSMs) of the 1970s and 1980s were rooted in the New Left sharing a concern for emancipatory politics and participatory democracy. They also emphasized the role of the individual, whose needs should not be subordinated to organizational concerns. However, the NSMs did not show much interest in the kind of (neo-)Marxist thinking that had preoccupied the New Left. Nor did they believe in revolutionary change. Instead they followed a pragmatic course of radical reform, seeking to build broad alliances and, in later phases, not shying away from combining extra-institutional and institutional politics.

Movement-controlled media

While the New Left integrated a number of issue domains without a distinct organizational specialization, the NSMs evolved around a range of issue domains such as human rights, women, peace, anti-nuclear, ecology, and Third World. Each of these domains became the focus of a particular movement, which developed its own organizational structure and means of communication (Stamm 1988). Most of the NSMs established their own journals, some of which still exist today. For example, the women's movement launched journals such as *Courage* and *Emma* in Germany and *Ms* in the USA. In addition, journals for more specific groups, for example lesbian feminists, were created. To the extent that large membership organizations existed or became revitalized due to the rise of the NSMs, internal newsletters produced by NSMs such as the National Organization of Women (NOW) and the Sierra Club in the USA also became important means of communication. Because the various movements had a common ideological background and organizational overlaps, they developed some overarching structures, for example educational centres and meeting places, but also print media that were not focused on a particular movement. In Germany a host of local political city magazines (*Stadtzeitungen*), usually published fortnightly or monthly, were created (Hübsch 1980). They included political essays and commentaries, reports on local movement activities, and practical hints (addresses, helplines, announcements of meetings, etc.). Because of the multitude of local groups, directories were published in most large cities. They were called *Stattbücher*, a play on words that emphasises the alternative character of this local scene but also refers to the idea of a 'city book'. In Berlin, for example, six different issues of the *Stattbuch* were published in the period from 1978 to 1999. In the prime time of the alternative milieu in Berlin, several thousand groups were represented in this directory.

The most significant step in terms of a communicative movement infrastructure in Germany was the establishment of the Berlin-based daily newspaper *die tageszeitung* in 1979, realizing a long-held dream of some New Left activists. The initiators of the paper clearly considered it as a mouthpiece of left-alternative movements which was set up with an alternative structure with little or no hierarchy, collective ownership, and the like. Over time, however, the newspaper, which currently has a circulation of roughly 60,000, became more professional, more independent from the movements, and less 'alternative' in its organizational structure (Flieger 1992). For instance, after long internal debates, an editor in chief was introduced. Nevertheless, it is still a paper close to, and widely read within, the NSMs. It has maintained, though somewhat softened, its leftist leaning. For instance, it is unlikely that the paper would accept an advertisement from, say, the chemical or automobile industry, let alone corporations engaged in the production of military weapons. Also, the paper occasionally surprises the reader with unconventional ideas. For example, when George W. Bush visited Berlin in May 2002 and was expected to give a 'historical speech' in the German Bundestag, the next day the paper came out with an empty front page entitled 'Bush's speech.'

The establishment of the German *tageszeitung* was not unique. The French daily, *Libération* had a similar background.[13] At least in its early days, this paper of the non-orthodox Left was meant to be a critical corrective and complement to the established media which were predominantly conservative or, in the case of *L'humanité*, an organ of the Communist Party. More than the German *tageszeitung*, however, its French counterpart became an 'established' left-liberal newspaper over time. Other attempts to create a daily paper as part of, or close to, the NSMs failed. For example, the Spanish paper *Liberación* had a short existence during the mid-1980s but was not economically viable, particularly because *El País*, a strong competitor on the Left, was already in place since 1976–77. By contrast, the French monthly *Le monde diplomatique* was a success story not only in its home country but also abroad. Today, this left-wing and movement-oriented journal is published in more than ten countries with a total circulation of 1.2 million copies, of which one quarter is sold in France (*Le monde diplomatique/die tageszeitung*, June 2002, p. 16).

Interactions with the 'establishment'

The examples of the *tageszeitung* and, especially, the French *Libération* indicate that groups and projects of the NSMs have changed considerably. In their period of formation, the NSMs considered themselves as outsiders who besieged the system of established politics as though it were a kind of fortress. As a consequence, they eagerly tried to build their own infrastructure and insisted on provocative action. Over the years, however, the majority of NSM groups have become less anti-systemic, more pragmatic, and more oriented towards problem-solving, thereby not shying away from *realpolitik* and co-operation with established actors. At the same time, the political and social context around the NSMs has changed – partly due to the aggregate impact of various movements that influenced people's minds, achieved some policy impacts, and triggered moderate reforms. As a consequence, the gap between the challenging groups on the one hand, and the established political actors on the other, narrowed (Rucht, 2003). The two sides began to talk to each other and, in some instances, even to cooperate. A telling indicator for this rapprochement was the debate about 'Staatsknete' (a casual term for state subsidies) in the early 1980s. When administrations discovered that some NSM groups were quite instrumental in reducing the burden of the welfare state, they offered financial and other support. This carrot triggered internal conflicts about whether or not it was politically correct to accept state money. Eventually, the large majority of the groups involved agreed to receive state subsidies in principle and, in part, even proactively asked for such state subsidies.

Another opening towards segments of the NSMs occurred in the mass media. To the extent that it became clear that most groups were far from being a bunch of mindless rascals who sought to overthrow 'the system', these groups were met with more fairness, if not open sympathy, by some in the mainstream media. Greenpeace is probably the best example. Although this group did not shy away from illegal activities, these were mainly symbolic and strictly non-violent. Above all, they were in full accordance with the media's news values. As a result, Greenpeace not only received tremendous media attention but also was treated by most media in a friendly or even supportive manner. Other groups had similar experiences with some mainstream media. Growing interaction with mass media led to an increasing professionalization of movement activists who learned to frame and stage their actions according to the needs and expectations of the mass media.[14]

What has been described here as a general trend does not hold for all social movement groups. Not surprisingly, mass media treated the more radical strands of the NSMs with much suspicion and often open attacks. Also, these groups learned that some kinds of messages and certain kinds of action were likely to be ignored by the mass media. As a consequence, they not only had to rely on their usual means of internal communication but also made deliberate efforts to correct institutionally what they perceived as structural deficits of the established system of mass media. One of these attempts was to extend the kind of media controlled by social movements. For example, groups were set up to produce and distribute videos or set up free radio stations that, in their early phase, were mostly illegal. Radio Dreyecksland, for example, located in the South-West of Germany close to the French border, was quite successful in evading surveillance and prosecution before it eventually became legalized; it recently celebrated its twentieth birthday. Another example of compensating for the selectivity and biases of established media was the creation of the Frankfurt-based 'information service to distribute withheld news' (*Informationsdienst zur Verbreitung unterbliebener Nachrichten*) in 1973 (Oy 2001: 134–137). Similarly, the US news magazine *Lies of Our Times*, mentioned above, was published to correct reports that, according to movement activists, were grossly and deliberately distorting or misleading. Another attempt to compensate for deficiencies of the mainstream media was the development of a media advocacy strategy or, in some cases, a kind of subversive strategy according to the advice: 'Use the media to fight and remember that it is a fight and it's guerrilla warfare' (Tony Schwartz). In these cases, groups stage provocative actions that are calculated to get mass media coverage. Particularly in the USA, the underlying body of knowledge has been codified in a number of 'how to do' handbooks so that groups do not have to reinvent the wheel.

All in all, the NSMs differed considerably from the New Left in the way they dealt with the media. First, they built up a much broader and more varied range of media that were controlled by, or close to, the movements. Second, these media were not reserved for small groups interested in theoretical and intellectual debates. Rather, they covered a wide range of political issues that were close to the experiences and needs of the broader populace. Not surprisingly, they also dealt with daily politics and conflicts that were local issues or restricted to particular segments of the population. Third, the NSMs created links with established mass media, which, as compared to the case of the New Left, were much more open and fair in their coverage of movement activities. To some extent, this openness was due to journalists who previously had worked in movement media or the underground press (Peck 1985: 313). Quite a few of them, even when working in a different setting and having a more conventional lifestyle, sympathized with protest groups and helped them to make some inroads into the established press. In addition, many movement groups professionalized their media work and adapted to the expectations of the established media. As a consequence, the lines between 'alternative' and 'established' media blurred in that the former became more conventional. Some of the magazines that were established by movements developed into regular media, thus completely abandoning their heritage. From this general trend towards 'conventionalization' one has to exclude the most radical groups, which, for better or worse, had to rely on their own means of communication. Via their newsletters, flyers and journals they try to identify, and compensate for, the selectivity and biases of the mainstream media, but without reaching a significant readership beyond their immediate ranks.

Coming back to the quadruple 'A' strategies introduced above, it is clear that the NSMs basically pursued two strategies. In a first period, probably informed by the negative experiences of the New Left with the established media, they relied heavily on the 'alternative strategy' by creating their own communicative infrastructure. In a second period, when less confrontational interactions between the NSMs and 'the establishment' prevailed, the movements gradually shifted towards the 'adaptation strategy' by conforming more or less to the requirements of the established media.

Transnational movements against neo-liberal globalization

During the 1990s, a new generation of progressive movements emerged, hereafter called transnational movements against neo-liberal globalization (TMs). Although it is difficult to determine whether these represent a new type of movement or should be regarded as an extension of NSMs, it is clear that they exhibit traits that, even if existent before, have now become more distinct and more salient. One of these is the focus on the global economy and politics and the critique of neo-liberalism. Another feature is the focus on public campaigns in which public relations strategies play a key role. A third element is the transnational character of these movements and their embracement of new information and communication technologies (ICTs). As most chapters in this volume deal with these kinds of groups and their use of ICTs, I will restrict myself to highlighting these phenomena in more general terms, particularly as compared to earlier developments.

As far as relations with established media are concerned, it is difficult to see a truly new element. However, it appears that the TMs have intensified and deepened the course taken by the NSMs. In other words, they are extremely conscious of the crucial role of mass media and have developed a good understanding of how these operate. Also, the TMs are usually quite professional in their way of doing 'public relations'. They deliberately design their actions and broader campaigns to attract media attention and positive coverage.[15] Probably more than most NSMs, TMs tend to stage actions that perhaps would not take place, at least not in their particular form, without the existence of mass media. This applies not only to transnational groups such as ATTAC that are basically located in the northern half of the globe but also to southern-based groups such as People's Global Action.

Conventional print media produced by the TMs, e.g. newsletters, newspapers, and magazines, appear to be of less importance than for the NSMs. Instead, the use of electronic communication, in particular the internet, plays a crucial role for TMs and, to a growing extent, contemporary NSMs as well (Scott and Steer 2001). As other chapters demonstrate in more detail, the internet serves several purposes. First, it is a convenient, fast and cheap means to find factual information about processes, groups, institutions, and events. Second, the internet – mainly communication by email – serves as a tool for individuals and groups to exchange information, to coordinate, and to ally. Third, it is used to mobilize for conventional actions such as rallies and blockades. Finally, the internet becomes a site of 'virtual' action in which the technology itself is both a weapon and a target (Ayres 1999; Smith 2001a). For example, protest groups disrupt electronic facilities and services of their opponents, or produce fake websites of their opponents stuffed with subversive information.

Clearly, the advantages of the internet are most obvious in terms of transnational communication and mobilization, which otherwise would be more cumbersome and costly. The Zapatista movement, for instance, used the internet to build a worldwide network of support groups (Schulz 1998). In addition, the international attention this movement received served as a shield to prevent military repression by the Mexican government.

Not surprisingly, the internet has also become a tool for movement groups specializing in facilitating and distributing information similar to what, by conventional means, has been intended by the German alternative news service (Informationsdienst zur Verbreitung unterbliebener Nachrichten) mentioned above. Indymedia, a leftist political network of movement-related information providers, originated in the framework of protests against the WTO meeting in Seattle in 1999. It describes itself as a 'democratic media outlet for the creation of radical, accurate, and passionate tellings of truth' (http:// www.indymedia.org/2 July 2002). Today, the network includes around 50 separate media centres and serves as a communication platform, particularly when major transnational protests are taking place. Not surprisingly, it is also being watched by journalists from conventional mass media. During the Seattle protests, the Independent Media Centre website received tens of thousands of visitors, including many journalists. In the week of the Genoa G8 protests, Indymedia sites received 'an estimated 5 million page views'.[16]

Though it would be an exaggeration to characterize the TMs merely as a child of the internet, they are the groups that rely most extensively on the net. Because much of the internet communication of TMs is open to everybody, academic observers use it as their main source of information and therefore tend to overestimate the relevance of the internet to these groups.[17] It seems that the internet is an important facilitator of information and mobilization, but it cannot replace the personal contacts among the key organizers of protest campaigns. Precisely because the internet allows so many diverse groups to join a campaign, it becomes important to the core organizers of protest campaigns to be able to build trust and solidarity based on personal connections. Also, it would be wrong to assume that protest via the internet (e.g. standardized emails to appeal to a political leader) can replace the physical encounter of masses of protesters. First, opponents and the wider public are more impressed by forms of protest that require a personal investment instead of just a mouse click. Second, because electronic protest letters, queries, etc. can be produced in immense numbers by one person or group, electronic protest may also raise doubts about the nature of the senders and their accountability. Third, since the internet is open to everybody, it essentially lacks quality control and therefore may lack the credibility that is generally attributed to the mainstream media.

In sum, for today's movements the internet has become an important extension of their means to communicate their messages. However, whether or not this reliance on the internet is part of an 'alternative strategy', as presented above, remains arguable. On the one hand, the internet, at least in part, allows TMs/NSMs to circumvent the established media, and to communicate directly with social movement adherents and sympathizers. Interestingly, in the case of the internet, the convenient distinction between media that are internal and external to social movements is no longer valid. Unlike other mass media, the information offered on the net is not controlled by a few gate-keepers. On the other hand, unlike conventional newsletters (which continue to exist even in TMs), the internet neither has been created nor is being controlled by the movements (though it is not under the control of the 'establishment' either).

Progressive movements use the net for its convenience and efficiency, not because the conventional mass media (as in the period of the New Left) are perceived as hostile and inaccessible. On the contrary, the strategy of 'adaptation' occupies a central place for NSMs and TMs. However, this does not necessarily mean that the movements' impact has increased. Also, their opponents and adversaries have realized the importance of mass media and learned to play the media game. This applies to both the use of the internet[18] and the interaction with established mass media. Moreover, one should not forget that the traditional means of internal communication such as printed newsletters still play an important role in many movements, although certainly less so in most TMs.

Summary

Social movements have increasingly moved from the local to the national (Tilly 1984) and, more recently, to the transnational sphere (della Porta *et al.* 1999; Tarrow 2001). This also implies that more and more people can observe, or may even become involved in, social movement activities, provided that adequate means of communication and mobilization exist. Hence, in a long historical perspective we observe a shift from direct to mediated communication in which various kinds of mass media play a crucial role. Mass media, though to different degrees, were and are an important reference point of social movements. Depending on the circumstances, the movements could follow different strategies that have been typified as the quadruple 'A': adaptation, attack, alternatives, and abstention.

Communication among groups of the New Left was heavily based on physical encounters so that movement-controlled media were of minor importance. This is also indicated by the fact that for many New Left activists, reading and digesting information was part of a collective enterprise. Another important factor was that the established media showed little sympathy with the New Left and, for the most part, was considered a tool in the hands of the movement's adversaries. Consequently, attack became the overriding strategy as a response to frustrating experiences with the mass media.

Compared to the New Left, the NSMs of the 1970s and 1980s were more numerous, socially more diversified, and more pragmatic in their overall attitude. Also, they raised issues that were closer to the daily experiences of ordinary people and did not need much theorizing. These properties have also influenced the movements' communicative structures. On the one hand, the NSMs built their own and self-controlled media – thus applying the *alternative* strategy. Thereby they could reach groups beyond their immediate ranks. On the other hand, the NSMs increasingly engaged in exchanges with the established mass media, which, at least in part, sympathized with the more moderate strands of the movements. As a consequence, the movements' critique of the established media was generally more moderate and the initial idea, borrowed from the New Left – to create some kind of counter-publics – gradually waned. The media's more open attitude to the

NSMs was another factor to broaden the basis and reach of the movements, which, particularly in a second phase, shifted towards the strategy of *adaptation*.

With the rise of *transnational movements* against neo-liberalism, the sophistication and professionalization of media work further increased, thereby making the strategy of adaptation even more pronounced when compared to the NSMs. However, the internet was more important in facilitating the exchange of information and mobilization for protest, particularly for this kind of movement. The net relativized, but did not replace, the traditional means of both internal and external communication of the movements.

Table 2.1, drawing on the media-related strategies of attack, adaptation and the creation of alternatives, summarizes these basic features. Abstention, the fourth option, is ignored because it hardly occurred among the movements investigated here. They were simply too committed to their cause to give up their struggle.

What do these changes mean for the self-understanding, the structure, and the effects of movement politics? Overall, it appears that today's protest groups are in a better position than their forerunners to reach their adherents and sympathizers across large territories. The range of media they use has broadened, and internal communication has become easier, more effective, and cheaper. Also, large segments of these movements have professionalized their ways of dealing with the established media and have partly won the latter's sympathy. Nevertheless, easily available channels and pieces of information create a situation where the average citizen risks drowning in a sea of 'noise' produced by an immense number of groups and issues. Hence, even with improved technical means, the 1960s' idea of creating a counter-public (*Gegenöffentlichkeit*) is far from reality. Instead, we witness a fragmentation of the public sphere that cannot be observed, let alone controlled, from any one particular vantage point. Moreover, the sophistication of media-related strategies was not restricted to progressive movements but also became a weapon in the hands of these movements' opponents.

Finally, coming back to the theoretical issues discussed in the introduction, it is important to note that the relationship between protest movements and conventional mass media has remained fragile and asymmetric in spite of the media's greater openness to the movements and the latter's better understanding of the media's modes of operation. It would be wrong to characterize this relationship as symbiotic, though remarkable exceptions such as the White March in Belgium (Walgrave and Manssens 2000) and the pro-East Timor movement

Table 2.1 Progressive movements' attitudes to the media

Type of movement	Attack	Adaptation	Alternatives
New Left	Strong critique of the established media; occasionally direct action against such media	None, but recognition of the media's attention for spectacular action	Importance of own (intellectual) journals; no daily newspapers
New social movements	Generally moderate	Gradual adaptation; partly professional media strategies	Importance of local movement media (weeklies and monthlies, free radios, etc.); creation of daily nationwide newspapers in some countries
Movements against neo-liberalism	Generally moderate, but strong critique by some radical groups who felt criminalized by the media	Professional media strategies; staging of spectacular action	Streamlining of alternative presses; growing importance of the internet; creation of the worldwide news service, Indymedia

in Portugal (Chapter 7) can be cited. The mainstream media basically select groups, issues, and actions according to their own criteria, and the movements get (positive) media coverage only to the extent that they respect these criteria. Groups that deliberately or inadvertently ignore these requirements are condemned to negative coverage or no coverage at all.[19] Some of them therefore resort to violence, which guarantees coverage. However, this coverage usually comes at a cost, namely social isolation.

What follows from these reflections is that social movements would be wrong to ignore the established mass media as a potential sounding board or, in rare cases, even as an ally. However, social movements would be equally mistaken in assuming that, in learning about the rules and mechanisms of the mass media, they could rely on, let alone instrumentalize, the mass media. These follow their own logic, which is markedly different from that of social movements. Therefore, the maintenance of movement-controlled media remains essential to secure autonomy and operational flexibility.

Notes

1 Social movements do compete with each other for scarce resources, e.g. attention, financial contributions, and activists' time.

2 This asymmetry, which is also emphasized by Gamson and Wolfsfeld (1993), escapes Molotch (1979: 92) when he concludes: 'Media and movements are dialectically bound, always in motion and alert one another's motion – be it embrace, flight, or thundering blow. The most appropriate metaphor to describe their relationship is dance – sometimes a dance of death.'

3 'Notes of Readers' in *New Left Review* 11 (1961). Cited according to Gilcher-Holtey (1995: 88).

4 Later, the journals *Il Manifesto, Lotta Continua, Quotidiano dei lavoratori, Quaderni Rossi, Classe Operaia, Quaderni Piacentini* and a few others became important forums of intellectual debate for the Italian student movement (Kurz 2001: 24–25; Tarrow 1989: 157).

5 For details on the intellectual background of both French journals, see Gilcher-Holtey (1995: 50–72).

6 Note that there was a journal *Studies on the Left* (founded in 1959) which, however, remained fairly insignificant.

7 This is captured by Rayna Rapp, an SDS activist from the USA: 'I think all our flamboyant "politics and culture" and "politics as confrontation" and "politics as theatre" stretched the boundaries in the U.S. and was useful – but it wasn't a strategy for reaching people who were different from us, who were either older or more ensconced in the working-class or even middle-class jobs. That was a tremendous mistake' (quoted in Fraser 1988: 358).

8 The obvious exceptions to this rule were major newspapers close to the communist parties in some European countries, for example *Il Manifesto* in Italy and *L'Humanité* in France.

9 *Leicester Mercury*, 6 November 1969, cited in Halloran *et al.* (1970: 311–312).

10 With some support of liberal-minded magazines, in particular *Der Spiegel* and *Stern*, an 'Institute for Press Analysis and Research on the Public Sphere' was created in 1968, though this remained essentially a symbolic act. In this context also, the idea of a radical left daily newspaper emerged but did not materialize before 1978–1979 with the *tageszeitung*. Another initiative was the plan to organize a critical evaluation of the Springer press corporation in February 1968. However, the organizers and potential contributors were divided over the question of whether this should be more a scientific hearing or a political tribunal, so that the event was cancelled on short notice (Oy 2001: 128–129).

11 See the 'Basic Declaration on the Campaign to Expropriate the Springer Corporation', SDS, 14 April 1968.

12 Note that the movement also inspired some journalists in the established press. For example, in 1969 an action group of critical journalists of *Der Spiegel* (the weekly magazine) distributed a flyer calling on people to fight 'against exploitation and incapacitation at the workplace' and for 'democratic participation'. These were also the journalists who wrote critical articles about the power of corporations, concentration in the press sector and the US war crimes in Vietnam in the following years, but gradually became silenced within the paper (Braun 1992).

13 The driving force behind the foundation of the paper was *La Gauche Prolétarienne* (*The Proletarian Left*), a non-orthodox group with its roots in the 1968 movement (Dupuy 1998). Before, the group had published *La Cause du Peuple* (*The People's Cause*) which, when declared illegal, was supported by Jean-Paul Sartre. In a symbolic gesture, Sartre also became the first director of *Libération*.

14 For an excellent account of how this can be achieved, see Ryan (1991).

15 This, of course, is not new. Already the peace activists organizing the Easter marches in Germany in the 1960s were evaluating and assessing their resonance in the media. However, it was, to my knowledge, ATTAC that organized the first crash course to instruct movement organizers on how to deal with the media in Germany in summer 2002.

16 Indymedia's Frequently Asked Questions. URL: http://process.indymedia.org/faq.php3 (4 July 2002).

17 Meyer and Tarrow (1998), for instance, praise the internet as a source to study computer-based political activism: 'Perhaps the most attractive feature of these computer networks is the accurate and easily traceable path left by activists'.

18 See, for example, Chroust's (2000) analysis of Taliban and neo-Nazis' use of the internet.

19 For a case of tremendous attention but unanimously negative coverage, see Rucht (2001) on the Mayday demonstrations in London in 2000.

3   Politicizing *Homo economicus*
Analysis of anti-corporate websites

Jacob Rosenkrands

Holding big business democratically accountable – this is the *raison d'être* of the new anti-corporate movement which has turned the market into a political battleground. This chapter explores the role played by the internet in the targeting of corporations. A number of popular anti-corporate websites are analysed and the following questions addressed: Which kinds of goals are pursued? Which types of organizations and groups run anti-corporate websites? Who are those who are targeted? How are the special functionalities and features of the internet utilized? Which types of organizational strategies do the websites reflect? How are websites linked to other websites?

The research outlined below indicates that anti-corporate websites are basically concerned with politics and societal change. The internet has facilitated the formation of new global alliances, bringing together well-established NGOs, so-called culture jammers, activists, and ordinary citizens. Individual companies are targeted as examples or symbols of general problems. The internet is used to increase the capacity of activists and organizations to disseminate information and mobilize support for their cause. Most of the websites studied link to other anti-corporate websites, which contribute to the notion of their being a significant movement on the internet, which I will outline below using examples of anti-corporate campaigns.

Let us begin with an example of consumer activism taking new forms in the information age as a result of internet use. In 1989, due to an initiative called 'The Barbie Liberation Organization', hundreds of children had a very special toy for Christmas. Families were confused when girls and boys opened their presents, which they expected would contain ordinary Barbie and G.I. Joe dolls. However, the voice boxes of the two types of dolls had been switched. Girls found their Barbies saying: 'Dead men tell no lies'. Boys were just as astonished to hear their G.I. Joes ask: 'Wanna go shopping?' The idea to alter these typical girls' and boys' toys was originally posted on the anti-corporate website of (R)(TM)ark. An anonymous person wanted to draw public attention to the sexist and violent images which Barbie and G.I. Joe represent. Soon, the idea found itself sponsored by a group of war veterans who were opposed to war-like toys. They invested $5000 in the project. The 'Barbie Liberation Organization' then turned the ideas, originally posted on a website, into a more concrete form of protest. They bought several hundred dolls, altered them, and put them back on the shelves in toyshops. By Christmas Eve and in the weeks to come, the action was first reported by local TV and newspapers, then taken up by national and international media which brought the message of the Barbie activists to hundreds of millions of people around the world (National Forum 2001).

On the internet there are now hundreds of websites for consumers who want to gather information on the activities of transnational firms, to build relations to other consumers and take action to hold companies to account. As a phenomenon this type of activism does not fit into the traditional categories for consumer action and political action, which are supposed to take place strictly in the sphere of the market or the domain of politics. Rather, it may be a manifestation of what in this chapter will be called the 'political consumer', but which is also referred to by terms such as the 'green consumer' and the 'ethical consumer' (Sørensen 2002). A political consumer can be defined as 'a person who seriously takes into consideration values when he or she deliberately buys or abstains from buying certain goods in order to achieve a political goal' (Andersen and Tobiasen 2001). What is stressed by this definition is that consumer action is not necessarily wholly self-oriented, but may in fact be based on concern for a larger community or society as a whole.

Whereas the 'political consumer' is a new concept, political consumerism is not new. Historically, the boycott, which is without doubt the best-known tool of the political consumer, was first described in 1880. The term was invented by the British newspaper the *Daily Mail* which covered a fierce conflict between the Irish National Land League and the British land-agent Captain Charles Cunningham Boycott. In recent years the public focus on the political consumer has been intensified due to a number of spectacular boycotts of specific countries and companies. Among these were the prolonged boycott of South Africa which was supported by United Nations (UN), and not the least the events of summer 1995 when consumers across the world took action against France, or rather its corporations, as a response to its testing of nuclear devices in the Pacific, and consumers also protested against Shell's dumping of the *Brent Spar* (Sørensen 2002).

Recent research suggests that the political consumerism should be considered as a form of democratic participation (Andersen and Tobiasen 2001). A study among Danish consumers found a significant correlation between a general interest in politics and political consumer behaviour. Political consumers express a higher degree of global orientation and sense of global solidarity than consumers who base their choices on economic criteria. On top of that, political consumers themselves consider patterns of shopping driven by political motivation to be an efficient means to influence politics. Interestingly, they rate that efficiency to be higher than a number of traditional forms of democratic participation, such as party membership, personal requests to politicians, public demonstrations and other forms of grassroots activities. Among political consumers, only voting is considered to be more efficient (Andersen and Tobiasen 2001). These results indicate that the boundaries between the consumer role and the role as a democratic citizen are less clear than they used to be. The question is how to describe behaviour that takes place beyond the political domain but nevertheless has political consequences. It has been suggested that political consumerism is an expression of what Ulrich Beck calls 'sub-politics', or is linked to Anthony Giddens' concept of 'life politics' (Sørensen 2002, Beck 1997, Giddens 1991). Indeed, as more people choose to take action on the market in order to bring about changes in society, researchers may need to develop a new ideal type – a mixture between *Homo economicus* and *Homo politicus*.

Clearly, the global marketplace seems to have become a new and rather significant political battleground. The now legendary public demonstrations against the World Trade Organization in Seattle in 1999 put into focus a large and diverse number of organizations, networks, movements and groupings from countries all over the world, which stand united when it comes to protesting against the power of transnational corporations and corporate globalization. Despite its heterogeneity it has been called an 'anti-corporate movement' (Starr 2000). Starr counts anti-free trade agreement organizations, organizations working for peace and human rights, environmentalists, groups supporting the Zapatistas in Mexico, explicitly anti-corporate movements and more as being the constituents of this movement. Although these organizations do not share a common identity – rather a common devotion to 'a politics of difference' – the links between most of the groups are so many that they may be seen as one movement.

In the core of this movement, and of special interest to this chapter, are the 'explicit anti-corporate movements', which are explicitly organized around limiting corporate power. Their strategic approach implies 'mobilizing existing channels of protest, seeking national legislation, mounting judicial challenges, mobilizing international agencies, boycotting and protesting' (Starr 2000: 45). Often individual companies are targeted by organizations aligned with this movement, but the cases are frequently presented to the public 'as just one example of the problem' (Starr 2000: 67). The intended target could just as well be whole industries or groups of companies engaged in genetical engineering or sweatshop production in the Third World. The Canadian journalist and activist, Naomi Klein, author of *No Logo* (2000), gives this explanation as to why activists address companies rather than politicians:

> It is a question of strategy. The corporations are not the real targets, but more like a doorway. The activists very deliberately choose corporations, which can be used to influence the public agenda and wake up politicians. They know very well that corporations are only the tip of the iceberg. Monsanto was targeted in the debate on genetic modification because it had a strategic value, because it was an industry leader and had the awareness of governments. In a way these big corporations are used as public education tools. Instead of discussing globalization the activists focus on a single company – how it does business, where in the world it has its activities, how it earns money and works with politicians. From this comes the understanding of the larger pattern.
>
> (personal interview, 2001)

Kenny Bruno, who is a project coordinator at CorpWatch, agrees that anti-corporate campaigning, even when it is directed against a single company, aims to reach a larger audience:

> I think the lesson gets sent to other companies when one company is hurt. I am sure that Shell is not the only company that has reacted to Shell's own problems. Other companies see that and say: 'Oh my gosh, that better not happen to me'. So I think it is worthwhile for our movement to target companies to make them examples.
>
> (personal interview, 2001)

Of course, neither political consumerism nor anti-corporate activism can be discussed in isolation from the general trends in business and the global market. Corporations are increasingly exposed to political scrutiny and criticism for a number of reasons. In the first place, liberalizations of trade and investment throughout the 1980s and 1990s – in the EU the Internal Market – have increased the liberties of corporations considerably. This, along with the ongoing concentration of power in ever-larger merged units, has paved the way for the commonly held view that corporations should be considered a political force and thus treated as such. Indeed, today among the 100 wealthiest economic units, less than half are nation states; the bulk is made up by multinationals. Secondly, corporations have themselves by their communication and marketing strategies invited the public to view companies as something more than mere providers of products. The focus on socially responsible behaviour and stakeholder relations is stronger than ever, which is also true of the corporate interest in branding. This notion refers to marketing processes linking the name of a company or a product to certain lifestyles or values such as freedom, healthiness, harmony. The growing importance of corporate image has clearly made the companies more vulnerable to even small groups of activists (Deegan 2001), as illustrated in this chapter and also by Bennett in Chapter 6. Activists themselves are very aware that the process of corporate branding can be turned around to the disadvantage of companies. This is what Naomi Klein describes as 'the brand boomerang'.

> It is the very idea of branding that has made these corporations so vulnerable. Branding is the idea that companies have to build a deeper relationship with the consumer. That they should sell a certain life style instead of a product. The criteria for success become how well the brand influences the identity of the consumer. But often this is a very hollow corporate model, in which the reality of production does not live up to the values which are marketed. So branding can be like putting a sign on your back saying: 'Kick me!' When consumers realize the mismatch between the ways goods are manufactured and the claims companies make about themselves, things can change quickly. What activists do is to systematically reveal juxtapositions between the grand, ambitious claims companies make about the meaning of their brand and the reality.
>
> (personal interview, 2001)

In their procedures for business intelligence, many companies will pay attention to the potential threats posed by internet-based activism. Thus, for example, the Danish medical company, Novo, constantly monitors the activities of animal rights groups on the internet. Novo is at risk of becoming a target of these groups because the company is highly dependent on animal experiments. The Novo researchers study their opponents: the rhetoric and storytelling techniques of specific organizations, the actual links and networks created between related activist groups, and the values which make up a social community among these groups (Advice A/S 2002).

The Coca-Cola Company also monitors its opponents, for example the CokeSpotlight website. The goal of this website was to make the company adopt a new refrigeration policy. 'Yes, we do monitor the internet for mentions of The Coca-Cola Company and its brands, using a variety of services', the company states in an official answer regarding the implications of the CokeSpotlight website. 'It did influence us, in the sense that it confirmed to us, a keen societal interest in HFC-free refrigeration and it probably affected the timing and place of the announcement concerning our public commitment', the statement says (email from Coca-Cola Company, June 2002).

The internet and the relation between citizens and corporations

In a European context the influence of new technology on the relationship between citizens and political parties, between citizens and administration and between citizens themselves – and the consequences for democracy – have been analysed (Hoff *et al.* 2000). In political science at least, the relationship between citizens and corporations has been less well documented, which is indeed also the case in terms of examining the influence of new technology on this relationship.

There are relatively few studies of the impact of the internet on the strategies and organization of movements operating in the field of anti-corporate activism. The American military think-tank, RAND, has documented the importance of the internet in international campaigns against political and economical institutions, and launched the term 'NGO-swarms'. This refers to situations when activists link themselves together on line in concerted actions, thus creating a multi-headed force, impossible to decapitate (Arquilla and Ronfeldt 1996, 2001). Both Starr and Deegan point to the internet as an important platform for interaction between activists in various countries (Starr 2000, Deegan 2001).

Kenny Bruno from CorpWatch has this to say about the role of the internet in the anti-corporate movement:

> It is obvious that the web is a tremendous tool because you can communicate with hundreds of people so easily and generate momentum among your colleagues and your allies and networks. The campaign against the Multilateral Agreement on Investment (MAI) is the classic example. But there are many more examples. I really believe that transnational campaigning is extremely important. Until recently it was very rare because of communication difficulties. Clearly the Internet has made transnational coordination and campaigning faster. In our campaign on UN [United Nations] in little more than a week we had over a hundred people signing letters for Kofi Annan. In the past that would have taken more than a month, and the whole issue would have moved on.
>
> (personal interview, 2001)

In the light of this statement the limited academic interest in this subject is in principle surprising. Hypothetically, the internet could play a very important role in empowering political consumers and anti-corporate activists, in such a way that they might become a true political force.

Empirical focus and research questions

Could the internet become a platform for developing a shared discourse among political consumers, activists or just concerned citizens? For mobilizing citizens across borders and independently of traditional mass media? For building new communities? This study will not bring the definitive answers, the modest ambition being to explore empirically the use of the internet by anti-corporate activists in order to find similarities and differences, from which new and more precise hypotheses can be derived about the possible effect of the internet in the relations between citizens and corporations. For this purpose a number of anti-corporate, but mutually diverse, websites were studied.

Included in the study are websites that explicitly address companies or markets in order to bring about changes in society. The selection of websites has been based on the search engine Lycos, which operates with a number of subgroups very useful for the purpose of this chapter, one of these being 'anti-corporation'.

The first step was a review of the brief summaries of websites provided in the sections concerning 'Activism' and 'Business'. This gives an impression of the prevalence of websites addressing the societal role of business: 'anti-corporation' 115 sites, 'anti-consumerist' nine sites, 'allegedly unethical firms' 326, 'corporate accountability' 43, 'ethical review' eight, 'sweat shops' 44 (December 2001). In comparison, the section 'Activism' totals around 1400 sites. The second step was to select websites from these groups to be analysed in relation to the research questions stated above. The websites analysed include sites that focus on individual companies as well as sites that cover other questions concerning business and democracy. Excluded from this analysis were a number of sites which had not recently been updated and sites which strictly focused on a national agenda, most of them American. Details of the websites are given in Table 3.1.

As suggested in the introduction to this book, analysis of social movements should address questions concerned with: the ideological or discursive frame within which a movement operates; the changes it works to bring about in society; the ways it mobilizes members and non-members to support its cause; and the larger network of social groups and organizations it may be part of. Hence, the following questions have guided the analysis.

- Methodological aim: How are the purpose, cause or values of the websites presented and justified?
- Agent: Who is the initiator and manager of the website?
- Target: Who is the object of the protest?
- Content and technological functionalities: How are the characteristics and opportunities of the internet utilized?
- Organizational purpose: What role does the internet play in the activities of the organization or movement?
- Links: Does the website link to other movements and organizations?

How are the purpose, cause or values of the websites presented and justified?

Not surprisingly, the wish to curb the power of big business is a common denominator of most of the anti-corporate websites. However, the focus varies slightly. Some websites, like CokeSpotlight, have such a well-defined mission that they cease to 'exist' the moment their specific goal is achieved, in this case the request that Coca-Cola phase out its use of greenhouse gas hydrofluorocarbons (HFCs) in refrigeration before the Athens Olympics 2004. In June 2000 the Coca-Cola Company announced that it would comply with this. Thus, Coke-Spotlight is the story of a single-cause campaign. But not many anti-corporate websites function like that. Most other sites are parts of ongoing ideological or value-based struggles – for example the struggle to secure workers' basic rights (Nike Watch) or to hold corporations accountable (CorpWatch). Remarkably, some websites simply state their mission to be to support the anti-corporate movement as such. This is the rhetoric of the No Logo site, of (R)(TM)ark which wants 'to further anti-corporate activism', and of Adbusters Foundation (www.adbusters.org), which strives 'to advance the new social activist movement of the information age'. This indicates that the anti-corporate movement is in fact considered a movement in its own right by these groups and organizations.

Most of the websites analysed assume that the user has some sort of interest in collectivist values and that he or she wants to be addressed as a citizen more than as a consumer. However, it should be noted that during the review of websites several were found which take another point of departure. For instance, the British site Ethical-consumer.org contains a database with differing kinds of information on the ethical behaviour of different companies. The impression is that this is a practical guide for consumers more than the face of a movement. This is definitely also the case for the American site, The Boycott Index (www.boycottindex.com). 'This site gives me the information I need to make informed choices at the local supermarket' is its self-description. This is a diffuse and divergent site displaying information supporting many different, and also mutually contradictory, points of view, e.g. pro-homosexuality as well as anti-homosexuality, and even links to sites about 'boycotting the boycotters'!

Who is the initiator and manager of the website?

At one end of a spectrum of transparency/anonymity are well-esteemed organizations such as Greenpeace and Oxfam, which have quite successfully integrated the internet into their existing strategies. At the other end of that spectrum are enterprises such as (R)(TM)ark, which does not describe itself as an organization in great detail, and Noamazon.com (www.noamazon.com), whose initiator is impossible to identify by looking through the website.

Without doubt, the perceived legitimacy of anti-corporate websites is dependent on who runs them. However, a track record as an established NGO seems to be secondary to the quality of the website and the ability to create activity on the site. A good example is the No Logo site (www.nologo.org), run by the Canadian Naomi Klein and a handful of activists, which in terms of content is very comprehensive and is

Table 3.1 Details of some anti-corporate websites

Website	Aim	Agent	Target	Functionalities	Organization's purpose	Links
Adbusters Foundation (www. adbusters. org)	To advance the new social activist movement of the information age. To run projects which counter consumer culture	Adbusters Foundation – a global network of artists, activists, writers, pranksters, students, educators and entrepreneurs	Business, the advertising industry, supporters of consumer culture	• Web version of *Adbusters* magazine • Personal statements and stories from users • Download of posters, stickers, postcards, etc. • Sale of Adbusters merchandise • Information on current campaigns and how to get involved	Information/ mobilization	To other anti-consumer websites and organizations
CokeSpotlight (www. cokespotlight. org)	To demand environmental responsibility from . . . The Coca-Cola Company	Adbusters Foundation and Greenpeace	Coca-Cola Company	• News about the campaign • Media center including facts and photos • Extensive information about global warming • Guide for individual action	Primarily mobilization	To other sites concerned with global warming
CorpWatch (www. corpwatch. org)	To hold corporations accountable and counter corporate-led	CorpWatch	Transnational corporations	• News, analysis and first-person accounts of corporate behaviour • Updates on CorpWatch campaigns	Primarily information	To sites related to a number of selected issues

| McSpotlight (www. macspotlight. org) | globalization through education and activism To oppose McDonald's as a symbol of multinationals pursuing their profits at the expense of anything that stands in their way | McInformation Network, an independent network of volunteers working from 22 countries | McDonald's and similar corporations | • Guide for users to do their own research on corporations
• Alerts and information on how to get involved in grassroots action
• Extensive information on the McLibel Trial
• News on latest activities and legal disputes of McDonald's
• News on previous and upcoming protest activities
• Discussion groups
• Sale of anti-McDonald's merchandise
• Media center with video, photos, extensive information
• Introduction to a large number of other anti-corporate issues | Information/ mobilization | To a large number of anti-corporate websites and organizations |

continued on next page

Table 3.1 continued

Website	Aim	Agent	Target	Functionalities	Organization's purpose	Links
Nike Watch (www.caa.org. au/campaigns/ nike/index. html)	To persuade Nike and other transnational corporations to respect workers' basic rights	Oxfam Community Aid Abroad	Nike	• News on corporate behaviour of Nike, resports about conditions in Nike factories, etc. • Action guide, including materal for teachers and information on 'nearest sweatshop campaign'	Information/ mobilization	To Nike and anti-sweatshop organizations
Noamazon. com (www. noamazon. com)	To oppose technology monopoly by Amazon (e-business software for 'one click ordering')	Unspecified	Amazon	• Specification of commercial alternatives to Amazon • News on the position of Amazon, including litigation against competitors • Guide on how to send protest emails to politicians and Amazon	Information/ mobilization	To commercial alternatives to Amazon products

Website	Aim	Initiators	Target	Content	Function	Links
No Logo (www. nologo.com)	To support the movement against big brands and corporate globalization	Author of *No Logo*, journalist Naomi Klein and individual activists	Corporate brands	• Information and debate on *No Logo* and related issues • Chatrooms • Questions and answers, user to user • Personal comments and articles by users • News on actions and events	Primarily community building	To a large number of anti-corporate websites and organizations
(R)(TM)ark (www. rtmark.com)	To further anti-corporate activism by channelling funds from donors to workers	The private enterprise, (R)(TM)ark – otherwise unspecified	Industrial and corporate interests	• Descriptions of previous and current projects • Discussion groups on specific projects	Primarily mobilization	To other anti-corporate websites and organizations
Sane BP (www. Sanebp.com)	To move BP from damaging oil exploration towards renewable energy	Umbrella group for BP investors concerned about climate change. Includes the project initiator, Greenpeace and the US Public Research Interest Group	BP	• Information on climate change and renewable energy • Information on Sane BP campaigns • Resolutions submitted to BP annual shareholder meetings		

also characterized by a high degree of user activity. New actors and new alliances play important roles behind the interfaces of anti-corporate websites. For Greenpeace, the coming of the information society has paved the way for interesting new alliances. In the Coke-Spotlight (www.cokespotlight.org) campaign, Greenpeace has worked closely with the Canadian Adbusters Foundation which is part of the Culture Jammers movement – a network of activists working in the area between pop culture, art and politics (Lasn 1999). In the 'Sane BP' campaigns an alliance has been formed between Greenpeace, the US Public Research Interest Group and many individually socially responsible investors. The idea is to encourage BP shareholders to bring societal concerns onto the internal agenda of the company. In BP's annual general meeting 2001 this led to a resolution being proposed calling for a shift from oil production towards renewable energy. Further, the diversity of involvement can be illustrated by the McSpotlight site (www.macspotlight.org), which is produced by a truly global network of activists and organizations consisting of volunteers working from 22 countries.

The relationship between activists and business is often described as a David–Goliath relation, which suggests that even small groups of activists can harm large corporations when conflicts evolve in the media. It seems that the internet opens up even more doors of opportunities for the underdog.

Who is the object of the protest?

Anti-corporate websites can be split into two groups: the ones that target individual companies, and the ones that characterize the opponent as being related to specific conditions within society, e.g. 'transnational corporations' or 'corporate globalization' or 'consumer culture'.

The review of Lycos website summaries shows that transnational corporations such as Coca-Cola, Exxon Mobil, Disney, Mattel, McDonald's, Monsanto, Nestlé, Nike, and Wal-Mart are among those most frequently targeted. They share this position with companies that produce computers, software or other solutions relating to the internet community, e.g. Adobe Systems, Amazon, Gator, and Microsoft.

The difference between websites that target specific companies and those that target specific conditions in society should not be exaggerated. Most of the websites focusing on individual companies cannot be reduced to single-cause enterprises since they often place themselves in a discourse which is much broader and very similar to the less focused – some would say more political – anti-corporate websites.

At the McSpotlight website, the reason for targeting McDonald's is said to be that the corporation is 'a symbol of all multinationals and big business relentlessly pursuing their profits at the expense of everything that stands in their way'. The site contains a section named 'Beyond McDonald's' which is a guide to how to protest against other big corporations which allegedly are out of line in terms of animal abuse, production of weapons, workers' rights, etc. The larger perspective of the specific campaign is also explicitly described at Noamazon.com. This site opposes the aggressive effort of e-commerce giant, Amazon, to defend its innovative software solution for 'one-click ordering'. In the absence of protest there is a risk that Amazon will 'achieve a technology monopoly across all internet commerce sites', that 'internet commerce will drown in a sea of litigation', that 'innovation will cease', and independent retailers 'will be squashed', it says. The message is that corporations are targeted because they epitomize general problems in the market or in society.

How are the characteristics and opportunities of the internet utilized?

Technically, most of the sites are quite simple. Sound and video files are rare, and these are primarily found on sites that have advanced media centres. In terms of interactivity, on most sites real-time chatting between users is not an option. The exception is the 'No Logo' site, which has a number of interactive features, one being the chatroom, another the research section where users can pose and answer questions about corporate power. Conferences and debates are a little more common. Several websites invite users to contribute their own views and stories. Lively debates, however, are hard to find. More emphasis is generally put on the unique storing capacity of the internet. Sites are used to document the work done and progress made by the organization or movement in question. McSpotlight, for instance, contains extensive information on the McLibel Trial between McDonald's and three activists, the longest trial in UK history. (R)(TM)ark (www.rtmark.org), which is an organization that does not publish much information about itself, in contrast offers rather detailed descriptions of previous activist projects supported by (R)(TM)ark. On the other hand, sites also offer news and information about their target or cause. McSpotlight, Noamazon.com, and Nike Watch (www.caa.org.au/campaigns/nike/index.html) systematically track information on their opponents; CorpWatch (www.corpwatch.org) serves as a watch dog following a wide range of multi-national corporations. CokeSpotlight does contain information on the Coca-Cola Company, but also focuses on topics such as climate change, global warming and cooling gases. Many websites offer news by email. From its website Adbusters Foundation presents a web version of its magazine, *Adbusters Magazine*.

In spite of the general low degree of interactivity, most websites offer plenty of possibilities to get involved. Users are invited to take part in specific campaigns, not only by sending financial donations, but also by means of a number of tools specific to the internet. On several sites it is possible to show support by downloading web banners, stickers, and posters, and to forward electronic campaign postcards to friends. Common to many of these forms of participation is that they do not require the user to register or be a member. Neither do they require much time and effort. As the CokeSpotlight site says: 'Getting involved in the Coke Challenge Campaign is simple – everything you need is right here'. Lists of upcoming street action in various countries and neighbourhoods are frequently used. On some sites it is possible to take immediate action, for example by using prefabricated protest letters directed at corporations and politicians, or by using prefabricated material targeted at groups such as the press or schoolteachers.

A special feature of some websites which align themselves with the Culture Jammers movement is the use of subversions of corporations' images of themselves or their products. Adbusters Foundation (which, apart from running its own website, is involved in the CokeSpotlight campaign) uses this technique, as does McSpotlight. These anti-ads exploit the graphic potential of the internet to deliberately ridicule the big brands which put so much effort into building and protecting their image (Bennett expands on this theme in Chapter 6). In summary, the anti-corporate websites – individually and taken together – provide a wide range of opportunities to get involved on different levels. This is very explicitly expressed on the American website Badads.org (www.badads.org), which opposes the ubiquity of ads. Here the user can choose action in accordance with how much time he or she has for democratic action. Whether this is one, five, ten, 90 minutes or more, the website has a suggestion for what to do.

What role does the internet play in the activities of the organization or movement?

The websites described above give different priority to their functionalities and characteristics. Whether this is due to deliberate organizational strategies could not be determined from this type of analysis. Similar studies of political parties' use of websites suggest that these often end up reflecting the culture of the mother organization, intentionally or otherwise (Löfgren 2000).

From the studies of websites it is possible to identify three strategic approaches, which are not mutually contradictory, and are in fact combined by several of the websites studied.

- *Information-oriented sites* seek to inform the user so that he or she can make more deliberate choices as a consumer on the market or as a citizen or voter. The sites which fit this model best are CorpWatch and, to some extent, Adbusters Foundation, which is basically about presenting an alternative vision of the world. Since these sites are typically up to date in terms of news and rich on information, they practically serve as alternative independent media bypassing the traditional media channels. In a micro-economic perspective this can be seen as an effort to diminish the problem of imperfect information which consumers experience in a global and changing market.
- *Mobilization-oriented sites* try to raise public support in favour of a pre-defined cause (example: CokeSpotlight). These sites are typically managed top-down, with little chance for users to change, comment upon or criticize the site's agenda. This is reflected by, among other things, the frequent use of prefabricated letters. Even so, these websites seem to offer a wider range of opportunities for citizens to participate than traditional campaigns run through print media, TV and radio. Here, people are often left with the choice to remain a spectator, send money or join as a full-time activist. An interesting website which is oriented towards mobilization but does not seem to be managed top-down is (R)(TM)ark, which resembles a modern project organization striving to bring together sponsors, ideas and people so that they can solve problems defined by themselves.
- *Community-oriented sites* seek to build relations and shared visions between citizens. Only the No Logo site comes close to this model, since this appears to be the only site with a high degree of inter-activity between users. In contrast to the bulk of the other sites

analysed, the No Logo site reflects a bottom-up approach with users themselves influencing the agenda of the site. Both the well-developed chatting and debating functionalities and the detailed bulletins on upcoming street action reflect an overall vision of bringing users together – virtually or in real life.

Does the website link to other movements and organizations?

Only a few of the analysed anti-corporate websites do not link to related sites and organizations. Generally the number of links is quite impressive. McSpotlight, for instance, forcefully encourages the user to subject other multinationals to public scrutiny and debate, and has hundreds of links. Also the No Logo site and CorpWatch have links covering a wide range of organizations affiliated with the anti-corporate movement. Other sites seem to be more selective, only including sites which relate rather narrowly to the agenda of the web-site. Sane BP (www.sanebp.com), which has been put up by, among others, Greenpeace, does not have links; the CokeSpotlight site, in which Greenpeace also has a share, includes only a few links. This may be due to deliberate editing in order to make one – and just one – overall statement, or it might reflect a top-down approach whereby the website is seen as just one of several levers to bring out the message of an existing campaign.

Conclusion

Even though they take place in the domain of the market, anti-corporate activities and campaigns can be seen as expressions of political orientation. The majority of anti-corporate websites do not restrict themselves to dealing with questions concerning consumers' preferences or the quality of goods provided by companies. Instead these sites reflect a determination to bring about certain changes in society and a concern for the rights of human beings and the condition of the globe. The anti-corporate websites do not focus on single causes and single companies, but on clusters of problems. The targeted companies are merely used as examples of problems and as levers that enable activists to make a clear public statement.

Most anti-corporate websites operate within the same frame of meaning. In this discursive universe 'big business' is seen as a bully that threatens social, ethical, and environmental core values, and thus needs to be held democratically accountable by citizens and consumers.

Several websites refer to themselves as part of an anti-corporate movement. In general, these movements do not push alternative epistemologies or political programmes, even though several sites in the environmental area discuss the potential of 'green' solutions in production and consumption. The anti-corporate websites reflect a logic of protest more than a logic of project.

Due not least to the internet, the anti-corporate movements are just as globalized as their opponents among the multinationals. Several of the websites studied are run by networks connecting and addressing citizens and consumers across borders. Some websites are also products of spectacular alliances between NGOs, culture-jammers, small groups of activists, opinion leaders, or just ordinary citizens with the skills and credibility to succeed in the attention game on the world wide web. This could be called network politics – a process in which people, organizations, and groups are included not because of formal status, but because they have specific resources needed in the process.

A question that deserves further research is the factors that give an anti-corporate website legitimacy. Does it depend primarily on who is behind it, the quality of the website – or something else?

Generally the anti-corporate activists do not fully exploit the potential of the internet. Technologically, the sites are not very advanced. Nor have the websites generally moved from one-to-many communication towards many-to-many communication. Functionalities for chatting and debate are not well developed on these sites. Most of the sites should not be considered virtual communities: such an appellation would presume at least some level of interactivity between users, so that personal relationships could be formed and maybe, as a next step, shared identities developed.

This study suggests that the activists and organizations behind the websites consider the internet primarily a means to bring down transaction costs as regards agenda-setting and campaigning. In the first place, websites are used to distribute information. Perhaps the most important accomplishment of anti-corporate websites is the fact that they significantly facilitate the free flow of information, internally within the anti-corporate movement, and externally in relation to the press and ordinary citizens. The monitoring of multinationals and publishing of such findings on the internet has made it less possible for them to hide from citizen protest by moving from one part of the world to another. This role of websites, obviously, also challenges the information monopoly of traditional media. Yet it remains to be seen whether this will in fact increase the legitimacy and influence of the anti-corporate movement on a global scale.

In the second place, websites are being used to mobilize people in favour of the cause of the mother organization. Websites literally 'bring activism to a computer near you'. By giving users the chance to participate according to time, skills, and personal interest, these websites may have some advantages in comparison with non-virtual movements. Anti-corporate websites seem to be in line with the general shift in citizen orientation and participation – away from institutionalized politics and towards more individual and *ad hoc* forms of participation which can be integrated to everyday life.

It should be interesting to investigate whether websites like these attract people who do not take part in traditional politics, or who are not even members of grassroots organizations. One could expect that anti-corporate websites would appeal to the political consumers who have so far been expressing their ethical and political concerns individually on the market. Until recently, the political consumer was left with the option to buy or boycott. That has been changed by the internet. Time will show whether more citizens – instead of just being selective in the supermarket – will take action against corporations on the internet.

4   Informing, communicating and ICTs in contemporary anti-capitalist movements*

Steve Wright

This chapter seeks to offer an insight into the role played by information and communications technologies (ICTs) within current movements against global capital. It offers examples from a number of social movements across the globe and seeks to identify common themes, opportunities and potential drawbacks in the integration of ICTs into the communication repertoire of social movements. It concludes not with a blueprint for 'success' but with a series of questions or areas that need further investigation in order to appreciate fully the impact of ICTs on the notion of protest. These reflections are prompted by my own passing involvement in a number of such online projects from the mid-1990s onwards. Is the nature of information and communication technologies and their use in such scenarios something self-evident, or instead might they be too often taken for granted, and perhaps be deserving of broader discussion?

While social movements have in recent years become significant actors on the global stage (Castells 2000b), the debate around their political meaning and social effects has been fractious indeed (Lacey 2001). Movements once deemed 'anti-systemic' (Arrighi *et al.* 1989) – for example, the official communist parties and their various auxiliary organizations – have long mutated into pillars of the global capitalist system or else declined altogether, while new movements have emerged to challenge them. In order to place the debate into context, perhaps it is wise to remind ourselves of the definition of a social movement offered by Mario Diani (1992: 13):

> A social movement is a network of informal interactions between a plurality of individuals, groups and/or organizations, engaged in a

---

* An earlier version of this chapter was presented as 'Issues surrounding the use of ICT by social movements' at 'Electronic Networks – Building Community. 5th Community Networking Conference', 3–5 July 2002, Monash University, Australia.

political or cultural conflict, on the basis of a shared collective
identity.

Social movements thus seek to alter the relations of power within
which they find themselves, by constructing their own meaning –
and, if possible, imposing that meaning within and upon social practices. As Diani's definition reminds us, however, the movements' own
ability to accomplish this is premised upon their capacity to engender
communication among their constituent parts, along with the social
forces with which they seek to engage.

Mass actions by social movement networks that identify themselves
as anti-capitalist have prompted both extensive mainstream media
coverage and broad public interest in recent years. Not all of this attention has been drowned out by what Matthew Fuller (2002) calls the
current 'war over the monopoly on terror': indeed, existing movements
against global capital have often played a central role in contemporary
opposition to war. As is proper, the anti-capitalist potential (or otherwise) of such movements has been widely debated. Among other things,
this has involved an assessment of their engagement (or otherwise)
with contemporary class composition, and the risks within many of
them of particular understandings of political practice: above all, the
'activist' syndrome (see, amongst others, Aufheben 2002; RTS 1999).
The ideological leanings of the new anti-capitalist circles have not
always been clear, even if the presence of left libertarian, as opposed
to Leninist, sensibilities is one common marker. Even making sense
of the terrain and parameters of these movements is not always an
easy task. While formally constituted organizations play an integral
part within them, in certain cases these movements' experiences of
'organizing' may not take the form of 'organizations' but of 'an ebb
or flow of contact at myriad points' (Cleaver 1999). Indeed, some
have argued that their very confluence may lend a number of today's
movements their anti-systemic edge, to the point where 'current
struggles for particular changes are linking up into a collaboration
whose impact may wind up being much larger than the sum of the individual influences' (Cleaver 1999).

An earlier article by Harry Cleaver points out that a primary means
by which movements against capital communicate within and among
themselves is through the circulation of struggle. By this term he under-
stands

> The fabrication and utilization of material connections and com-
> munications that destroy isolation and permit people to struggle

in complementary ways – both against the constraints which limit them and for the alternatives they construct, separately and together.

(Cleaver 1993; see De Angelis 1993)

Michael Hardt and Antonio Negri (2000) state in their book *Empire* that one of the most distinctive aspects of anti-systemic movements in the decade before the Seattle days of 1999 was precisely their inability to establish such a circulation of struggle. From Tiananmen Square onwards, social movements emerged in dramatic circumstances while 'fail[ing] to communicate to other contexts'. This, Hardt and Negri contend, was due to the absence firstly of 'a recognition of a common enemy against which the struggles are directed', and secondly of a 'common language of struggles that could "translate" the particular language of each into a cosmopolitan language' (Hardt and Negri 2000: 54, 56, 57). Only with Seattle, Negri has since asserted, has a new cycle of struggle truly emerged, albeit one fundamentally different in nature to that captured in Marx's metaphor of the 'old mole' burrowing away beneath the surface of daily routine (Cocco and Lazzarato 2002).

In reality, the picture is not nearly as simple as the one painted in *Empire*; indeed, in one important case – that of the Zapatista uprising in Chiapas – Hardt and Negri are completely mistaken (Cox 2001; Dyer-Witheford 2001). In part, this inability to pay full heed to the communication between anti-systemic movements before the events of Seattle 1999 may well stem from an undue emphasis placed upon the most spectacular, visible aspects of the circulation of struggle. Criticizing Negri on this score, Sergio Bologna has argued that

> Conflict as the moment of identity, as 'the' moment of constitution, of politics, of class constitution . . . this for me is a forced understanding. Amongst other things, this conception still attributes great value to visibility. The 'other', in order to be such, must be visible, manifest, and the more clamorous the conflict, the greater the identity it confers . . . This is the back door through which the traditional logic of politics is returned to play. I prefer the image of beams eaten from within by termites, I prefer a non-visible, non-spectacular path, the idea of the silent growth of a body that is foreign to the sort of visibility that leaves you hostage to the universe of mediation.

(Borio *et al.* 2001: 14)

Modes of communication

There are many ways in which social movements communicate both among themselves and with the social forces they seek to influence, and if we are to make sense of their use of ICTs, we first need to address this broader picture (Diani 2000: 388–391). An easy mistake would be to assume that such forms of communication are always either verbal or direct. Take the movement of Italian industrial workers known as the Hot Autumn of 1969, which had its origins in modes of communication peculiar to the work regime of Fordist mass production techniques (Wright 2002). As Negri himself once noted of that movement's origins in the workplace unrest of the early 1960s:

> We began to follow a whole series of dynamics of sabotage: in fact no-one had set out to commit sabotage, yet there existed a continuity of imperfect operations such that by the end the product was completely useless . . . What is spontaneity? In reality it is my inability to establish an organisational, i.e. voluntary, precise, determinate relationship with another worker. In these conditions spontaneity acts through the very communication, which the labour process as such, as a machine foreign to me, determines.
>
> (Negri 1979: 64–65)

Beyond such subterranean channels, social movements have often relied on corporate and state media as a means of communicating with other sections of society, with all the attendant risks that this reliance brings. Such 'guerrilla tactics' (Fiske 1989: 19) were again demonstrated as recently as the Melbourne S11 blockade of the World Economic Forum in 2000; for example, with the mock adoption of a John Farnham song as the protest anthem, and the media furore that this provoked. At the same time, this attempt to detourn* corporate media also indicates a fundamental weakness:

* See Debord and Wolman (1956). Ken Knabb's translator's note to that article is as follows. 'The French word *détournement* means deflection, diversion, rerouting, distortion, misuse, misappropriation, hijacking, or otherwise turning aside from the normal course or purpose. It has sometimes been translated as "diversion", but this word is confusing because of its more common meaning of idle entertainment. Like most people who have actually practised *détournement*, I have chosen simply to anglicize the French word.'

The old media was important in publicising and drawing attention to the new, highlighting the fact that, although the Net is an important new tool, activists still largely rely on coverage in the traditional media and cannot rely solely upon the emerging communications networks.

(Gibson and Kelly 2000)

More than this, such dependency also offers space for the social ventriloquism of self-defined vanguard formations. While left libertarian circles argued the case as to whether, and in what circumstances, corporate media can be instrumentalized, 'The tensions within the autonomous networks regarding media representation have allowed for an easy capitalisation by more media hungry and obedient groups' (Aggy and Andrew 2002).

Modest though it may appear to be in scope, movement media has been on the rise in many places over the past few years, in many cases building upon an already existing undergrowth of communication channels, from print to radio (Downing 2001). Nonetheless, opinions differ as to the moment when computer-mediated communication became fundamental for global social movement activities. Cleaver (1997, 1998, 1999) has written eloquently of the 'electronic fabric of struggle' woven around the Zapatistas, while himself playing a pivotal role in establishing and maintaining that fabric. Peter Waterman (1992) and Eric Lee (2000) have traced the online activities during the 1980s of rank-and-file and dissident union members in the West, as well as those of 'official' unions. At the same time, others (Frederick 1993; Myers 1998) have sketched the development of organizations such as the Association of Progressive Communication in the years before the internet was opened up to a mass audience beyond US defence and academic circles.

If the enthusiastic embrace of ICTs has been the norm within the social movements that aim to challenge global capital, their use has not been without controversy. Some, working from a Green perspective, are critical of those who hold that 'technology is "neutral" and could be made to serve social justice' (Starr 2000: 177). Beyond this, the criticism of the place of ICTs within radical politics has been couched in terms of how time and energy invested in the 'virtual' relates to activity in the 'real' world. For example, some participants have feared the possibility of a situation in which 'information circulates endlessly between computers without being put back into a human context' (ECN 1992). In a related manner, others have argued that the unconsidered application of electronic communications may serve to undermine more traditional forms of linkage. In the words of Randy Stoecker (2000), not only is there the risk that 'the internet is isolating us in front of our monitors, keeping us off the streets', but many of the relationships that are established online will by their very nature remain superficial – 'faceless one-dimensional stranger to stranger interaction'. Then again, if Mario Diani is right, this risk may be overstated. Diani (2000: 393–394) makes the point that different kinds of social movement networks use ICTs in different ways, consistent with their broader approach to marshalling support and effecting social change. More than this, he suggests that 'the most distinctive contribution of CMC [computer-mediated communication] to social movements', particularly those premised upon a participatory organizational structure oriented towards direct action, has been 'of an instrumental rather than symbolic kind'. In other words, the use of ICTs in such circles has largely been to 'reinforce face-to-face acquaintances and exchanges' (Diani 2000: 397, 391).

From Indymedia to the European Counter Network

It is with projects such as the Indymedia network (IMC, www.indy media.org) that it becomes possible to talk of the emergence of a distinctly social movement electronic communications forum. The first Indymedia site was established as part of the Seattle days of protest, where it proved effective in relaying images, audio recordings and written accounts of the mass blockade (Weingartner 2001). Since then, Indymedia sites have been formed across Western Europe, the Americas, and Australasia (Shumway 2001) – and most recently, in the Middle East. Aiming for a broad participative management structure (Halleck 2002), Indymedia is powered by 'open publishing' software that allows users both to upload materials and to offer commentaries on the stories, opinions and images provided by others. In the words of one of its architects, Indymedia can be seen as part of a broader internet phenomenon of sites fuelled by 'the creativity of their users, *not* [by] professional producers as was the tradition with earlier electronic media' (Arnison 2002). At the same time, Arnison has argued, one of the issues at present being debated within the Indymedia network of websites is precisely 'what to do when they are *not* covering a major event'. One response to this dilemma has been to mentor new ventures into 'real world' media. In Melbourne, for example, there is *The Paper*, a fortnightly publication that began around the S11 protests, and has since carved out its own identity independently of the local Indymedia collective. Meanwhile, the Indymedia network continues to grapple with the trolling* that has plagued many affiliated sites in the lulls between big actions. According to one web media activist, this will remain a serious problem so long as

> The liberal free speech attitudes of most IMC volunteers . . . paralyze them from implementing consistent moderation . . . I've been a free speech advocate for many years and often considered myself to be a free speech zealot, but not even I would argue that our websites should provide any space for right wing and racist views. The racists have their websites – we don't need to use our limited resources to promote their hideous and offensive views.
>
> (Chuck0 2002)

Different issues arise from the experience in Italy of the European Counter Network (ECN). In a country where anti-capitalist politics have assumed strong regional identities, the ECN emerged at the end of the 1980s as a network within which the character of individual local bulletin boards (BBs) remained marked. Like the libertarian Cyberpunk network, with which it overlapped in part, the ECN was tied closely to the movement of occupied social centres, itself the heir of the autonomist and anarchist politics of an earlier generation (Wright 2000). Within a few years, the ECN in that country had expanded to encompass nine BBs running under Fido protocol, although formally outside Fidonet itself. Of these nodes, at least two (Turin and Padua) provided their own regular hard-copy edition of postings circulated on the network, while others contributed items to local autonomist publications. Indeed, by the mid-1990s, the relationship between cyber and 'real world' cultures had become a heated topic of discussion among the sysops ('system operators') running the ECN's various bulletin boards.

In an article he had written for the left daily *Il Manifesto*, and then reproduced as part of the debate, Sandrone had made two central points about the ECN. The first of these was that it expressed 'the desire to create a forum [piazza] open to all', unlike the regulated atmosphere which pervades Fidonet and similar systems. Much more than this, however, the role that he and others had sought to develop in Milan was that of 'a human interface' between various social subjects – he cited a range of examples, from AIDS activists to militant workers – who themselves showed little interest in using the network.

---

* Mike Slocombe (2003) suggests that 'a Troll's basic mission in life is to mischievously manufacture inflammatory opinions in an attempt to stir up disharmony and discord'.

This notion of the network as 'a crossroads between subjects' that 'first of all, connects realities outside' itself, was one that he would return to again and again over the course of the debate.

Marta's position was rather different. More than a simple interface between humans in the 'real' world, she stressed that computer networks represent 'a new medium' fast becoming an important place of 'struggle and resistance' in its own right. As a consequence, attention had to be paid to 'the features peculiar to [computer] networks – anonymity, the loss/construction of ascribed relations and identity, socialisation, the possibilities of experimentation', to see whether these might generate new ways of destabilizing power. In other words, it's not a matter of simply seeking to use computer networks as a means to connect the struggles of social subjects in the so-called real world, but rather of exploring the subjects that are forming *within* the networks themselves (Margin 1995).

Issues raised by the ECN's migration to the internet some months later (www.ecn.org) would soon overshadow this particular discussion, yet its terms have resurfaced again and again within Italian anti-capitalist circles. A recent case concerns the website of Radio Sherwood (www.sherwood.it), a Venice-based movement transmitter intimately connected with the historical autonomist movement of the region and its successors (Ya Basta, Tute Bianche, Disobbedienti). In that instance, differences as to whether the Sherwood site should privilege the production of a webzine directed at internet 'prosumers' (Rosati and Prieur 2000), or instead serve primarily as the online emanation of the radio station, would ultimately end with the victory of the latter, and the departure of those most keen to rethink the meaning of political communication in a digital age.

Information overload

Is more media always better, even if it is alternative media? Can there be such a thing as too much information? The problem of information overload in electronic environments has been a topic of periodic discussion over the past two decades or so (Valovic 2000; Hiltz and Turoff 1985). With the West's embrace of the internet, David Shenk (1997: 30–1) sees growing 'data smog' as the dark reality at the heart of today's so-called information society. As the volume of information accelerates relentlessly, 'noise' overshadows 'signal'. Communication may be speedier thanks to the internet, but it is increasingly coupled with 'bad decision making' (Shenk 1997: 137) that serves only to strengthen existing relations of power (Shenk 1997: 15). Far from levelling social inequities, Shenk concludes, 'cyberspace is Republican' (Shenk 1997: 174). Developing aspects of Shenk's argument, Tim Jordan (1999: 118) has identified two kinds of information overload: that which arises from excess volume, and that arising from information so 'chaotically organized' as to be useless. Together, he argues, these aspects of information overload fuse in a 'spiral' (Jordan 2000: 128) that constantly reproduces the existing power relations of the internet.

The practical implications of information overload for those seeking to challenge the powers that be have been clearly articulated by Anne Scott's (2001: 417) reflections on feminist activism:

> Expectations are being raised, moreover, in regard to the quantity and quality of information needed before a plausible case can be said to exist. As one respondent noted, people want more and more information before taking action. But there is a point at which one has enough information to act; the acquisition of more information beyond this point can be confusing and paralyzing – and can actually block the taking of effective action.

Jim Walch (1999: 72) has noted the range of strategies for dealing with information overload that he has observed in social movement circles. For the most part, these tend to involve shifting responsibility elsewhere (into electronic folders, onto other people, or blocking certain information flows altogether through the use of filtering software). While conceding that these are understandable coping strategies, he argues that such efforts to 'manage' information flows also carry risks, in terms both of the construction of meaning and of denying access to 'new and unexpected information and contacts'. Walch's concerns here echo those of Howard Besser, who has asserted that

> One of the identifying characteristics of the information age is to get people directly to the information they need without exposing them to tangentially interesting or relevant material.
>
> (Besser 1995: 70)

Although ultimately inconclusive, a debate on information overload within social movements that took place around the Second Intercontinental Encuentro of 1997 helps throw further light on the question. The First Encuentro, held the previous year in Chiapas, had brought together some 3,000 activists from a range of circles – above all in North America and Europe – linked by a sense of affinity with the Zapatistas of Southern Mexico. One of the proposals arising from the First Encuentro was for an international network of communication, able to circulate news and views of the 'One "No" and Many "Yeses"' opposed to global neo-liberalism. Consideration of how best to achieve this was placed on the agenda for the follow-up gathering in Spain.

The debate began with a long reflective piece penned primarily by Monty Neill (1997a), an editor of the US-based journal *Midnight Notes*. Following a considered account of the Zapatistas' significance for other movements seeking to challenge global capitalism, Neill (1997b) turned to the specific proposal for a communications network:

> Abstractly this is fine, but it begs essential questions: what is to be communicated, by whom, to whom? In the 'information age,' it is all too easy to be deluged with information. This is not helpful unless the information is well organized for some use – which only raises the question, who will organize the information? The EZLN and its supporters have been marvellously inventive in using networks, but multiply Chiapas by even ten, never mind the thousands needed: how many channels can the mind consider? This is not the individual's problem. Sorting information requires political collectivity. It implies calculated division of labour and aspects of centralization: someone else will decide for you (presumably with your consent) what reaches you and what is the most important information. It also poses the related problem: what struggles deserve what attention, and who decides?

In other words, any discussion of how to process the volume of information circulating within and between the various movements engaged with the Zapatistas immediately raised questions about the nature of the power relations existing within and between the various class forces with which they were associated. For his own part, Neill (1997b) saw no simple solution to the problem; any real answer, he believed, would only follow from a serious exploration of how to challenge the more general problem of 'hierarchy – of race, gender, nation, work, wages – within the [global working] class'.

The most detailed response to Neill came from Stefan Wray (1997), who argued that what might at first seem to be political issues were often instead technical problems with software solutions. Criticizing a push-based model for a global communications network (RICA 1996) that threatened to bury recipients under what he termed 'a mountain of information', Wray argued instead for a 'user-based information retrieval system'. In his model, email would be deposited at an archive, where automated software residing on subscribers' computers could interrogate it by keyword, selecting only those files identified as relevant to the individual user.

Tim Jordan (1999: 122), at least, is sceptical that technical approaches to information overload do anything more than exacerbate the problem. This is because clearing the decks of unwanted and/or irrelevant information simply provides more space for other sources of information to take their place – much as freeway extensions or widenings commonly only increase the volume of automobile traffic. In any case, as one participant in the Encuentro debate pointed out, something like the system proposed by Wray already existed in the form of Usenet groups (Kerne 1997). On the other hand, as another list member based in the South reminded everyone, 'Although we are living in a new era, although globalism presents us every opportunity of technology in every country, it is not for everyone' (Sungu 1997).

Any discussion of global activism and the internet quickly raises questions about the distribution of resources between the North and South. Here again the volume of information is a pressing issue. As Walch (1999: 55) has indicated, ICT access can be expensive for many living in Asia and Africa, and all but inaccessible for others. Connections to groups elsewhere can bring not only new affinities, but also the risk of 'information dump', with local channels clogged by electronic messages originating from locales where bandwidth may not be an issue. Nevertheless, Walch is optimistic about the possibilities of electronic connectivity between social movements, arguing that even as simple a step as linking websites can enhance the 'inter-organizational transfer of information' (Walch 1999: 74). Har and Hutnyk (1999) point to the obverse of Walch's problem: that connections to North-based social movements frequently force 'activists from South East Asia to continuously send information to (careerist?) activists in the west', when that time might be better spent in other activities. While they do not call for the abandonment of electronic communication, Har and Hutnyk (1999) reiterate Stoecker's (2000) concern that ICTs be understood in a properly instrumental way, as tools that are useful only so long as they facilitate efforts at social change. They conclude with a call for more reflective moments within activist practice:

> The beast of capitalism takes such forms that require more than documentation. The danger would be if the internet encourages

only an information rich, but analysis poor edification. More education is more important than more information.

Can knowledge be managed in social movements?

There is a certain irony in suggesting a need to explore the place of knowledge management within social movements – particularly within those openly in opposition to global capital. After all, knowledge management as a discourse has commonly concerned itself with how best to 'capture' those insights and abilities that workers have to date failed to surrender to the organization that employs them. In this respect, it stands firmly within a managerialist tradition that stretches back to Frederick Taylor's time (Braverman 1975; Day 2001b).

Not surprisingly, then, few studies to date have attempted to ascertain what, if anything, social movements might usefully learn from knowledge management as a discipline. One such attempt, by Karen Nowé (2001), argues that knowledge management itself has too often concentrated on technological fixes when trying to think through information flows within organizations. Noting that social movement organizations are typically poor in terms of finances and physical resources, she adds that they face the additional problem of peaks and troughs in membership and activity as a consequence of the very ebbs and flows of cycles of protest:

> It is important that the knowledge . . . can be kept alive through the periods of low activity. How do social movements manage that? It is clear that this has more to do with cultures and people than with simple information technology solutions.

In other words, Nowé returns us to the same questions raised among others by Neill (1997a, 1997b) and Har and Hutnyk (1999). Like them, she freely admits that for now, such problems remain unresolved, while arguing that information flows within social movements that aspire to self-managed organizational practices may well conflict with what knowledge management as a discipline would deem to be 'a rational decision-making procedure'.

The nature of information itself has been talked of in a fairly unproblematic way throughout this chapter. In many ways, the circulation of information has indeed been one of the success stories in social movement use of ICT to date. As Cleaver (1999) has pointed out, ICTs have been used with effect:

1 'To obtain accurate information on a given situation and then circulate it widely';
2 To facilitate 'the circulation of interpretation and evaluation' of such information through 'discussion and debate', so as
3 To enable 'various kinds of off-line activities'.

Just the same, Har and Hutnyk (1999) are correct in arguing that more thought needs to be given to our understandings of the nature of information itself. After all, the standard metaphor of the communication of information via value-free 'conduits' (Day 2001a: 38–46) is unable to grasp that

> Not everything can be collapsed into the realm of representation and transmission. Some 'content' cannot be expressed; some will always be misrepresented because of inequalities and interpretation.
>
> (Har and Hutnyk 1999)

Seeking a critical – that is, self-reflexive, historically specific – definition of information, Ron Day (2001a: 120) has offered the following:

> Information is the quality of being informed. But this is a highly ambiguous – 'theoretical' and affective – state of affairs, one that leaves the nature of knowledge, as well as of the world and the subject, still to be formed and discovered.

Day's definition suggests rather more than 'transmission', and is far away from notions that see information as indifferent to its medium. At the same time, it also provides a useful starting point for making sense of the ways in which information is handled in organizations and movements that claim commitment to participatory decision-making processes.

Being 'informed' implies relationships of trust. The matter of trust has arisen forcefully in an interview that Anita Lacey and I recently conducted with one Melbourne-based activist, Colin, as part of a small, ongoing enquiry into the use of information and ICTs in local anti-capitalist politics. Part of a network that seeks to open up space for an ongoing dialogue between environmental and workplace activists, Colin defined useful information as 'what can facilitate the process of building bridges and crossing borders'. Sceptical of the notion that trust – 'the most important question' – could be established 'through the screen', his biggest concern was that the enormous quantities of information available online may blind us to the knowledge and wisdom available from face-to-face encounters with those who have experienced and learned from earlier struggles against capital and the state. For Colin, instead, broaching the question of trust in this way meant thinking through the whole purpose of communication within and between social movements, and the place within this of listening and learning. As Cleaver (1997) has noted,

> One of the great lessons that the Zapatistas have learned within their communities and which they have shared first with other Mexicans and then with the world is the fundamental importance of listening. Of listening, and understanding, before you speak.

This then leads us on to conclude not with answers but with a series of further questions that deserve attention in rethinking the place of information and communication within contemporary anti-capitalist movements.

1   The first of these concerns analysis. ICTs have sometimes played a dramatic role in communicating rich, multiple impressions of particular events as they unfold (witness Indymedia's coverage of the global antiwar demonstrations of February 2003), but they have been used less successfully in promoting a coherent, collective assessment of what these events mean within the overall process of social change. In conventional politics of the left and right, judgement on such matters is ultimately deferred to specialist leaders or their advisers. In a halting fashion, some contemporary anti-capitalist movements have begun to experiment with a different approach, in which it is recognized that many participants have relevant specialist knowledge to contribute to a shared understanding, without this granting them any final word on the decision-making front (Wright 2004). Here use of the internet has entailed something of a paradox. On the one hand, it has provided ready access to a rich source of materials able to help frame the collective process of sense-making (for one example, see the discussion of shifting global power balances in Arrighi 2002 and Wallerstein 2001). On the other hand, the soundbite nature of email-based discussion has meant the continual risk of sloganeering over analysis. Then again, this may have less to do with the internet as such, and more with the ongoing presence within anti-capitalist movements of a mindset that holds 'action' and 'theory' as separate (perhaps

even performed by mutually exclusive circles), while always privileging the first over the second.

2   On the other hand, ICTs have sometimes played a dramatic role in facilitating the organization (in real time) of certain forms of direct action. A spectacular recent example has been the phenomenon of 'train-stopping' in Italy, where thousands mobilized themselves in the weeks before the invasion of Iraq to block the movement by rail of US military *matériel*. Perhaps the most striking aspect of this action was the combined use of a range of ICTs old and new – the internet, mobile phones and movement-aligned radio stations – both to monitor the movement of the trains in question and to coordinate their physical disruption (Oliveri 2003; Casarini 2003). This suggests that Dorothy Kidd (2002: 22) may well be right in arguing that

> The greatest shock to the status quo has not been from sophisticated computer networks, but from the social organization and networking among a myriad of social forces, using all the new and old communications available.

Thus one might argue that it is the integration of ICTs into the web of existing communication tools and the networks in which they are operative that marks any change in facilitating action of any kind.

3   Another point concerns social roots and linkages. Much of the left debate over contemporary movements against global capital has raged over their connection – or otherwise – to overtly working class forms of organization and conflict. If much of this debate has really been about something else (above all, the claims of various political forces for a leadership role within the new movements), it is also true that anti-capitalist circles have been most effective where links have been consolidated with workplace-based organizations. In Italy – a country that seems once again to be assuming a 'laboratory' role in matters of social conflict (Virno and Hardt 1996) – opposition to the 2003 Iraqi war included a million-strong one-day stoppage on 2 April, organized by alternative unions and rank-and-file groups long active in networks against global capital. Other examples can be seen throughout this volume.

4   A fourth point concerns language. How likely is the production of a 'cosmopolitan language' (Hardt and Negri 2000) able to facilitate the circulation of struggles between social movements?

How might such an entity be formed? And can such a project begin without wrestling with the problem of translation, and all that this implies for the generation of information and knowledge (Day 1994)? For, as Walter Benjamin (1969: 69) pointed out long ago, 'any translation which intends to perform a transmitting function cannot transmit anything but information – hence, something inessential'. This in turn raises another matter beyond the prospects for the shared vocabulary of a 'cosmopolitan language': namely, the linguistic barriers to communication that at present separate many around the world. While internet uptake is growing among those outside North America and Western Europe, internet-based communication within and between anti-capitalist movements continues to be dominated by English language users. Not only does this situation marginalize those unable to use English, it also deprives members of the net's dominant language group of insight into some of the most important developments around the globe. After 1993, a small band of internet-based translators played a significant role in popularizing the situation in Chiapas, and so helped to consolidate links between a number of circles later prominent in global anti-capitalist protests. To date, however, we have yet to see any comparable circulation in the English-speaking world of information concerning social movements operating in circumstances such as the equally dramatic events unfolding since 2001 in Argentina, with its complex network of neighbourhood assemblies, occupied factories and organized unemployed groups (Jordan and Whitney 2002).

5   The sort of instrumental approach to ICTs described in this chapter, where cyberspace is seen primarily as an ether through which to connect to other realities rather than a domain worthy of consideration in its own right, may carry costs of its own. Opting to be the online wing of radical movements, rather than the radical wing of online cultures, is probably a false choice, but it is one that has nonetheless been made by many involved in anti-capitalist movements. As Enda Brophy (2002) reminds us, however, 'the political struggle for the future of the electronic commons' holds significant portents for the future. What, for example, are the implications for anti-capitalist politics of peer-to-peer online cultures (Moglen 1999; Richardson 2001)? For this reason alone, perhaps it is time to go back and review the work of Geert Lovink (2002) and others who have refused to submit to ready-made dichotomies between engagement with the 'real' as against the 'virtual'.

6 Finally, and at the risk of once again stating the obvious: movements, anti-capitalist or otherwise, can easily become victims of their own apparent success. Here there is much to learn from the experience of Italian self-managed social centres, within which so many important political–cultural experiments were conducted in the 1990s. As I have argued elsewhere (Wright 2000: 131):

> Dynamism tends to bring unforeseen consequences. The second half of the 1990s has signaled the less than comfortable discovery that, like the universe itself, the movement's expansion may only have increased the distance between its constituent parts.

Marx (1973: 539) once suggested that capital's quest for its own expanded reproduction led it to attempt 'to annihilate . . . space with time'. So-called globalization has made this tendency seem very real for millions of people today, often to their cost. Nick Dyer-Witheford (1999: 238) has described what is now at stake:

> There are now visible signs of an emergent collectivity refusing the logic of commodification, uprising at the very moment that the world market seems to have swallowed the entire planet. Deepening and expanding this process of recomposition depends on interconnection between many and disparate movements at different points along capitalism's circuits. Ironically, the conversations necessary for creation of the new combination are now being conducted across the world-spanning communication networks that information-age capital has itself created.

As we move into a period where the reality of war hangs over everything, our ability to sustain such conversations – offline no less than online – is likely to be as sorely tested as it is indispensable.

Part II

Changing strategies and stratagems

Action and activism in the
information age

5 New media, new movements?

The role of the internet in shaping the 'anti-globalization' movement

Peter Van Aelst and Stefaan Walgrave

This chapter maps this movement-in-progress via an analysis of the websites of anti-globalization, or more specifically anti-neo-liberal globalization organizations. It examines the contribution of these sites to three different conditions that establish movement formation: collective identity, actual mobilization, and a network of organizations. This ongoing, exploratory research indicates signs of an integration of different organizations involved and attributes an important role to the internet. However, while both our methodology and our subject are evolving rapidly, conclusions, as our initial results show, must be tempered. The enormous growth of the internet since the mid-1990s has placed debate about the potential consequences of this new media on the political process, on the top of the research agenda (Johnson and Kaye 2000; Bimber 1998; Barnett 1997; Castells 1997; Hague and Loader 1999; Lax 2000; Norris 2001). Most observers of the 'digital democracy' are quite subtle about the impact of this evolution. They don't believe it will radically transform democracy in either a positive or a negative way. While both political insiders and outsiders can use these new information and communication technologies (ICTs), the balance of power and the existing political structure are not likely to change. Research shows that people who are politically active on the web were already 'political junkies' (Johnson and Kaye 2000; Norris 2002). However, we argue that participation in politics will have been facilitated through the use of ICTs. Political action is made easier, faster and more universal by the developing technologies. ICTs lower the costs and obstacles of organizing collective action significantly. Bimber (1998) argues that this will be particularly beneficial for those groups outside the boundaries of traditional public institutions or political organizations. These new, more citizen-based, groups – which cannot depend on formal support or funding – will benefit relatively more from the internet than, for instance, political parties or labour movements.

Social movement watchers agree that the new media offer new opportunities for international collective action, but are more sceptical on the development of stable, long-lasting movements in the future. According to McAdam *et al.* (1996b), the expanded capacity for transnational communication will not automatically lead to international social movements. They believe that indispensable interpersonal networks cannot simply be replaced by new virtual contacts created by the internet. van de Donk and Foederer (2001) also doubt that virtual demonstrators can do without the emotions and thrills of participating in real direct action. Etzioni and Etzioni (1999) address the same problem: can virtual contacts be as real as face-to-face contacts for building a community? On the basis of their exploratory research they conclude that a combination of the two is best to create and maintain some sort of community. In the formation of a (transnational) social movement this would mean that when groups of people meet in person, e.g. at a protest meeting, and have some shared values, they can maintain or even improve bonding by what Etzioni and Etzioni call 'computer-mediated communication'. Interaction solely based on internet communications usually lacks the necessary basis of trust for building permanent relations (Diani 2001).

In this chapter we focus on the impact these new media have and will have on the success of the recent anti-globalization protests and the plausible formation of a new social movement. To speak of a social movement, generally four elements should be present: (1) a network of organizations, (2) on the basis of a shared collective identity, (3) mobilizing people to join, mostly unconventional[1] actions, (4) to obtain social or political goals (Duyvendak and Koopmans 1992; Diani and Eyerman 1992). In this case we would broaden the concept of social movement to that of a 'transnational social movement organization' (TSMO) (Smith *et al.* 1997; della Porta *et al.* 1999), or even further to a 'global social movement' (GSM) (O'Brien *et al.* 2000). This concept refers to a network of organizations that are not bound by state barriers and that connect people and places 'that were formerly seen as distant or separate' (O'Brien *et al.* 2000: 13). Tarrow, who uses a typology to indicate different forms of transnational collective action, argues that the conditions for a sustained transnational social movement 'that is, at once, integrated within several societies, unified in its goals and organization, and capable of mounting contention against a variety of targets' are hard to fulfil (Tarrow 1998: 185).

It is not our intention to find out whether the anti-globalization coalition is a true movement or rather a temporary (international) outburst of dissatisfaction with global economic and political governance. Our research is too limited and the actions too recent to go into this discussion. We confined ourselves, by means of an analysis of websites, to the contribution of the internet to three different elements or conditions that establish movement formation: a shared definition of the problem as a basis for collective identity, actual mobilization of participants, and a network of different organizations. These three dimensions of social movements constitute the theoretical framework of our study. The fourth element of the definition has not been the major focus of this research and thus will be dealt with in less depth.

Before elaborating on these research questions, we will give a brief overview of the transnational protest actions against globalization. Special attention will be devoted to the role of the internet.

Global protest against globalization

Globalization means different things for different people. In the business community it refers to a 'free world' for trade, commerce and money; for political scholars and politicians the disappearing or at least challenging of state borders is central; while globalization for the average man or woman means he or she can eat the same food, wear the same shoes or watch the same television programmes as someone living on the other side of the planet (Dodds 2000). It would be wrong to state that what are called anti-globalization protesters are against 'globalization' *per se*. In that case they wouldn't try to create a global network of organizations, or use a tool for global communication like the internet. It is rather the neo-liberal way the globalization is shaped and the negative (side-)effects it has on human beings and the environment that are contested (Ayres 2001). The international economic institutions that are created to regulate the globalization process, like the WTO and IMF, are especially in the protesters' spotlight. Both their form (structure, decision-making procedures) and the content of their policies (free market, deregulation of trade, and environmental degradation) are fiercely challenged (O'Brien *et al.* 2000). The discussion about a more apt name to label the movement is ongoing, and important because the movement has regularly been attacked on the basis of its anti-globalization label (Smith, 2001b).

Other names are being used, such as 'anti-neo-liberal', 'anti-corporate' or 'democratic globalization', but since their use is, as yet, not widely spread, we will keep with the traditional 'anti-globalization' label, despite its shortcomings.

The demonstrations at the WTO congress in Seattle at the end of 1999 have become a major symbol of the anti-globalization struggle (Van Aelst 2000, Smith 2001c). However, it would be incorrect to reduce the protests to the 'Battle of Seattle'. Seattle was neither the beginning nor the end of this (plausible) movement.

Before Seattle: the MAI and the first signs of virtual resistance

Protest against certain aspects of globalization isn't new. Third World organizations have been posing questions on the unequal distribution of wealth and the dubious role of international organizations such as the IMF and the World Bank for several decades.[2] But their concerns received a new, more international *élan* with the protest against the Multilateral Agreement on Investment (MAI) in 1998. From May 1995, trade ministers and economists from the leading industrialized world had secretly worked on the MAI. These talks should have led to a treaty by the end of 1998. However, they did not. The internet-based campaign of an international network of organizations (600 in the end) from 70 countries was the villain in this play. The protest they created by informing and mobilizing people against these new plans in favour of free trade, led to the end of the negotiations and the failure of the agreement. Although traditional protest means such as demonstrations and petitions were not absent, the internet 'provided the glue to bind the opposition that had begun simultaneously in a variety of developed countries' (Ayres 1999: 140).

It is difficult to prove that without the internet opposition the MAI would be in use today, but there are indications that this might be the case. Peter Smith and Elizabeth Smythe (2001) studied the role of the internet in this case, and although they point to political delays and disagreements as important factors, they conclude that it was the social groups, armed with internet technology, that successfully exploited these political opportunities. According to Ayres (1999), the fact that similar campaigns ten years earlier, using more costly and time-consuming methods, did not have the same result shows the internet's crucial role.

The battle of Seattle: 'We win'

Encouraged by this success, the global coalition started preparing for a bigger event: the ministerial meeting of the World Trade Organization (WTO) scheduled for the beginning of December 1999 in Seattle. The hometown of Boeing and Microsoft was eager to show itself off as a successful example of free trade to the representatives of 135 countries. The outcome was not exactly what the representatives of the city and the WTO had expected. A mixture of established NGOs and direct action groups engaged in colourful marches, road blockings and confrontation with the police. The media let a worldwide public enjoy what has become known as 'the battle of Seattle'. The almost complete obstruction of the opening day of the conference and the fact that their concerns were global news left the demonstrators with a feeling of victory that was best indicated by one of the graffiti slogans left behind: WE WIN (*Newsweek*, 13 December 1999). There were of course multiple causes for the failure of the meeting, such as the North–South divide and the agricultural conflict between the USA and Europe, but, as Jackie Smith stated: 'It would be hard to argue that the Seattle Ministerial would have failed as miserably as it did without the tens of thousand of protesters surrounding the meeting site' (2001c: 3). In Seattle activists took part in the conference, even if they were not invited.

Although this was not a virtual action in cyberspace – ask any inhabitant of Seattle – the internet yet again played a vital role in the anti-globalization protest. Throughout 1999, thanks mainly to the internet, people got plenty of chances to join the anti-WTO campaign. A main rallying point was the StopWTO Round distribution list. This list enabled many to receive detailed information on different aspects of the WTO (George 2000). The communication was facilitated further by various sites on the internet, the umbrella website of the anti-WTO coalition being the most famous. The new media contributed to an international division of work between different organizations both prior to (George 2000) and during the protests (Smith 2001c). While groups with local ties concentrated on mobilization and direct action, more transnationally based groups provided information and frames to feed the action.

Not only activist and movement scholars but also Western governments are impressed by the internet as a mobilization facilitator. As evidenced in an official report on the website of the Canadian Security Intelligence Service devoted to the anti-globalization protests: 'The Internet has breathed new life into the anarchist philosophy, permitting communication and coordination without the need for a central source of command, and facilitating coordinated actions with minimal resources and bureaucracy' (Canadian Security Intelligence Service 2000: 8).

Besides being a mobilization tool, the internet and other new means of communication in Seattle were used as means of action on their own. This virtual activism is intended to 'attack' the opponent from the inside rather than on the streets. Those who could not make it to Seattle could therefore engage in a virtual 'sit-in', blocking access to official sites, or send collectively an email or fax to disrupt the target's information flow (Smith 2001c). However, these forms of electronic activism were not used massively and were far less important to the movement's success.

After Seattle: from WTO to IMF, EU, G8 . . .

Since the WTO débâcle in Seattle, almost every summit of a transnational (economic) organization has led to street mobilizations. This was also the case for the meeting of two other symbols of globalization: the International Monetary Fund (IMF) and the World Bank in Washington.[3] Again the internet was used for mobilizing 'anti-globalization' activists to join the protests, and again a heterogeneous mixture of activists from over 200 groups and 55 nations (*USA Today*, 17 April 2000) tried to prevent the world's finance ministers from gathering. They failed, mainly because of better police organization, and the members of the IMF achieved a major breakthrough: they met (*New York Times*, 17 April 2000). But at the same time the impact of this embryonic movement was acknowledged. In a communiqué both institutions admitted that their role had become a subject 'of growing public debate' and that the benefits of free trade and international capital markets were not reaching everyone. Similar sounds could be heard half a year later in Prague when the two institutions met again: talks on 'debt relief' and 'the fight against poverty' were more prominent than before. However, the protests in Prague did not leave the activists in a victorious mood. There were fewer participants than expected and media reports focused on the violence and the damaging of property by anarchists, leaving the public with a rather negative image of the movement. In Prague, the media platform that the 'anti-globalization' coalition received in Seattle, and that brought worldwide attention to their cause, did not work in their favour and certainly obscured their main message.

Discussion on the peaceful versus more obstructive strategy was still hot half a year later, when the same organizations joined forces once more, this time against the summit of the FTAA.[4] In Quebec, leaders of countries from across the Americas negotiated on setting up the world's largest free-trade zone by 2005. Information and calls for action on the internet were again numerous. For example, 'The Field Guide to the FTAA Protest in Quebec City' provided a mass of detailed suggestions for joining different actions. This 27-page alternative 'travel guide', with links to all the relevant allies and opponents, leaves very little room for improvisation.

Not only the WTO and the IMF meetings, but top gatherings of the European Union (Nice, Göteborg, Brussels) and the G8 (Genoa) have witnessed outbursts of protest that are linked with the globalization issue. Besides their subject, all these actions have in common that they are mainly 'orchestrated' via the internet. An action that is also linked to this issue but which followed a different strategy was the 'World Social Forum' held for the second time in Porto Alegre. Parallel with the World Economic Forum, members of social organizations met in Brazil to discuss the effects and alternatives for neo-liberal free trade and globalization. Porto Alegre was not chosen at random. The city has become a 'social laboratory' for civic engagement in politics. People are informed, can make suggestions or complaints, and can vote on local issues using the internet (*Le Monde interactif*, 7 February 2001).

In addition to extensive use of the internet, these actions have something else in common: they are 'summit-related'. Probably unwillingly, the advocates of globalization have created with their conferences and meetings a (media) platform for its opponents. According to Ayres (2001), these international summits have stimulated new political opportunities for transnational activism. It is therefore hardly surprising that the last WTO meeting has taken place in the oil-state Qatar, where protest opportunities were reduced to an absolute minimum, and that after the tragedy in Genoa, where a young Italian protester was killed in a violent confrontation with the police, the next G8 summit took place in a remote venue in the Rocky Mountains.

Research on the internet: limitations and opportunities

Data reduction: from ICTs to websites

The decision to confine our study to an analysis of websites has to lead to tempered conclusions on the role of new information and communication technologies for social movements. Perhaps email or mobile phones are more important for activists and insight into their users would perhaps teach us more about transnational networks, but this type of research would cause problems even for Sherlock Holmes! However, websites are an interesting starting point for several reasons.

1   They contain lots of information on the actual organization(s). How are they organized? What do they stand for? What issues do they stress? A content analysis should point out whether the different organizations are on the same track, or, in movement terms, whether they share the same frame of reference.
2   We also wanted to examine to what extent these sites are used as a means for mobilization. Do they actively motivate people to engage in unconventional actions? How detailed is the information on these actions? Is the internet used as a means for action on its own?
3   Perhaps most importantly, by analysing their 'links' to other groups and organizations we can learn something about their network function. Is there one big virtual network among organizations involved in the anti-globalization struggle? Or are there still geographical or other kinds of barriers that prevent a global movement from evolving?

As stated above, the enormous growth of the internet has made it an attractive research subject for social scientists. However, research strategy and methodology are almost unexplored (Wakeford 2000) and, to the best of our knowledge, only a few pioneers have studied websites. van de Donk and Foederer (2001) made a quick scan of some environmental-organization websites without using a research instrument. Hill and Hughes (1998), who sampled 100 politically oriented websites in the USA, 'quantified' their study by using more objective parameters such as the number of web pages, graphical elements and hyperlinks that were found. Chandler (1998) developed a sort of coding scheme for his study on personal homepages.

More useful for our analysis are the examples of research on political websites. Pippa Norris (2001) made a list of criteria to classify websites on their information and communication function. Similar, but more elaborate, is the work performed by scholars of the Amsterdam School of Communication Research (De Landtsheer *et al.* 2001a, 2001b). They created a coding scheme to study political websites in terms of political participation: in other words, to determine whether political websites are 'participation-beneficial' characteristics such as

information, interactivity, user-friendliness and aesthetics were quantified. This scheme was used as a source of inspiration for our own
study, but needed, in view of the different research subject and question, serious rethinking – particularly in view of the need to add a
part on the mobilization function of the sites.

Before explaining our coding scheme and the results that were
found, we need to go into the data selection and analysis. This part of
the research process faced numerous difficulties and pitfalls.

Data selection: 17 websites

Probably the trickiest part of this study was the criteria for the selection of the websites. First of all, there is no such thing as one master
list of all the organizations involved in the anti-globalization struggle.
It is even unclear how many organizations or sites can be linked to
this subject. Moreover, search engines on the net did not give a good
overview.[5] Hill and Hughes (1998) used the subcategories (politics
and interest groups) made by search engines to reduce their population: however, anti-globalization is not focused upon and relevant
sites are spread among numerous categories (anti-corporation,
environment, labour, Free Trade Area of the Americas, etc.) A normal
sampling procedure therefore was not possible. Another option was
to use external links from the sites of the most important organizations
to other organizations. But this would have manipulated the results
strongly because the network function of these sites is a primary
research question.

Finally, we chose to select the sites of organizations that were
mentioned in the different national and international news reports on
the major anti-globalization protests. In this way we ensured that we
would analyse the actors that played some kind of role in the effective
actions that took place. Among these organizations a sample selection
was made, because an analysis of both the content and structure of
sites is rather time-consuming. The number of sites was therefore
further reduced on the basis of practical factors such as language
(only English and French speaking) or because the site was no longer
operational. This was the case with some sites that were created
especially for one protest event. The fact that the actual research
took place in the months March till May 2001 therefore influenced
our selection. In particular, the Summit of the Americas, which took
place in April 2001, contributed to the fact that 15 of the 17 selected
websites had a North American hometown. If, for example, Prague
or Genoa had been the centre of these protests, more European sites

might well have featured in our study. Despite these careful considerations, we can hardly claim that this limited selection of websites is truly representative of all the organizations involved, and we accept the limitations of our approach.

The 17 websites that were finally selected can roughly be ordered in three different subgroups (Table 5.1). The first group is of sites devoted to single events; in this case it concerns the FTAA meeting in Quebec and the World Social Forum in Porto Alegre. The second group is social organizations or action groups that were fully or partly engaged in the anti-globalization struggle. Some of them, such as WTOaction. org or 50 Years is Enough, were founded as a direct reaction against globalization; others, such as Friends of the Earth, were active long before globalization led to contention. A last group is labelled as 'supportive organizations'; they delivered a service to others that could facilitate their actions.

Each site was accurately analysed by two graduate students, who made this their 'homepage' for a month (29 March–3 May). They received careful instructions, especially on the interpretation of the coding scheme. Elaborate justification of the codes made it possible to compare and adjust their fieldwork afterwards.[6]

Mapping anti-globalization on the web

The analysis of the sites focuses on three diverse parts of the discussion on social movement theory and ICTs. First of all we try to find out whether the 17 organizations gave a similar interpretation of the anti-globalization theme. Secondly, attention was given to the mobilization function these sites fulfil. Finally, the links between the organizations were examined in detail. On the basis of these three elements, the '*movementization*' of the anti-globalization protests and the role of the internet in this process should become somewhat clearer.

Content analysis: what is anti-globalization for different organizations?

As the concept of identity, including feelings of identification and solidarity (Diani 2001), is broad and difficult to quantify, we restricted ourselves to a study of the shared 'frames of reference' of the different organizations. Without collective frames or 'shared meanings and definitions that people bring to their situation', it is unlikely that people will form a collective identity and permanently join forces (McAdam *et al.* 1996a). This does not mean that all activists have identical opinions or ideas regarding specific facts or persons, but rather that they use the same references or interpretations. The concept of frames in the context of social movements was introduced by Snow *et al.* (1986) and further applied and developed by many others (Gamson and Meyer 1996; Gerhards and Rucht 1992; Walgrave and Manssens 2000). A 'master frame' consists of different elements or dimensions. In this contribution, we focus on the first dimension of diagnostic framing, which is the identification of problems and causes (Snow and Benford 1988; Gerhards and Rucht 1992). To this end, we looked at how the websites conceive and define globalization. Do they hold a common view on the problem? Or, as critics assume, do all organizations focus on different aspects of a complex phenomenon?

Websites could possibly sustain the formation of such a shared (diagnostic) frame by giving information (a), stressing the same elements of the issue (b), and organizing discussion and interaction on the subject (c).

(a) As mentioned above, we developed a coding scheme to map different functions of the websites. Codes varying from nought to two were attributed to various aspects of information. In Table 5.2 the scheme and the motivations for the codes is presented in detail. In general, code 1 refers to a minimal presence of the characteristic while code 2 represents a more extensive one. Table 5.3 gives an overview of the codes and a standardized 100-point sum score of the 17 sites.

As one might expect, most sites are coded highly on their information function. It is quite normal for a website to say who its '(web)master' is and what it stands for. It is notable that while all organizations gave some information on their own organizations, in half of the cases this was done in a minimal or insufficient manner. Often they remain vague on their precise composition or structure.[7] Although this could be a deliberate strategy, it raises questions on the representativeness of some of them. Their views and opinions were generally clearer. Perhaps more remarkable than the high scores on internal information are those for external information. Especially, the number of websites with links to other organizations is significant. This is not always the case among movements, as for instance van de Donk and Foederer (2001) found an absence of external links among environmental organizations. In our selection there is only one organization that doesn't refer to others: the environmental organization Friends of the Earth.[8]

Table 5.1 Websites of organizations linked to the anti-globalization protests

ANTI-GLOBALIZATION EVENT SITES

A20
http://www.a20.org/

An 'umbrella site' against the meeting of the FTAA (April 2001).

Anti-Capitalist Convergence (CLAC)
http://www.quebec2001.net/

Gives information about organizing activities against Summit of the FTAA in Quebec City (April 2001).

World Social Forum
http://www.forumsocialmundial.org.br/

Site of the 'alternative Davos' in Porto Alegré

SOCIAL ORG. – ACTION GROUPS

WTOAction.Org
http://wtoaction.org/

Continues to engage people in opposing trade agreements, such as the WTO and FTAA.

50 Years is Enough
http://www.50years.org/index.html

Activates for economic justice plus profound transformation of the World Bank and IMF.

ATTAC
http://www.attac.org/

Association for the Taxation of Financial Transactions for the Aid of Citizens.

The International Forum on Globalization
http://www.ifg.org/index.html

An alliance of 60 leading activists, scholars, economists, researchers and writers.

Global Trade Watch
http://www.tradewatch.org/

A part of Public Citizen that focuses on action against free trade.

Corporate Watch
http://www.corpwatch.org/
Provides news, analysis, and action resources to respond to corporate activity around the globe.

Global Exchange
http://www.globalexchange.org/
A human rights organization dedicated to promoting environmental and social justice around the world.

Friends of the Earth
http://www.foe.org/
A national environmental organization and part of an international environmental network.

Infoshop.org
http://www.infoshop.org/Welcome.html
Has lots of information of interest to anarchists, anti-authoritarians, and other activists.

The Institute for Agriculture and Trade Policy
http://www.iatp.org/
Promotes resilient family farms, rural communities and ecosystems around the world.

SUPPORTIVE ORGANIZATIONS

Protest.Net
http://www.protest.net/
A collective of activists who are working together to create a public record of protest actions on the web.

Ruckus Society
http://www.ruckus.org/
Provides training on the skills of non-violent civil disobedience to help environmental and human rights organizations achieve their goals.

Indymedia
http://www.indymedia.org/
A collective of independent media organizations and hundreds of journalists offering grassroots, non-corporate coverage.

The Association for Progressive Communications
http://www.apc.org/english/index.htm
Advocates for and facilitates the use of ICTs by civil society in a variety of ways.

Table 5.2 Coding scheme for the information, interactivity and mobilization functions of websites

Information	Score

1   Self-presentation (1 = minimal information on the organization; 2 = extensive info on the history, goals, structure, members . . .)
2   Views of the organization (concerning social and political issues) (1 = minimal or unclear info on the views of the organization; 2 = extensive explanations of views and opinions, certain info can be downloaded . . .)
3   External information (links) (1 = minimal info on other organizations and no links; 2 = extensive info or several links to other organizations)
4   Background information (1 = the issue is briefly placed in its context, other ideas and arguments are referred to concisely; 2 = an extensive overview is given of the debate with attention to different views (newspaper articles, scientific studies, reports of organizations . . .)

Interactivity

1   Feedback opportunities (1 = there is an email address for further info, suggestions or complaints; 2 = visitors are encouraged to react by email, the email button is not placed only on the homepage)
2   Electronic correspondence (1 = occasional info via email; 2 = regular info via an electronic newsletter)
3   Online debate (1 = one general forum or chat group where visitors can join the discussion; 2 = numerous debate opportunities on different issues)
4   Personal contribution (1 = visitor can react to specific info on the site (for example to a columnist); 2 = visitor can make his/her own contribution on the site)

Mobilization

1   Support/membership (1 = possibility to become a member, to donate money, or to buy supportive products)
2   Action calendar (1 = calendar with an overview of activities; 2 = accompanied by a call for participation, or more detailed info (further link/contact address); 3 = 2+ opportunity to put your action online)
3   Online actions (1 = (sort of) online petition; 2 = extensive computer actions (a call to pin down servers . . .)
4   Training (1 = limited info on how to organize actions or references made to other organizations/sites; 2 = detailed, concrete info – manuals – on different action techniques (e.g. how to block roads, how to influence the media . . .)

Table 5.3 Codes and standardized scores of 17 websites on their information function

	Code 0	Code 1	Code 2	Standardized score
Self-presentation	0	8	9	76
Views of the organization	1	4	12	82
External information (links)	1	0	16	91
Background information	2	11	4	56
Subtotal				76

(b) To further explore the content of each site, a 'checklist' of 12 subjects related to the 'anti-globalization' protests was used. If it concerned a main subject on the site it received code two, a minor subject was coded one, and if the subject wasn't mentioned at all, code nought was attributed.[9] With an average of eight of the eleven subjects coded as minor or main subject, most of the sites were very broad in their view on (anti-)globalization. An exception is the Ruckus Society, which supports other organizations in using non-violent action techniques and gave hardly any information on globalization or themes linked to it. The fact that most organizations have a frame that defines a multitude of problems is not necessarily problematic. Gerhards and Rucht (1992) also found that the coalition behind an anti-IMF demonstration in Berlin addressed a very wide range of issues and still managed to connect them to each other.

As Table 5.4 shows, most important are the contested economic aspects of globalization. Free trade and, to a lesser degree, economic dominance are given full attention on most websites. Although, as noted above, this outcome is probably influenced by the research period, it shows a consensus on globalization as a primary economic matter. This confirms Cecilia Lynch's earlier findings that among progressive contemporary social movements economic globalization is seen as 'the primary obstacle to the fulfilment of their goals' (1998: 149). Further, most organizations state that this economic matter has important side-effects on other issues such as the environment (sustainable development), the unequal distribution of wealth between the North and the South, human rights, and the labour conditions of many.

Table 5.4 Codes and standardized sum scores of 17 sites on themes linked to the anti-globalization issue

	Code 0	Code 1	Code 2	Sum score (/100)
1 Free trade (against the liberalization of trade, against the WTO, pro fair trade . . .)	1	2	14	88
2 Economic domination (the market dominates political and social life)	4	1	12	73
3 International democracy (undemocratic international institutions)	3	5	9	68
4 Unequal North–South distribution (Third-World debt relief, IMF programmes, Tobin tax . . .)	5	2	10	65
5 Sustainable development (environmental problems, animal rights, respect for the planet . . .)	1	10	6	65
6 Human rights (protection of minorities, poverty reduction . . .)	2	8	7	65
7 Labour (employee-rights, wages . . .)	3	7	7	62
8 Civil society (cooperation between NGOs, movements, action groups . . .)	3	7	7	62
9 Participative democracy (improving the participation of citizens in policy in general)	5	7	5	50
10 Decentralization (taking decisions on a lower level, smaller communities . . .)	9	6	2	29
11 Cultural homogenization (against Americanization, pro cultural autonomy . . .)	8	8	1	29

Besides being regarded as an economic problem, globalization is also seen as a political one. Particularly, the problem of an international government led by 'undemocratic' international institutions was discussed on several websites. Many of them referred to a stronger civil society and a more participative democracy as plausible solutions. Decentralization as such was less explicitly mentioned.

The cultural aspect of globalization was clearly the least important. Only the more intellectual International Forum on Globalization saw it as a main part of the issue.[10] However, it is not unthinkable that for organizations in the South this is a more crucial part of their struggle.

(c) Finally, views and ideas on the globalization issue might be further elaborated by an extensive discussion. When a medium like the internet is used by a 'citizen-based' organization, one would assume that is in a highly interactive manner. However, this was not shown to be the case (Table 5.5). Most sites offer the 'basics', such as a feedback possibility or a newsletter, mostly via email. More sophisticated ways of interaction and debate, such as forums or chat groups, are limited. Only four sites host some kind of online debate.[11] The opportunity for members or visitors to have a personal contribution on the site, for instance by reactions to articles, is more widespread.

We can conclude that most of the organizations inform about different causes and consequences of globalization, which is defined in general as being primarily an economic problem that has created a problem of democratic governance. While the information is elaborate, the possibilities for debating that information are rather limited. We must also point out that the consensus on such issues says little about the way this global economy should be altered. This study did not allow for more than a surface study of the second, 'prognostic' dimension of framing. Prognostic framing implies the formulations of solutions for the problems defined earlier (Snow and Benford 1988). At first sight, most sites leave big questions on the ideal strategy unanswered. For instance, the site of the World Social Forum asks: 'Is it necessary to abolish the World Bank, the IMF, and the WTO or can they be reformed?' At this moment, it seems to be a NO-consensus: most organizations know what they are against but little is said about what they are in favour of. At the same time we can see how the final statement of the second World Social Forum in Porto Alegre (2002) remains awfully vague when it comes to formulating alternatives.

Yet a strong prognostic frame is something most movements lack. But since, unlike political parties, they are not immediately expected to offer clear solutions, this shortcoming is not too problematic (Gerhards and Rucht 1992). The anti-globalization movement first needs to de-legitimize the dominant views on globalization before it can legitimize others (Lynch 1998). Further research on the variation in goals and strategy should improve our view on the master frames of these organizations.

Websites: a new means for real or virtual mobilization?

We stated above that the selected websites assist the process of informing their members or participants. They can learn about the organization and what it does or does not stand for. More crucial for a social movement is the fact that these websites could also facilitate the actual mobilization of activists. The mobilization process, getting people onto the street, has always been a difficult and unpredictable element in the movements' success (Klandermans 1984). In the literature different methods of mobilizing people are distinguished, varying from direct mail, mass media, and formal organizations, to more informal networks of friends and relatives, or what McAdam calls 'micro-mobilization contexts' (Klandermans and Oegema 1987; McAdam 1988; McCarthy *et al.* 1996; Walgrave and Manssens 2000). It is clear that after the recent 'anti-globalization' protest, ICTs should be added to this list.

Without guessing how many people actually showed up in Seattle or Prague thanks to the internet, we can take a look at the way these websites are 'action mobilizators'. In the WWW area, the concept of mobilization should perhaps be extended from (former) 'unconventional' street actions such as demonstrations and sit-ins to new virtual actions varying from an online petition to pinning down the enemy's server (see Table 5.6).

As mentioned above, we use a coding scheme that is explained in detail in Table 5.2.

A first, more passive way, of mobilizing people for the good cause is to give them the opportunity to join or to support the organization. Two-thirds of the sites offered such online registration forms to become a member, donate money or buy promotional goods. With a bit of creativity, organizations like Corporate Watch were even willing to support 'a small fundraising party that will be fun for all and help CorpWatch gain new supporters'.

Table 5.5 Codes and standardized scores of 17 websites on their interactive function

	Code 0	Code 1	Code 2	Standardized score
Feedback opportunities	0	9	8	73
Electronic correspondence	2	3	12	79
Online debate	13	3	1	15
Personal contribution	5	7	5	50
Subtotal				56

The more active elements in Table 5.5 confirm the role of the internet as a medium for promoting and organizing protest activities. Only two organizations did not host a calendar with the upcoming activities to contest globalization. Visitors were mostly encouraged to participate and given detailed information on how to do so. Some sites gave practical information (on transport, sleeping accommodation, hours, places), while others referred to external links or email addresses. Above we gave the example of 'The Field Guide to the FTAA Protest in Quebec City' as a document that took the activist by the hand and guided them through all the obstacles to effective participation. To make a friendly impression on the inhabitants of Quebec, some words of French are even taught to the English-speaking participants. So, after reading it they knew that 'prison' and 'police' mean the same in French as in English.

On seven websites activists had the possibility to add protest activities, and on a more specialized site like 'Protest.net' you could ask to be sent an email reminder. And finally, for the ones who weren't able to join the actions, 15 sites also reported on previous events.

Most sites gave some information on how to use or improve certain action techniques, or referred to manuals or other organizations for more activist 'training'. The advice given was quite diverse and varied from techniques on how to climb a building (Ruckus Society) through to dealing with media attention (Global Trade Watch). The Association for Progressive Communication even devoted a great deal of its website to improving ICT skills for other organizations and activists (using email effectively, website development).

The websites were clearly a means of support in the mobilization process for all sorts of 'real' protest actions, but were used far less as an action tool on their own. Barely half of the organizations used some form of online action, for the most part online petitions. Only

Protest.net, promoting a 'netstrike', and Friends of the Earth, offering all kinds of protest emails to politicians, took a step further in the virtual direction.

Linking websites: one network?

Social movements are often conceived as social networks of informal and formal organizations (Diani and Eyerman 1992; Diani 1997). Certainly in a transnational context the network perspective seems most applicable. A network of different social organizations or action groups is, as Tarrow (1998) states, not necessarily a social movement but it can become the basis of one.

Earlier it was shown that globalization is a very complex and diverse issue that attracts different organizations for different reasons. Besides the ideological 'nuances' (Greens, labour unions, anarchists, Third World movements . . .), there are strong geographical differences that have to be bridged. Can the world wide web overcome all those cleavages? The mobilization successes of Seattle, etc. of course prove some kind of collaboration, but it is hard to say how far this network reaches and how stable it is. We have examined the connections between the 17 selected organizations by analysing their links to other sites (Table 5.7). Hypertext links set the web apart from other media channels such as television, newspapers or magazines. Virtual links are used in other research too, for example a study on the relations between US Congress members (Cha 2001), as a way of exploring networks. For activists and social organizations it is a unique facility

Table 5.6 Codes and standardized scores of 17 websites on their mobilization function

	Code 0	Code 1	Code 2	Standardized score
Support/membership	6	11	–*	64
Action calendar	2	3	5–7†	66
Online actions	9	6	2	29
Training	4	9	4	50
Subtotal				52

* This chaacteristic could be coded from 0 to 1; see Table 5.2 for an explanation of the codes.
† This chaacteristic could be coded from 0 to 3; see Table 5.2 for an explanation of the codes.

Table 5.7 Number of external links on and to 17 websites

		Number of external links	Number of links to anti-globalization sites (max. 16)	Referred to by anti-globalization site (max. 16)
1	A20	66	6	5
2	CLAC (Quebec 2001)	26	2	5
3	World Social Forum	41	1	2
4	WTOaction.org	260	13	2
5	50 Years is Enough	83	7	5
6	ATTAC	88	6	3
7	Global Trade Watch	63	4	7
8	Corporate Watch	249	7	7
9	IFG	40	5	5
10	Global Exchange	393	9	7
11	FOE	1	0	8
12	IATP	48	0	6
13	Infoshop	400	9	3
14	Protest.net	126	3	3
15	Ruckus Society	46	2	3
16	Indymedia	94	8	10
17	APC	29	1	2
Average		126	5	5

for referring to like-minded groups or to sites of the opponent.[12] Smith and Smythe (2001) found that most of the anti-MAI websites linked to the website of the OECD, the organization responsible for the secret trade negotiations they opposed. The reason behind this was that the draft text of the MAI that was released on the OECD site was considered a major source of information. Therefore, a link does not necessarily prove a relationship but can be seen here as a basic form of alliance, certainly when it is a link to a like-minded group or organization. The more 'missing links' there are, the weaker the social movement network becomes.

Most of the 17 websites were strong advocates of hyperlinks. When we compare with the study of Hill and Hughes (1998) on politically oriented websites, which found an average of 28 links, our average of 126 is relatively high.[13] Still, in the dynamic life of the internet it remains hard to evaluate data from 2001 compared to a study dated from August 1997.

This high number of links does not automatically imply a connection between the selected websites engaged in the anti-globalization struggle. An average of five links out of 16 prevents us from speaking of a close-knit network. The practice of linking is clearly not always a reciprocal one, which means that not all relations are equally strong. The Canadians of WTOaction.org are, for example, the most 'bonding' organization with no fewer than 14 links, but are referred to by only two others. Conversely, Friends of the Earth, which has only one link to its umbrella organization, is referred to by half of the other sites.

If we do not focus on the missing links between some organizations, but look instead at the visualization of the network (Figure 5.1), we could interpret the results in a different way. All websites are in fact indirectly linked to one another. So if an activist starts intensively surfing the web, he or she can visit all 17 websites (and probably a few hundred like-minded more). Central in the network are WTOaction. org (4 in Figure 5.1), Corporate Watch (8), Global Exchange (10), 50 Years is Enough (5), and Indymedia (16). With ten incoming and eight outgoing links, Indymedia appears to be the most crucial for the coherence of the network. This independent medium is, since its foundation for the Seattle protests, a fast growing network of its own with almost 60 centres in 20 countries. If these 'local' divisions of Indymedia were added to the analysis of links, the central role would be even more pronounced.[14]

Only the World Social Forum (3) and the Association for Progressive Communication (17) fall a bit out of the centre. For the WSF this could be due to the fact that the conference took place more than a month before our research started, and some temporary links might have disappeared. The link from Corporate Watch to the WSF was found in their article archive. Sites that do not keep information stored, like Protest.Net, are therefore less connected to others. Another explanation involves also the only other non-North American organization in our study, the French organization ATTAC. Both have, besides their mutual connection, only one or two other incoming links. This means that they are a little isolated from the organizations located in the USA and Canada. Does this suggest a geographical, linguistic gap? We must refer to the finding that 'local' divisions of, for instance, Indymedia do have links to ATTAC and the WSF, so 'gap' is probably too strong. Further research seems necessary to answer this question properly. On the other hand, there seems to be no cleavage on issues or strategy. No separate subgroups or clusters could be identified. An anarchistic site like Infoshop (13) is only 'two steps' away

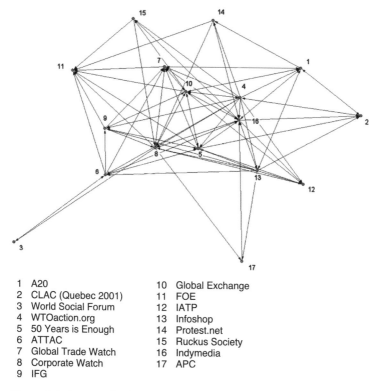

1	A20	10	Global Exchange
2	CLAC (Quebec 2001)	11	FOE
3	World Social Forum	12	IATP
4	WTOaction.org	13	Infoshop
5	50 Years is Enough	14	Protest.net
6	ATTAC	15	Ruckus Society
7	Global Trade Watch	16	Indymedia
8	Corporate Watch	17	APC
9	IFG		

Figure 5.1 A network of seventeen websites on the basis of external hyperlinks

from more moderate organizations like FOE (11) or Global Trade Watch (7). Perhaps recent violent clashes between militant protestors and the police at summits in Göteborg and Genoa will lead to a clearer division in the movement.

We can conclude that although the network is not complete on the basis of external links, it is highly integrated. On the basis of Figure 5.1, the social movement condition 'a network of organizations' seems to be no problem in this case. However, the arrows in the figure suggest a real connection but do not guarantee it. You can easily link to other organizations without having real contact. What does a hyperlink signify? Is it a way of providing more information, irrespective of approval, or just a way to show that others are fighting for the same cause? At the moment we know little on the network value that can be attributed to the use of hyperlinks. Is a temporary link, for instance in an article, as important as a permanent one in a separate 'links' page? On the other hand, some organizations have worked together or have intensive contacts, but for unknown reasons have no mutual hyperlink on their websites. Are these contacts, as some assume, mainly sustained by email and mailing lists (Smith and Smythe 2001)? Do they wish to keep the visitors on their own site and fear losing members to other, similar organizations? Is there a kind of thematic or territorial competition for website visitors and potential donators? This could be an explanation as to why established environmental organizations were not linking to each other (van de Donk and Foederer 2001). Other aspects, such as the individual role of the webmaster(s), can also explain the presence or absence of certain links. It is clear that further research is needed, but for the time being the value of hyper-links to construct a network of organizations is questionable, particularly in this case when sites refer to hundreds of others.

Conclusion: globalization, social movements and the internet

In this chapter we have evaluated three social movement conditions of the coalition against neo-liberal globalization by analysing a limited selection of 17 relevant websites in March–May 2001. On all three, relatively positive conclusions can be drawn. First of all, there is a sort of consensus on the globalization issue they contest, by framing it primarily as an economic problem that has negative consequences on human beings and the environment. Also, the political aspect of globalization, the lack of democratic legitimacy of the international organizations, is usually contested. Besides giving general information on the issue, the sites actively mobilized people to demonstrate against the symbols of economic globalization. By following detailed guide-lines, all supporters can easily become real participants. Finally, all 17 websites were directly or indirectly 'hyperlinked' to each other, creating a kind of network of related organizations.

This positive judgement of the anti-globalization coalition becoming a social movement, and the contribution of the internet, has to be tempered as both movement and medium are in full evolution and hard to quantify. In the fight to alter the process of economic globaliza-tion, new events take place, new organizations join the protest, new coalitions arise while others disappear, and few can predict what will happen next. Therefore, at this point in time, it is difficult to state categorically that this mix of 'anti-globalization' protesters is evolving towards a transnational social movement. However, it is clear that they, like other protest movements (Castells 2001), prove that globali-zation is contestable and that the protest is becoming 'as transnational as capital' (Smith and Smythe 2001).

Is this all due to the technological evolution? Have the new forms of communication, in this case, changed the 'logic of collective action' or just the speed of protest diffusion? We are not sure. The internet brings new opportunities for everyone, but at the moment international activists are benefiting more than their opponents. It seems that the fluid, non-hierarchical structure of the internet and that of the international protest coalition prove to be a good match and that it is no coincidence that both can be labelled as a 'network of networks' (Scott and Steer 2001). On the other hand, the role of the internet is often exaggerated. For instance, during the 'Carnival against Capitalism' that took place in cities around the world in 1999, while *The Guardian*, a UK-based newspaper, reported that the demonstration in London was entirely dependent on the web, according to Stephen Lax (2000), who found a range of posters, leaflets and graffiti advertisements, the internet was used alongside other mobilizing means. There is, as this and others studies confirm, little evidence that the internet is becoming a substitute for traditional forms of protest (Smith and Smythe 2001; Pickerill 2001).

Within the movement, the role and importance of the internet are also regarded in different ways. This was revealed when we interviewed two Belgian representatives of involved organizations. Han Soete, of Indymedia Belgium, was convinced that the movement could not exist in its then state without the internet, which made the exchange of information and creation of contacts in a global context both easy and cheap. Nico Verhaegen of Via Campesina, an international organization of small farmers, had a more modest view on the new media: 'If the same globalization would have occurred without the existence of the web or email, the same transnational protest movement would have founded. Perhaps with a bit more tension, and not that fast, but the movement would have come there for sure.'

Again it is difficult to say who has the more accurate vision on the contribution of the new technology in this case. Our explorative research can perhaps inspire others to improve our knowledge on this increasingly important aspect of social movements. At this moment we can't say it better than the Canadian Security Intelligence Service: 'The internet will continue to play a large role in the success or failure of globalization protests and demonstrations. Groups will use the internet to identify and publicize targets, solicit and encourage support, organize and communicate information and instructions, recruit, raise funds, and as a means of promoting their various individual and collective aims' (Canadian Security Intelligence Service 2000).

Notes

1 Although peaceful forms of protest have become a rather normal or conventional form of politics, the term 'unconventional' is still used to define all sorts of protest action varying from petitions to violent demonstrations (Van Aelst and Walgrave 2001).

2 As an example we can refer to a heterogeneous coalition of 133 groups that organized a demonstration against the IMF and World Bank meeting in Berlin in 1988, which attracted up to 80,000 people (Gerhards and Rucht 1992).

3 A lot of websites were devoted to the event labelled as A16, referring to the protests on 16 April 2000.

4 The Canadian police reduced the opportunities for activists to disturb the meeting by building a six-kilometre chain link and concrete wall around the conference centre. The 1000 protesters who tried to 'break down the wall' received much more media attention than the 25,000 others that took to the streets peacefully.

5 Just typing the word anti-globalization in the search engine Google resulted in 8,300 web pages in no useful order.

6 After careful comparison of the codes, only a handful of justifications seemed necessary. This was the case when the students gave similar explanations but different codes.

7 For instance, the Canadian site WTOaction.org claims to present the Common Front on the World Trade Organization (CFWTO), which brings together over 50 national organizations and regional networks, but fails to name members.

8 We should be careful not to generalize the absence of links on environmental sites, while we found hundreds on the site of the UK department of Friends Of the Earth. In this study we analysed only the main US site of FOE.

9 A main subject is mentioned several times or as a priority of the organization, while a minor subject is mentioned only occasionally.

10 In their words: 'Worldwide homogenisation of diverse, local and indigenous cultures, social and economic forms, as well as values and living patterns that reflect the efficiency needs of the new global monoculture' (www.ifg.org).

11 Also Pippa Norris (2001) found in her analysis of political websites limited debate opportunities for visitors. Only 35 per cent of the websites hosted some kind of online debate.

12 Many of the organizations referred also to the websites of the WTO, IMF or World Bank.

13 This average is probably an underestimate, because the links are spread all over the site and easily overlooked. We only counted the links on this website and not on separate sites of divisions in other cities or countries.

14 Divisions of Indymedia referred to ATTAC, The World Social Forum and the 50 Years is Enough network. And the website of the Anti-Capitalist Convergence only linked to a Canadian department of Indymedia.

15 The network was drawn using Pajek, a program for social network analysis (http://vlado.fmf.uni-lj.si/pub/networks/pajek/).

6 Communicating global activism

Strengths and vulnerabilities of networked politics

W. Lance Bennett

Networks of activists demanding greater voice in global economic, social, and environmental policies raise interesting questions about organizing political action across geographical, cultural, ideological, and issue boundaries. Protests against world development and trade policies are nothing new. For example, Rucht (1999) has documented such action in Germany dating from the 1980s. However, social justice activism in the recent period seems to me different in its global scale, networked complexity, openness to diverse political identities, and capacity to sacrifice ideological integration for pragmatic political gain (Bennett 2003a). This vast web of global protest is also impressive in its capacity to refigure itself continuously around shifting issues, protest events, and political adversaries.

The 'Battle in Seattle', referring to the demonstrations against the 1999 World Trade Organization ministerial meeting, has become recognized as a punctuating moment in the evolution of global activism (Levi and Olson 2000). Seattle, like most subsequent demonstrations, primarily attracted local and regional activists. However, there is growing evidence that a movement of global scope is emerging through the proliferation of related protest activities (Lichbach and Almeida 2001). Observers note, for example, that activist networks are engaging politically with non-state, transnational targets such as corporations and trade regimes, and that there is growing coordination of communication and action across international activist networks (Arquilla and Ronfeld 2001; Gerlach 2001; Lichbach and Almeida 2001; Rheingold 2002).

It is clear that personal digital media are important to these activists. One indicator is the expansion of a web-based communication infrastructure, marked, for example, by the growth of the Indymedia activist information network (www.indymedia.org) from one outlet to more than 100 in the three years following Seattle. Many activists cite the importance of personal digital media in creating networks and coordinating action across diverse political identities and organizations (see online interviews at http://www.wtohistory.org). A key issue is whether these communication practices merely reduce the costs or increase the efficiencies of political action, or whether they change the political game itself. My interest in this chapter is to explore some of the ways in which digital communication networks may be changing the political game in favour of resource-poor players who, in many cases, are experimenting with political strategies outside of conventional national political channels such as elections and interest processes.

Observations reported in this chapter indicate that digital communication practices appear to have a variety of political effects on the growth and forms of global activism. These effects range from organizational dynamics and patterns of change to strategic political relations between activists, opponents and spectator publics. In addition, patterns of individual participation appear to be affected by hyperlinked communication networks that enable individuals to find multiple points of entry into varieties of political action. Moreover, the redundancy of communication channels in many activist networks creates organizational durability as hub organizations come and go, and as the focus of action shifts across different events, campaigns, and targets. Finally, there appears to be a relationship between communication practices and the evolution of democracy itself. One of the important subtexts of this movement is *media democracy*, centred on the conversion of media consumers into producers, with the introduction of open publishing and collective editing software – all channelled through personal digital networks.

While there are many indicators that digital media have become important organizational resources in making this movement, there are also potential problems or vulnerabilities associated with these communication-based networks. For example, the ease of joining and leaving polycentric (multi-hubbed) issue networks means that it becomes difficult to control campaigns or to achieve coherent collective identity frames. In addition, organizations may face challenges to their own internal direction and goals when they employ open, collective communication processes to set agendas and organize action. Some organizations even experience internal transformation when they become important hubs in networks and must accommodate demands by other network members. These vulnerabilities are, of course, in constant creative tension with the strengths outlined above, making this movement an interesting case of large-scale applications of networked communication as foundations for political organization and action. This analysis attempts to examine both strengths and vulnerabilities associated with various communication practices that make transnational activism possible.

Talking about such substantial digital media effects flies in the face of the conventional wisdom that internet and other digital media typically do little more than amplify and economize communication in political organizations (Agre 2002; Davis 1999). For example, Agre (2002) argues that in most cases the internet is subordinated to the existing routines and patterns of the institution using it, and that internet applications either amplify and economize areas that already define the institution. One observer has even gone so far as to assert that 'the Internet is less applicable [to] the creation of new forms of democratic public spheres than [to] the support of already existing ones' (Buchstein 1997: 260, discussed by Agre 2002). The problem with these accounts of the internet and politics is that they generally look at how established political institutions and organizations adapt the internet to existing routines.

It is easy to see how conceptual confusion surrounds the political impact of the internet and other digital media. When political networks are viewed at the level of constituent organizations, the implications of internet communications can vary widely. Political organizations that are older, larger, resource-rich, and strategically linked to party and government politics may rely on internet-based communications mostly to amplify and reduce the costs of pre-existing communication routines. On the other hand, newer, resource-poor organizations that tend to reject conventional politics may be defined in important ways by their internet presence (Graber *et al.* forthcoming). In this analysis, I contend that the importance of the internet in networks of global protest includes – but also goes well beyond – gains that can be documented for particular resource-poor organizations. For example, effects at the network level include the formation of large and flexible coalitions exhibiting the 'strength of thin ties' that make those networks more adaptive and resistant to attack than coalitions forged through leader-based partnerships among bureaucratic organizations (Gerlach 2001).

The implication here is not that the distributed (multi-hub, or polycentric) structure of the internet somehow causes contemporary activists to organize in remarkably non-hierarchical, broadly distributed, and flexible networks. Digital media applications can take on a variety of forms, from closed and hierarchical to open and broadly distributed. Preferences for the latter pattern reflect the social, personal, and political contexts in which many global activists define their mutual relationships.

The social contexts of internet activism

One idea upon which most observers agree is that applications of the internet, like the uses of most communication media, depend heavily on social context. As Castells (2001: 50) puts it: 'The Internet is a particularly malleable technology, susceptible to being deeply modified by its social practice, and leading to a whole range of potential social outcomes.' Polycentric (socially distributed) networks that display the flat, non-hierarchical, flexible, and resilient characteristics of much global activism are well supported by various digital technologies (Gerlach 2001), but the inclination to construct such networks in the first place reflects at least two defining qualities of their makers: the identity processes and the new politics that define many younger generation activists.

Identity in distributed social networks

Various theorists have discussed the transformation of social structures and identity processes associated with economic globalization in the so-called post-industrial or late modern societies (Giddens 1991; Bennett 1998; Beck, 2000). In these visions of 'late' and 'post' modern society, identity becomes a personally reflective (and reflexive) project that is organized and expressed through often elaborately managed lifestyles. Through this process, personal identity narratives replace collective social scripts as the bases for social order. These narratives become interpersonal linkages as network organization begins to displace hierarchical institutions as primary membership and social recognition systems for individuals.

A defining quality of the *network society* is that individuals are likely to form political ties through affinity networks based on repertoires of these narratives. This quality of networks contrasts sharply to the 'modernist' tendency to forge social and political order through mutual identifications with leaders, ideologies and memberships in conventional social and political groups. Castells (1997) has documented how these highly individualized identity processes find creative forms of empowerment through diverse organizational capacities of the internet. In many ways, the organizational, personal, and cultural diversity of global activism reflects what Wellman calls 'networked individualism': the ease of establishing personal links that enable people to join more diverse and more numerous political communities than they would ordinarily join in the material world (Wellman 2000, paragraph 1.6). I explore these social and identity processes in greater detail elsewhere (Bennett 2003b). The present analysis is focused on the ways in which identity-driven communication practices characterize and organize the politics of these activists.

One might argue that various longstanding social movements – feminism and environmentalism come to mind – have displayed similar horizontal and segmented patterns of network organization. Indeed, one of the classic accounts of such movement network organization is the SPIN model developed by Gerlach and Hine (1970). SPIN stands for segmented polycephalous integrated networks. However, when Gerlach (2001) applied the SPIN model to contemporary global protest networks, he made two interesting conceptual adjustments, which he passed over without the fanfare that I believe they deserve. First, he replaced the idea of *polycephalous* organization with *polycentric* order, indicating that, like earlier SPIN movements, global activist networks have many centres or hubs, but unlike their predecessors, those hubs are less likely to be defined around prominent leaders. In addition, he noted that the primary basis of movement integration and growth has shifted from ideology to more personal and fluid forms of association. In my view, these changes in the SPIN model reflect the identity processes of fragmented social systems that make electronically managed affinity networks such essential forms of political organization.

A new politics suited to distributed communication networks

Beyond identity processes, a second impetus for creating such broadly distributed communication networks is that the targets of global activism are numerous, and they are slipping off the grid of conventional national politics. Many activists believe that labour, environment, rights and other policies of their governments have been weakened by pressures from global corporations and transnational economic regimes such as the World Trade Organization. The neo-liberal drift and rebranding of labour parties in Europe and the Democratic Party in the United States provide some evidence for these concerns. The resulting capacity of corporations to escape regulation and win concessions from governments has created a political sphere beyond normal legislative, electoral, and regulatory processes – a sphere that Beck (2000) calls subpolitics. The subpolitics of corporations and transnational economic regimes has been countered by activist sub-politics that includes global demonstrations, campaigns against companies and economic development regimes, and the creation of epistemic networks to gather and publicize information on global issues (Keck and Sikkink 1998).

The place of government in the activists' political calculus clearly varies from nation to nation and from organization to organization. However, newly emerging forms of political action are being aimed beyond government nearly everywhere in the post-industrial North. These politics include creative experiments with publicly monitored labour, environmental, food, and trade standards regimes designed to hold transnational targets directly accountable to activist networks and their publics (see examples at www.globalcitizenproject.org, under labour standards, fair trade, and corporate social responsibility). These nimble campaigns aimed at corporations and transnational trade and development targets lend themselves to the repertoires of digital com-munication: lists and action alerts, swarming responses (e.g. denial of service attacks on corporate websites), and the continuous refiguring of web networks as campaigns shift focus and change players.

Tarrow touches on these subpolitics and their organizational effects in describing global activism:

> as unlikely to sustain high levels of confidence in government and may trigger less trusting attitudes in the public by demonstrating the inadequacy of governmental performance; but on the other hand, neither do they create enduring negative subcultures. Their variform and shifting organizations, their tendency to produce rapid and rapidly-liquidated coalitions, their focus on short- and medium-term issues rather than fully fledged ideologies do not produce standing activist commitments or deeply held loyalties.
>
> (Tarrow 1999: 30)

The emergence of a politics that is shifting away from organizational conventions such as leadership, ideology, and government processes invites a fresh theoretical perspective. The goal of this analysis is to begin explaining how webs of contentious transnational politics oper-ate on such a large scale, particularly among groups and individuals joined by little binding leadership or ideology, and whose protests cover such diverse political issues.

Rethinking the organization of protest networks

The features of global activism outlined above raise interesting challenges for thinking about movements and protest politics. One of the best-known models of contentious politics refers to the diffusion of protest networks and the accompanying transformation of collective identities as 'scale shift' (McAdam *et al.* 2001; Tarrow 2002a). According to this view, scale shift depends on the existence of several mechanisms of human agency: *brokerage* (creating social links among disconnected sites of protest), *diffusion* (transfer of information across those links), and *attribution of similarity* (mutual identification) (McAdam *et al.* 2001: 331–339). As I understand it, this process generally involves face-to-face agency (brokerage) in the recruitment of protesters and in the negotiation of new identity frames to accommodate the expanding coalitions of groups. A now classic formulation of the identity framing process at the core of this theory of scale shift is Snow and Benford's (1992) account of the continuous redefining of 'interpretive schemata' to provide common meaning as movement coalitions grow.

Most of the cases that illustrate this process are instances of national and cultural mobilization. In order for scale shift to occur transnationally and cross-culturally with the magnitude and diversity of contemporary global activism, the process seems to require mediation by digital communication networks. More importantly, the ease of linking to these digital networks (aided by activist preferences for an inclusive politics) also eases the demand to continually renegotiate collective identity frames as movements shift in scale. The idea here is not that communication networks replace social transactions or dispel the identity issues of collective action. Rather, the nature of social transactions, themselves, is changing due to the capacity of distributed communication networks to ease personal engagement with others. In thinking about 'computer networks as social networks', Wellman and his colleagues describe a variety of ways in which digital communication can initiate, enhance, and in some cases even replace direct social relationships (Wellman *et al.* 1996). In addition, Castells (1996, 1997) argues that we must grasp the transformations of space, society, and identity that are associated with digital communication networks. Thus, an inseparable mix of virtual and face-to-face communication defines many activist networks, and contacts in these networks may range far from activists' immediate social circles if they can be sustained in terms of the cost and scale offered by digital communication applications.

All of these features of scale shift in the absence of ideological integration, clear collective identity framing, and strong organizational leadership reflect important degrees of organization via communication systems – as opposed to communication merely reflecting or amplifying political organization. The following analyses suggest how the same communication practices that serve strategic political purposes can also operate as social organizational resources.

Communication as political strategy and organizational resource

This analysis is based on observations of various protest activities aimed at trade and development organizations and corporations. Materials developed by the research teams in these projects can be found at the Global Citizen Project (www.globalcitizenproject.org), and in the civic engagement, issue campaigns, culture jamming, and digital media sections of the Centre for Communication and Civic Engagement (http://www.engagedcitizen.org). These studies support a number of generalizations about the internet and activist politics, four of which are reported here. The intriguing feature of each generalization is that communication practices are hard to separate from organizational and political capabilities, suggesting that personal digital communication is a foundation of this identity-driven subpolitics. The patterns of communication that both reflect and reproduce global activism are briefly summarized here and elaborated in the remainder of the chapter.

Permanent campaigns

Global activism is characterized by long-running communication campaigns to organize protests and publicize issues. Campaigns in activist politics are not new, but the campaigns of the current generation are more protracted. They are less likely to be run by central command and coordinating organizations such as unions or environmental NGOs, making them less centrally controlled, and more difficult to turn on and off. The networking and mobilizing capacities of these ongoing campaigns make campaigns, themselves, political organizations that sustain activist networks in the absence of leadership by central organizations.

Communication in diverse networks is ideologically thin, but rich in terms of individual identity and lifestyle narratives

In recent years, songbirds have been linked to the fair trade coffee campaign in North America, and clothing brand logos have been attached to sweatshop labour campaigns in Europe and North America. Such communication formulas travel well across broad electronic networks and often reach spectator publics, but they do little to advance common movement ideology or identity framing.

Internet use patterns affect the organizational qualities of networks, and can affect the internal development of member organizations

Networks can be reconfigured rapidly as organizations come and go. In addition, hub organizations that become resources for others can be changed by their place in the flow of communication.

New media can alter information flows through the mass media

The creation of a public sphere based in micro-media (email, lists) and middle media internet channels (blogs, organization sites, e-zines) offers activists an important degree of information and communication independence from the mass media. At the same time 'culture jams' and logo campaigns initiated in micro-media and middle media have attracted surprisingly positive coverage of activist messages in the mass media (Klein 2000; Lasn 1999; Bennett 2003c).

Permanent campaigns and political organization

It is often said that we have entered the age of permanent political campaigns, whether waged by elected leaders in order to govern after they win office, or by interest groups to mobilize publics and promote their policy agendas. Campaigns increasingly do more than just communicate political messages aimed at achieving political goals. They also become long-term bases of political organization in fragmenting late modern (globalizing) societies that lack the institutional coherence (e.g. strong parties, grassroots or bottom-up interest organization) to forge stable political identifications. In the American case, the model for activist issue campaigns can be traced to 'corporate' campaigns pioneered by labour unions in the early 1980s (Manheim 2001). These corporate campaigns have now spread throughout activist and advocacy circles, being adopted by environmental, health, and human rights as well as anti-globalization and sustainable development groups and coalitions. For example, a small global network of NGOs stopped Monsanto's plans to develop genetically engineered seed with a successful media campaign labelling the sterile seed strain 'the Terminator'. The small human rights organization Global Witness also successfully targeted the diamond giant De Beers, which ultimately agreed to limit the market for the 'bloody conflict' diamonds that motivated mercenary armies to establish regimes of terror in crumbling African states (Cowell 2000).

Some of these campaigns resemble traditional boycotts in the sense that they are run by relatively centralized organizations or coalitions, and they can be turned off when specified goals are accomplished. However, an increasingly common pattern is for whole activist networks to latch onto particularly ripe targets such as Nike or Microsoft because their heavily advertised and ubiquitous logos stick easily to lifestyle meaning systems among consumer publics. This 'stickiness' of logos helps activists get political messages into the mass media, reaching audiences whose attention is often limited in matters of politics. Thus, unlike boycotts, many contemporary issue campaigns do not require consumer action at all; instead, the goal is to hold a corporate logo hostage in the media until shareholders or corporate managers regard the bad publicity as an independent threat to a carefully cultivated brand image.

Success in publicizing hard-to-communicate political messages may bring new players into campaigns even as others leave a network having declared their goals met. The influx of large and unwieldy networks of activists running through political territories once occupied in more orderly fashion by a small number of rights, environmental, consumer protection, labour and development NGOs presents an interesting strategic dilemma for movement organizing. One attraction of centrally run campaigns is the ability to stop them, which reinforces the credibility of activist organizations by rewarding the compliance of campaign targets. The attraction of decentralized campaigns is the ease of joining them and adding new charges against targets.

The vulnerabilities of these networked campaigns are often inseparable from their strengths. Thus, the decentralized webs of thin ties that make for unstable coalitions, communication noise, lack of clarity about goals, and weak idea framing, also enable networks to refigure themselves after losses and disruptions. For example, the San Francisco-based social justice organization Global Exchange (www.

globalexchange.org) left the long-running campaign against Nike after generating enough negative publicity (see below) to induce company president Phil Knight to promise to take greater responsibility for poor labour conditions in Nike's contract factories. However, other players (e.g. United Students Against Sweatshops, and Press for Change, Jeff Ballinger's founding campaign organization) contended that a key unresolved issue was creating an effective labour standards monitoring system in the absence of reliable government regulation (see Bullert 2000 and Bennett 2003c). As a result, the network reconfigured after the loss of the Global Exchange hub, and student activist organizations became the central hubs. The campaign focus shifted to verifying Nike's claims of greater corporate responsibility.

Observations of long-running campaigns suggest several hypotheses. Campaigns are likely to continue over time, and change in terms of networks and goals to the extent that: (a) the target is widely recognized and newsworthy; (b) the target can be connected to various lifestyle concerns (consumer protection, endangered species, environmental quality, human suffering, political corruption); (c) weblogs, lists, and networked campaign sites create an epistemic community that makes the campaign a source of knowledge about credible problems, while making the target an exemplar of both problems and solutions.

Beyond their many applications in issue activism, continuous campaign networks also organize the steady stream of public demonstrations against transnational targets. For example, Lichbach and Almeida (2001) note that on the dates of the Battle in Seattle, simultaneous protests were held in at least 82 other cities around the world, including 27 locations in the United States, 40 in other 'Northern' locations including Seoul, London, Paris, Prague, Brisbane, and Tel Aviv, and 15 in 'Southern' locations such as New Delhi, Manila, and Mexico City. Not only were these other protests not organized centrally by the Seattle campaign coalition, but information about timing and tactics was transmitted almost entirely through activist networks on the internet. In addition to extending the global reach of single protest events, internet campaigns also enable activists to create and update rich calendars of planned demonstrations. Lichbach and Almeida (2001) discovered wide internet postings and network sites for no fewer than 39 scheduled protests between 1994 and 2001. This suggests that Seattle was just one of many events in a permanent protest campaign organized by different organizations in the global activist network.

The point here is that sustained issue and protest campaigns on a global scale cannot be explained by leadership commitments from centralized organizations with large resource bases or memberships. Coordination through polycentric (distributed) communication networks marks a second distinctive feature of global activism. In keeping with our 'strengths and vulnerabilities' analysis, the next section suggests that, while networked communication may help sustain the campaigns that organize global activism, these leaderless networks may undermine the thematic coherence of the ideas that are communicated through them.

Communication in diverse networks is ideologically thin

Both the strengths and weaknesses of loosely linked, ideologically thin networks are illustrated in the permanent campaign against Microsoft. This campaign began with labour activism in the early 1990s, and has since expanded to include trade, consumer protection, product innovation and many other issues, with campaign fronts in North America, Japan, and the European Union. During the years of the most rapid growth in the network (1997–2001), an important hub was Netaction (www.netaction.org), an organization created explicitly as an internet campaign hub to archive information and mobilize activists (Manheim 2001; Bennett 2003c). The richness of Netaction reports and papers reflects the rise of epistemic communities promoting diverse causes of consumer protection, product innovation, electronic privacy, business ethics and practices, and open source software and internet architecture, among others. Netaction later evolved to occupy similar hub positions in other digital democracy campaigns, and it has reappeared as a hub in the Microsoft network as the campaign entered different phases.

Such networks that do not produce common ideological or issue frames allow different political perspectives to coexist without the conflicts that such differences might create in more centralized coalitions. On most days, conservative United States Senator Orrin Hatch and consumer activist Ralph Nader would not find themselves in the same political universe. Yet they have comfortably occupied network space for years in the anti-Microsoft network. The network of opposition to Microsoft includes businesses (Sun, Oracle, Netscape and others), consumer protection organizations, Computer Professionals for Social Responsibility, the Government Accountability Project, labour organizers, and thousands of direct 'hactivists' (Manheim 2001; Bennett 2003c). These diverse campaign members can coordinate attacks or wait until the company becomes vulnerable from one attack and open a new front, as happened when labour began a union organizing effort aimed at Microsoft's many temporary workers in the midst of the company's antitrust trial with the US government.

Ideologically weak networks can reduce the conflicts often associated with diverse players entering campaigns; they also may harbour intellectual contradictions. Thus, when the moment arrived to adopt solutions for the Microsoft 'problem', there was considerable disagreement among key players about what a proper settlement of the antitrust charges might look like. And when the legal ordeal began to take a toll on Microsoft stock value (which fell in the wake of an initial judicial ruling calling for extreme penalties), the union campaign on labour issues was undermined by company cutbacks.

Rather than trying to find an issue, identity, or ideology that joined so many different players in enduring battles on so many fronts against Microsoft, it makes more sense to think that the openness of the network itself is the defining quality – inviting diverse activists to use the visibility of the target company and its aggressive culture to raise the visibility of their many diverse causes. Such networks can give voice to member organizations without necessarily producing collective action frames of the sort that we generally associate with the growth of movements. Another example of this is the North American fair trade coffee campaign in which Global Exchange (former hub in the Nike sweatshop campaign) became an important hub in a diverse network of birdwatchers, anti-bioengineering groups, and sustainable development organizations. In this network each member could maintain its own identity, while adding value to the causes of others. For example, the Audubon Society provided a credible source for claiming that the failure of coffee companies like Starbucks to pay a fair price for their beans resulted in the disappearance of the small shaded coffee farms which provided habitat for the migrating songbirds that enlivened Northern back yards each summer. The songbird represented a more effective lifestyle symbol for communicating the fair trade message than trying to communicate more ideological discourses about world coffee markets and the plight of peasant farmers (Iozzi 2002; Bennett 2003a).

Ideological and identity thinning may also operate in single organizations that adopt open network designs to promote member equality or minimize bureaucracy. Le Grignou and Patou (Chapter 8, this volume) note this potential for open networks to diminish organizational identity in their analysis of the French organization ATTAC (Association for the Taxation of Financial Transactions for the Aid of Citizens). ATTAC (www.attac.org) is an interesting case because it began with a very specific organizational goal of creating a tax on global financial transactions and using the funds for sustainable development. ATTAC even formed a Scientific Council to guide the production of high-quality information. However, the organization also promoted the autonomy of local chapters through an open communication network that resulted in the posting of diverse concerns from the ATTAC activist membership. Le Grignou and Patou conclude that the easy communication of local interests quickly diversified the organizational agenda to include Commander Marcos, 'mad cow disease', human rights in Tunisia, and the labour struggles of Danone employees. Le Grignou and Patou explain that the 'click here' logic of the open network at once makes connections between such disparate ideas possible, and at the same time creates an intellectual dilemma for the organization. As one ATTAC officer they interviewed put it, 'the main problem for ATTAC today concerns the unification of the movement and the way to give it a more unified content'.

Several related hypotheses emerge from this analysis. In particular, the degrees of ideological discourse and identity framing in a network are inversely related to: the number and diversity of groups in the network; the churn, or turnover of links; the equality of communication access established by hub sites in the network; and the degree to which network traffic involves campaigns. This analysis suggests that it is not so much the internet as the network structures established through it that shape the coherence of communication content. This leads to our third generalization: uses of the internet may have important effects on organizational structures, both inside member organizations and in terms of overall network stability and capacity.

Internet applications as organizational processes

The uses of the internet may be largely subordinated to existing organizational routines and structures when dedicated to the goals and practices of hierarchical organizations such as parties, interest associations, or election campaigns. However, as noted above, the fluid networks of global issue activism enable the internet to become an organizational force shaping both the relations among organizations and, in some cases, the organizations themselves. Some organizations are even transformed by inter-networks as they take on new functions and partnerships. At least four distinct organizational dynamics have been identified in our case studies of organizational interaction with communication networks: (1) organizational transformation due to demands of network partners; (2) organizations that 'move on' to other networks to avoid transformation and to maintain their capacity as activist hubs in other campaigns; (3) network organizations created to perform specific tasks that produce successor networks; and (4) organizations that adopt open communication networks and then become transformed by the information exchanges among their members.

Organizational transformation through network demands

Because easy internet linkages can open organizations to unpredictable traffic patterns, obscure nodes can become more central hubs in networks. As discussed above, the Netaction organization in the Microsoft campaign became such a rich archive of reports and research information about the corporation and the campaign that it became a central hub in the campaign network (as measured, among other things by overlapping board of directors members). The early mission and identity of the organization were synonymous with Microsoft, even though the mission statement promised engagement with a wide range of electronic policy issues. As noted in the next section, Netaction reclaimed its broader policy agenda only by breaking with the Microsoft campaign and 'moving on' to hub positions in other campaign networks.

Another interesting case is the vast network of Jubilee debt relief campaigns. If one follows the origins of these organizations back into the 1990s, they began largely as religious networks proclaiming debt relief a moral and religious issue. For example, one of the largest contingents at the Seattle WTO protests was churches operating under the Jubilee banner. This coalition led the first large march on the evening of 29 November 1999, drawing 10,000–15,000 activists, and setting the stage for the even larger labour-led actions the next day. Although Jubilee chapters with religious agendas continued to appear in demonstration organizing networks after Seattle, the organization has evolved into a confusing array of different organizations in different national contexts. To some extent, the entry of diverse players into the debt relief game (from rock stars such as Bono of U2, to nations themselves) put pressures on weak church networks to open their political and religious frames to larger networks of activists. One result is considerable instability in the Jubilee organizational system, with various name changes, new coalitions in different nations, and most recently, very different political frames in North America and Europe. For example, the United States coalition (www.jubileeusa.org) retains more of its original religious grassroots identity and network structure, while the United Kingdom hub (www.jubilee2000uk.org) has moved so far from its religious origins that they are barely evident in its far-flung international think-tank and policy NGO network. Even the name of the latest incarnation of the UK organization has changed to Jubilee Research, although the URL remains the same as in the last incarnation.

Moving on to other networks as a protective strategy

Because of the potential to become redefined by location in a communication network, many organizations that provide coordinating or information functions in campaign networks adopt a strategy of periodically 'moving on' to new networks. As noted above, Netaction (www.netaction.org) maintained its identity as a multi-issue organization in the digital communication policy arena by moving on to other campaigns in areas of digital communication regulation and consumer protection. A recent inspection of the website revealed activities in the areas of broadband regulation, electronic privacy, the future of an open internet, and others.

As indicated in earlier in references to the Nike and fair trade coffee campaigns, Global Exchange is another organization that has been careful to leave campaigns before becoming defined by them. During its time as the main hub in the Nike sweatshop campaign (1995–1998), Global Exchange used creative communication strategies that produced a deluge of negative press for Nike based largely on a worker's own account of conditions in Indonesian factories (Bullert 2000; Bennett 2003c). Global Exchange left the campaign when Nike CEO Phil Knight admitted that Nike had a labour problem and would do something about it.

Just as the 'move on' organization protects itself from transformation by network dynamics, it also tends to make few identity demands on other network organizations. Since Global Exchange, Netaction, and other 'move on' organizations know they will leave networks, they are unlikely to broker collective identity frames or induce other organizations to transform in ways typically associated with movements when they are viewed from more conventional organization-centred perspectives.

Specific task organizations that produce successor networks

Internet umbrella organizations created to organize issue campaigns and demonstrations often take distinctive network forms based on how they allow users to access and communicate through the site. Many of these organizing networks have survived beyond the action that drew them together because they generally offer networking services and calendars that became useful for future communication and planning. In some cases, these secondary planning features of internet-only mobilizing networks helped to create successor organizations to mobilize future events. For example, the A16-2000 umbrella organization that coordinated the demonstrations at the Washington, DC International Monetary Fund meeting in April 2000 opened its website to announce a constantly changing roster of participants. The site enabled newcomers to post their own rallying messages at the top of the site (http://www.infoshop.org/octo/alb_a.html). The user interface emphasized the political diversity of participating groups, along with an amazing number of different political reasons for opposing the IMF. The list of endorsing and participating groups (692 and still growing at the time I captured the site) was indexed by geographical location so that organizations in different locales could be viewed on the same page. Another page of the site revealed an equally diverse core group of demonstration sponsors: 50 Years is Enough, Alliance for Global Justice, Campaign for Labour Rights, Global Exchange, Mexico Solidarity Network, National Lawyers Guild, Nicaragua Network, and Witness for Peace, among others.

In contrast to the diversity of the A16 organization, the organizing site for the demonstration against the Free Trade Area of the Americas (FTAA) meeting in Montreal in April 2001 had a much more focused agenda aimed at mobilizing people in localities and training them in direct action and street theatre tactics before they arrived in Montreal (http://www.stopftaa.org/oldsite/organize). The site listed a different and much smaller set of lead organizations than those involved in the IMF protests above. The Ruckus Society featured prominently in the training and local mobilizing, and the Montreal Anti-Capitalist Convergence was identified as the lead organization at the protest site. A tighter focus on specific protest themes, training, and coordinated action was maintained through much more restricted user features and cross communication opportunities than offered by the A16 site.

Despite these differences in the communication interfaces created to organize the two demonstrations, both websites offered user features that kept them alive and networked with broader communities of activists beyond those attending the specific demonstrations. For example, the FTAA protest site referred to the A16 site (which was still running), and contained its own extensive calendar of past and future demonstrations. In addition, the Montreal organization prominently featured links on its front page to several current issue campaigns against corporations (e.g. Nike and Monsanto) that needed support. Also posted were news reports from activists who had attended the recently concluded first World Social Forum (WSF) in Porto Alegre, Brazil. These user interfaces extend particular protest events forward in time, and give them broad connection to diverse protest communities in cyberspace. Embedding otherwise dated organization sites in these broader structures of time and space helps their successor organizations form with new networking patterns of their own.

Organizations transformed by their internal communication networks

Applications of the internet and other digital media may also affect the internal development of organizations themselves. As noted in the previous section, le Grignou and Patou's study of ATTAC in France (Chapter 8) found that communication practices affected the political identity of the organization. They also found that the structure of the organization is affected by those communication practices:

> Till January 2001, no one represented local groups at the administrative council . . . The structure of the association gives them a total autonomy, which sometimes verges on isolation. Local leaders happen to be in touch with National ATTAC only through the internet, while others hardly ever receive news from Paris. The electronic offer is sometimes the only link between local groups and other branches of the association, be it through discussion lists (ATTAC talk), work lists (ATTAC local), mailing lists (Grain de Sable or Lignes d'ATTAC), or electronic secretaries (site on the WTO or current campaigns). Internet is so seminal to the association life that Local Electronic Correspondents (CEL) have been created, as connected members would 'chaperone' non-connected members.

Thinking about how digital networks can transform the political capacities of both nodes and collectivities raises some interesting questions about measurement. Some combination of ethnographic observation, member narratives of organizational roles, and network link mapping seems appropriate. It is clear, for example, that link maps alone are often difficult to interpret. A study of websites linked to by other organization sites at the time of the Seattle protests showed that the official WTO site was the link leader (2129 links), followed by several protest hubs with impressive links: One World (348); Institute for Global Communications (111); Seattlewto.org, the sponsored site of the NGO coalition (92); and Corporate Watch (74), among others (Smith and Smythe 2000). Various accounts of the Seattle protests (www.wtohistory.org, Levi and Olson 2000) suggest that one could not easily derive the key mobilizing coalition players from these link patterns.

A promising approach is Van Aelst and Walgrave's (Chapter 5, this volume) analysis of organizations that received news coverage surrounding the 2001 protests against the Free Trade Area of the Americas in Montreal. They found that the top 17 organizations mentioned in the news also maintained substantial cross-communication channels on the internet, and that most of them maintained online calendars for the FTAA and other protest activities. By these measures, there was a mutually engaged political action network that operated with a high degree of coordination through digital channels. What is interesting is that the underlying coherence in the digital channels linking these organizations was also reflected in mass media attention to the individual members of the networks. This suggests that digital networks have found paths to jump their communication from relatively personalized digital channels to the mass media. It is important to begin understanding these crossover communication effects of digital networks as well.

New media can alter information flows through mass media

The public spheres created by the internet and the web are more than just parallel information universes that exist independently of the traditional mass media. A growing conventional wisdom among communication scholars is that the internet is changing the way in which news is made. New media provide alternative communication spaces in which information can develop and circulate widely with fewer conventions or editorial filters than in the mainstream media. The gate-keeping capacity of the traditional press is weakened when information appears on the internet, presenting new material that may prove irresistible to competitors in the world of 24/7 cable news channels that now occupy important niches in the press 'food chain'. Moreover, journalists may actively seek story ideas and information from web sources, thus creating many pathways for information to flow from micro to mass media.

An interesting example of micro-to-mass media crossover in global activism began with an email exchange between a culture jammer named Jonah Peretti and Nike (Peretti 2003). Peretti visited a Nike website that promised greater consumer freedom by inviting customers to order shoes with a name or slogan of their choice on them. He submitted an order to inscribe the term 'sweatshop' on his custom Nikes. Several rounds of amusing exchanges ensued in which Peretti chided the company for breaking its promise of consumer freedom. Successive rounds ended with Nike's awkward and less automated refusals to put any of Peretti's requests for political labels on its shoes. Peretti sent the exchange to a dozen friends, who forwarded it to their friends, and, so, the Nike-Sweatshop story spread in viral fashion, reaching an audience estimated from several hundred thousand to several million (Peretti 2003).

Based on the flood of responses he received, Peretti tracked the message as it first circulated through the culture jamming community, then the labour activist community, and then 'something interesting happened. The micromedia message worked its way into the mass media' (Peretti 2003). First it reached middle media sites such as weblogs (Slashdot, Plastic and others) where it began to resemble news. From there, it was picked up by more conventional middle media sites such as Salon, which are read by journalists. At that point, it was a short journalistic step to *USA Today*, *The Wall Street Journal*, NBC's *Today Show*, and dozens of prominent North American and European news outlets. Whenever Peretti was interviewed about his media adventure, the connection between Nike and sweatshop was communicated again.

Another flow from micro to mass media has occurred in the vast global network of anti-Microsoft protest (Bennett 2003c; Manheim 2001). Numerous derogatory images have travelled through internet chats, networked campaign sites, and webzines, and surfaced in mainstream news accounts indicating that the company was trying to 'crush competition', that it was known by opponents as 'the Seattle Slasher', or that Bill Gates was the latter day incarnation of Robber Baron icon, John D. Rockefeller. The difficulty of anticipating the rise of such images – and of using standard public relations techniques to combat them – has given activists new levers of media power in global subpolitics. This media activism has forced many companies to weigh the advantages of highly profitable business models against the damage inflicted on precious brand images. Canadian media consultant Doug Miller was quoted in *The Financial Times* as saying 'I visit seventy five boardrooms a year and I can tell you the members of the boards are living in fear of getting their corporate reputations blown away in two months on the Internet' (Macken 2001).

While many activist issue campaigns have secured remarkably favourable media coverage, disruptive public demonstrations – the other major power lever of protest politics – have generally received fairly negative coverage. The interesting exception is the Battle in Seattle, which produced fairly extensive coverage of activist messages about globalization (Rojecki 2002). The more favourable coverage of Seattle was due, in my estimation, to a combination of factors: its size and consequence took journalists by surprise, President Clinton made a public statement admitting the protesters had some valid concerns, and there was a strong presence of labour and church organizations which provided credible media sources. Since Seattle, it seems that a more familiar press pattern has emerged in both US and European media coverage of demonstrations: protesters have generally been cast as violent and anarchistic, and even equated with soccer hooligans in some European accounts. (My preliminary impressions will surely be tested and refined by the great volume of research in progress by scholars around the world.)

Beyond the characterizations of the activists, the predominant news framing of the overall protest movement is also negative, as in 'anti-globalization'. This is clearly a news construction that is at odds with how many of the activists think of their common cause. If movement media framing could be put to a vote among activists, I suspect that 'democratic globalization' would win over 'anti-globalization' by a wide margin. For example, here is how American labour leader John Sweeney put it: 'It's clear that globalization is here to stay. We have to accept that and work on having a seat at the table when the rules are written about how globalization works' (Greenhouse 2002). In another account, Susan George (one of the founding members of the French global social justice organization ATTAC) rejects the 'anti-globalization' framing as an insultingly poor account of global activism. In explaining the inadequacies of the 'anti-globalization' frame, she also reveals why better accounts are unlikely to be written by news organizations bent on producing simple narratives:

> The movement itself is, however, multi-focus and inclusive. It is concerned with the world: omnipresence of corporate rule, the rampages of financial markets, ecological destruction, maldistribution of wealth and power, international institutions constantly overstepping their mandates and lack of international democracy.
> (George 2001)

Mass media framing of movements clearly varies from case to case, depending on how activist communication strategies interact with media gate-keeping (Gamson 2001). Gitlin (1980) identified the demand of news organizations for movements to produce leaders and simple messages as part of the explanation why the American new left of the 1960s received considerable media attention, and also fragmented into disunity and internal conflict. A global activist movement that is committed to inclusiveness and diversity over central leadership and issue simplicity should have low expectations of news coverage of demonstrations that display the movement's leaderless diversity in chaotic settings.

Why has a movement that has learned to secure good publicity for particular issue campaigns and organizations not developed more effective media communication strategies for mass demonstrations? I think that the answer here returns us to the opening discussion of the social and personal context in which this activism takes place. Not only are many activists in these broadly distributed protest networks opposed to central leadership and simple collective identity frames, but they may accurately perceive that the interdependence of global politics defies the degree of simplification demanded by most mass media discourse. While issue campaign networks tend to focus on dramatic charges against familiar targets, most of the demonstration organizing networks celebrate the diversity of the movement and resist strategic communication based on core issues or identity frames. For example, Van Aelst and Walgrave (Chapter 5) found at least 11 political themes that were shared by substantial portions of the network involved in the FTAA demonstrations in 2001. Thus, demonstrations may be staged mainly as reminders of the human scale, seriousness, and disruptive capacity of this movement, while issue campaigns remain the stealth factor carrying radical messages through the gates of the mass media.

Conclusion

The internet is implicated in the new global activism far beyond reducing the costs of communication, or transcending the geographical and temporal barriers found in other communication media. Various uses of the internet and other digital media facilitate the loosely structured networks, the weak identity ties, and the issue and demonstration campaign organizing that define a new global politics. In particular, we have seen how particular configurations of digital networks facilitate: permanent campaigns, the growth of broad networks despite (or because of) relatively weak social identity and ideology ties, the transformation of both individual member organizations and the growth patterns of whole networks, and the capacity to communicate messages from desktops to television screens. The same qualities that make these communication-based politics durable also make them vulnerable to problems of control, decision-making and collective identity.

It is clear that personal relations remain important in the glue of this movement, giving particular meaning to the now trite slogan that the global is local. Interviews with Seattle WTO protesters make clear that personal contacts were essential to organizing such an effective large-scale demonstration (see online interview transcriptions at www.wtohistory.org). At the same time, the creation of digital information and planning networks eased personal frictions and strengthened fragile relations. More generally, the growing technical capacity of activists to report on their own actions has created unprecedented parallel public records of events, while permitting unusual degrees of organization within chaotic real-time situations (Rheingold 2002).

What can we conclude from weighing these strengths and vulnerabilities, and from the balance between the virtual and the material in these networks? Perhaps most importantly, it seems that the ease of creating vast webs of politics enables global activist networks to finesse difficult problems of collective identity that often impede the growth of movements. To a remarkable degree, these networks appear to have undergone scale shifts while continuing to accommodate considerable diversity in individual-level political identity. Moreover, the success of networked communication strategies in many issue and demonstration campaigns seems to have produced enough innovation and learning that keep new organizations emerging despite (and because of) the chaos and dynamic change in those organizations. In order to grasp these properties of communication-based politics, it is important to resist the temptation to view this scene from the perspective of particular organizations or issues. Instead, the dynamic network becomes the unit of analysis in which all other levels (organizational, individual, political) can be analysed most coherently.

The rise of distributed electronic public spheres may ultimately become the model for public information in many areas of politics, whether establishment or oppositional. It is clear that conventional news is withering from the erosion of audiences (more in commercial than in public service systems), and from the fragmentation of remaining audiences as channels multiply (Bennett 2003b). Perhaps the next step is a thoroughly personalized information system in which the boundaries of different issues and different political approaches become more permeable, enabling ordinary citizens to join campaigns, protests, and virtual communities with few ideological or partisan divisions. In this vision, the current organizational weaknesses of internet mobilization may become a core resource for the growth of new global publics.

7 Mass media driven mobilization and online protest
ICTs and the pro-East Timor movement in Portugal

Gustavo Cardoso and Pedro Pereira Neto

This chapter addresses the pro-East Timor movement in Portugal in 1999 and the role that ICTs and the traditional mass media played in its emergence and orientation. It aims to identify the pattern of use of these media by the agents directly implicated and, on the other hand, to ascertain changes prompted by such usage on the underlying organizational structure and communication fluxes. We do this through the intertwining of the constructive insights of different analytical approaches in the social movements field, thus shedding light not only on the societal context in which the protest evolved and the resources it mobilized but also on the cultural identity framing it promoted. We highlight the following aspects, all of which are staple features of our analytical objective: (a) that this movement qualifies as a networked social movement, i.e. a movement focused on cultural values, acting from the local in an attempt to influence the global, using ICTs as a fundamental tool (Castells 2001: 138); (b) that it illustrates an ability to integrate fruitfully different media, with a central axis on the internet; (c) that media agents themselves may be assuming a key role in the very orientation of some protests. Accordingly, the following hypotheses will be tested: on one hand, that ICTs facilitate traditional forms of protest; on the other hand, that ICTs are simultaneously a tool used by protesters and sometimes a target of their actions.

East Timor: think local and act global

Following its 1974 democratic revolution, Portugal initiated a process meant to give up its authority over several colonies, one of these being the territory of East Timor – north of Australia, bordered by land by the Republic of Indonesia – a territory Indonesia would later invade in September 1975. During the following 24 years of occupation a war was fought against the native Maubere people and the leader of the FALINTIL (Timorese Liberation Army), Xanana Gusmão.[1]

In August 1999 a United Nations-sponsored referendum was held in East Timor. Of over 400,000 voters, a massive 78.5 per cent rejected an administrative autonomy proposed by Indonesia, thus stating a preference for independence. But soon after the results became common knowledge a widespread wave of violence erupted, leading to the evacuation of all UN personnel and to the killing of several thousand people in East Timor.

At the same time, in order to act in support of the Maubere people, an unparalleled social participation movement developed in Portugal, comparable only to that which occurred following the Portuguese 1974–1975 revolution. There were 17 days, from 4 to 20 September, of intense diplomatic action by the government officials; more importantly, these were days of nationwide civic participation, solidarity and action towards the defence of human rights in East Timor. Anyone visiting Portugal at the time would have witnessed creative forms of protest: from painted murals and daily demonstrations at the UN and Security Council countries' embassies in Lisbon, to people wearing white clothing, to cars holding white flags and written messages of support. The country stopped for three minutes and flowers were thrown into rivers.

Traditional mass media – radio, television and newspapers – gave plenty of visibility to the protests, contributing directly to the achievement of the movement's goals. New media also became a protest ground: international fax lines were jammed by calls to the government representatives of the five permanent members of the UN Security Council; more than 100,000 personal emails were sent to the UN proclaiming a fierce opposition to the Indonesian actions; and dozens of websites were created to provide a public forum.

Why study the pro-East Timor movement and the use of ICTs in it?

Social movements, one of society's most common phenomena (Neveu 1996: 110), have increased in recent decades not only in terms of figures but also in terms of diversity (Rocher 1977–1979: 119; Crook *et al.* 1992: 140). However, if the forms assumed by collective action are this diverse, so are its possible approaches, from the ones inscribed in macro-historical trends to the so-called mid-range theories. In spite of such diversity it seems analytically useful to take into account the strengths of each of these approaches, much as Garner suggested (Garner 1996: 5).

In order to understand the pro-East Timor movement we need to understand the social structure that informs its action at both national and international levels and frame the protest in a socio-historical context, in terms of ongoing changes in the economic, social and cultural fields (Crook *et al.* 1992: 141–142). If social structures and cultural frames are, as Calhoun states, inseparable (Neveu 1996: 74), it seems all the more important to support an analytical crossover underscoring the relations between structure and agency.

Portugal, a relative newcomer to the world of democratic nations and a member of the EU since 1986, has made a hard transition from the mainly agricultural society of the 1970s (Viegas and Costa 1998: 17–43) to the Informational Economy (Cardoso 1999) of the late 1990s. Only recently has Portugal been able to draw closer to the European Union average standards of living. Following Veene and Inglehart's (Crook *et al.* 1992: 145–148) line of thought, some of the aims already present in other late modernity societies' collective action might be surfacing only now in Portugal. Until the events of September 1999 Portugal and its civil society political participation, in the shape of social movements, had been mainly concerned with national and local agendas, with the media, especially television and newspapers, feebly incorporated by movements such as trades unions and ecological groups. As far as the use of the internet is concerned, its involvement in the context of social protests before the events of September 1999 had also been somewhat low, with the exception of the Accessibility Campaign (Cheta 2002). Until 1998 the internet had essentially been used by students through a government-funded network, which serves schools from first grade to the university, and by a small number of households and companies. Political parties had started to incorporate the role of the information society in their discourse from 1996 onwards, and the first websites in political elections were conceived in the same year (Cardoso 1999).

In this context, the pro-East Timor protests may just have represented a turning point in civic participation in Portugal for several reasons: they introduced a new set of issues, namely the open defence of human rights; they developed around the need for a global reach, promoting the aim of collective action from the national to the global level; new social actors took political stands, from individual citizens to national companies; the ICTs – traditional mass media (McQuail 1998: 12–20) and new media (Silverstone 1999) – assumed a central role in the protests; and journalists participated actively in the mobilization of citizens and the coordination of the movement.

All things considered, we argue the pro-East Timor movement is not only of interest to the study of social movements in Portugal but also an interesting illustration of the evolution of such movements in what Giddens (1998) identified as late modernity.

The pro-East Timor movement: a social movement?

In his proposal of readdressing Alain Touraine's classic categorization of social movements, Manuel Castells (1997: 71) states two key ideas. First, that social movements must be understood in their own terms: namely they are what they say they are. Their practices (primarily their discursive practices) are their self-definition (1997: 69–70). Second, that the definition of a social movement stands on three principles: the movement's identity, the movement's adversary, and the movement's vision or social model, which Castells calls its societal goal.

The pro-East Timor movement identified an adversary, i.e. all those acting against the Maubere people – both those directly involved in the violence and those states which, by omission, were not helping to stop it – and had as a goal the request to stop the violence and achieve the presence of a multinational intervention force in the territory. Regarding its identity, the movement – the result of an informal coalition of Portuguese citizens, Maubere associations and refugees, NGOs, civic associations, private companies and members of the state apparatus – spoke on behalf of the Maubere people, which could not make itself heard outside East Timor.

Although assuming many different shapes, the pro-East Timor movement had a common objective: 'to end the suffering of the Maubere people', that is, to stop such abuses as the killing and wounding of people, the lack of freedom of expression and the sexual abuse of women. We should then consider it, from an analytical perspective, a social movement geared towards the defence of human rights (Garner 1996: 149) – even though, according to Cohen and Rai, the human rights movements have been poorly integrated into the social movements analysis, particularly the new social movements literature (Cohen and Rai 2000: 10). But this is a challenge rather than an obstacle: not only is the very development of human rights simply inconceivable outside the dynamic of new social movements (Baxi 2000: 36), but the socialization of 'grievances' into causes of social praxis should be a staple theme of the social movements theory (Baxi 2000: 37).

The role of traditional and new media in the pro-East Timor movement

Most of the events in our lives take place within contexts decisively influenced by information (Melucci 1995b: 434). The role of ICTs is then of particular interest for the understanding of the particularities of the pro-East Timor movement: they were a precious organizational resource, both in their traditional mass media and new media dimensions, in the emergence, organization and development of this movement. Not only did they become the organizational tools that made actions at the national and international levels easier, but it was through the traditional mass media that the cultural and political context of opportunity for the emergence of the East Timor protest was laid.

The role played by the traditional mass media and journalists

As Eder states, when approaching collective action we should take into consideration that it is inevitably mediated by culture (Pakulski 1995: 67; Gibbins and Reimer 1999: 96–97; Tarrow 1998: 106). Both as a precondition for and as a result of social movements, action frames – conceived as carriers of meaning – are created, translating strains, conflicts and grievances into social action patterns (Maheu 1995: 11) by resonating them with a population's cultural predispositions (Tarrow 1998: 110). However, although consensus formation can emerge concerning a given subject, only consensus mobilization will orient individuals to action (Tarrow 1998: 113), not only by summoning the 'right' individual identity but also by prompting it to become connected to practices as well as ideas (Garner 1996: 374).

It was thanks to the work of two freelance journalists (ETAN 2002) that the Portuguese population became truly aware of the drama of the Maubere people. On 12 November 1992 the massacre in Santa Cruz cemetery, Dili, was videotaped and smuggled outside the territory, allowing it to be broadcasted worldwide. If it had a significant impact outside Portugal, it had a tremendous effect within its borders, because during the shootings one could hear and see people praying in Portuguese. These images did to the collective identity what the political parties and NGOs hadn't been able to achieve since the invasion of East Timor in 1975: the establishment of a cultural link between the suffering of the Maubere people and the Portuguese people. It should be noted, then, that unlike the White March event in Belgium (Walgrave and Manssens 2000), the pro-East Timor activism in Portugal largely preceded the media leverage of the social movement we have portrayed. There existed, for instance, the CDPM, an NGO created in 1981 to ensure constant small, volunteer-based protests, and which was at the genesis of some of the demonstrations that took place following the Santa Cruz cemetery massacre; also several organizations of Catholic inspiration had acted in support of Maubere refugees living in Portugal since the mid-1970s. University students constituted another example of civic involvement in the East Timorese cause: from informal groups acting at the student union levels they evolved to a formal group, MEUDH (University Students for Human Rights), that promoted several demonstrations in Portugal and raised funds nationally to install a giant TV screen displaying the Santa Cruz massacre during the EU Treaty signing in Maastricht.

Credit should, then, be due to the catalytic power of images: just as in the case of the cultural link established in the Los Angeles riots, prompted by the broadcasting of video footage showing the beating of Rodney King, again the ICTs seem to make one activist as important and effective as a large group of activists; since camcorders are everywhere, suddenly everybody is a potential reporter.

Traditional mass media are nonetheless the means through which the majority of citizens establish contact with the political sphere (Gibbins and Reimer 1999: 106). Not only are social problems often the result of media assimilation and interpretation of specific situations (Neveu 1996: 97–98), but the media give visibility to certain facts, including them in the political agenda, thus creating new modes of political discourse (Crook *et al.* 1992: 148) and changing the political field itself (Gibbins and Reimer 1999: 106).

Although media became a tool that movements cannot easily replace in reaching out to their potential supporters, such usage poses specific problems. First of all, it sets media world-related boundaries for the framing of movement discourse if movements are to get adequate coverage (Garner 1996: 31). Secondly, because of the specific list of media issues – where competition for visibility is fierce, making such usage limited (Tarrow 1998: 116) – movement actions often have to turn into more emotional 'performances' (Neveu 1996: 93; Tarrow 1998: 107; Touraine 1981a: 137). Social movements have to manage information strategies in order to capture the attention of the media and use the acquired broadcasting time, or articles in a newspaper, in order to mobilize support and interact with the powers on the public arena. Those information strategies try to gain the attention of the media through emotional performances: such was the case of the pro-East Timor protest. However, in this case those strategies were initiated and promoted by the media system itself, namely by journalists, in a way that should not be underestimated.

To understand the real importance of the Portuguese media in this process we must return to the analysis of the structural constraints and cultural–political opportunity context under which the movement grew. Portugal, although a member of the EU, is a country with medium to low diplomatic influence in the international scene, and could not immediately deploy any military forces to East Timor due to a set of institutional limitations. Those constraints were known to the public, because the media had for a long time dealt with the question of the human rights abuses towards the Maubere people. So the question people wanted answered was: 'if the politicians can't solve the problem, what can we do to help?' The media gave the answer by establishing an agenda destined to amplify the protest movement up to the point where it could reach international decision-makers. In an analysis of the role of the radio in the pro-East Timor movement, Proença argues that the TSF radio station, during non-stop broadcasting – the first 100 hours without any commercial jingles, from 7 p.m. on 5 September to 11 p.m. on 9 September – acted not only as a news radio station but as a grassroots radio station (Proença 2000). Further,

> if the news director wanted to generate 'street effects' capable of capturing the attention of the international news media in order to be able to reach worldwide audiences and influence the political decision centres, particularly the countries with veto in the security council of the UN, that could only be achieved by promoting initiatives of highly emotional nature, that is, aimed at television broadcast.
>
> (Proença 2000)

Among the initiatives promoted by TSF, and later embraced by the national television broadcasters and newspapers, we can identify the following as being more effective in the mobilization of individuals and enhancing the human rights movement: 'A day dressed in white!' 'Throw a flower into the river!' and 'Stop the country for three minutes!' Proença, in his analysis of the role of TSF as a grassroots radio station, describes how the choice of those initiatives was tied to the symbolic meaning and degree of media attention they could promote (Proença 2000).

In the 'A day dressed in white!' initiative, the objective was to promote a common element to the different protests that were emerging: the colour white. White was chosen because it could be understood by different cultures, allowing for its message to be internationally amplified – white standing for purity in western cultures, for joy and happiness for Asians, and a symbol of respect for Muslims. White was adopted as the colour of protest, and from TV anchors presenting news dressed in white to people with flags on their windows and cars, a unified element was incorporated by the protesters.

The second initiative was put forward by the need to mourn all those being killed in East Timor. In the absence of bodies to mourn in traditional senses, people were invited to throw flowers into rivers so that they could symbolically unite the two countries in their suffering. In order for the action to become more media-oriented, people were also invited to gather in front of the US Embassy in Lisbon.

The last event, again coordinated with other media and this time joined by unions, was to 'Stop the country for three minutes!'. This last event was widely publicized in the international media, since people stopped their cars on the streets, stopped walking, left their jobs to come out into the streets. The idea was simple: not to get just a moment's silence but to achieve a total stoppage to all activities in Portugal.

These forms of protest had two objectives: first, to give a unified structure to the protest movement and secondly, while doing so, to build the necessary synergies to make the abuses occurring in East Timor known to international public opinion. The radio news directors and radio journalists played an important organizational role in the mobilization process around East Timor and, more importantly, they gave people the resources to express their solidarity through participation in the actions promoted by the media. That role was amplified from the moment newspapers and television joined the mobilization process.

In September 1999, the two leading daily national newspapers, *O Público* and *Diário de Notícias*, published, respectively, 399 and 350 articles about East Timor. The weekly newspaper *Expresso* gave Timor 176 articles in four weekends. The national news agency Lusa transmitted, on average, 100 reports per day on the Timorese issue. To the agenda-setting promoted by the newspapers we must add the publicizing of daily lists of hundreds of small-scale initiatives promoted by individual citizens, identifying companies selling goods imported from Indonesia, or the bank account numbers for donations for humanitarian aid.

From the analysis of the empirical data available about the production of news in the month of September 1999, we can say that journalists chose to break away from the traditional impartiality of their editorial lines, which tended to promote political parties' and interest groups' agendas (Gibbins and Reimer 1999: 114), and gave priority to the defence of cultural values, namely human rights. This decision was of essential importance because their knowledge of how the media system works gave the civil society the means to express their feelings into a collective action of high media visibility; this know-how became a fundamental organizational asset.

Having chosen to follow this path, journalists through the media took the role of catalysts for a feeling already shared by the Portuguese population: being pro-East Timorese. As Carlos Andrade (1999), the news director of the TSF (the leading Portuguese 24-hour commercial news radio station), stated in a interview, 'regarding the relationship between Portugal and East Timor and in order to understand the protests, there are three paths worth paying attention to: the politicians, who lived the situation without many hopes for its resolution; the press, which sooner than everyone else understood the true issue; and the people, who kept Timor close to their hearts'.

Many of the actions promoted by journalists and the editorial stances of the Portuguese press during that period seem to qualify as what Shah designates as development journalism: a kind of journalism that is concerned with social, cultural and political aspects of development, in addition to economic aspects; a kind of journalism that is democratic and emphasizes communication from the 'bottom up'; that is pragmatic and unconventional in its approach to reporting and that can encourage action, can help create, maintain and strengthen a mobilization space with news (Shah 1999: 176–178).

Shah, therefore, envisions journalists as possible substitutes for the intellectuals' role in social movements: to provide energy for collective action by helping create a space for awareness and action (Shah 1999: 176–178). Their identities, as the identity of the social movement they gave impulse to, were interactively created (Shah 1999: 176–178). We should, therefore, consider that journalists, during the East Timor protests, played the leverage role of the latent social movement.

The role played by new media

We have so far acknowledged that communication and traditional mass media, as in other social movements (Downing 2000: 26), have played a fundamental role in the pro-East Timor movement trajectories. However, social movements often seem to be striving for the establishment of new platforms of communication (Garner 1996: 375). Manuel Castells states that the most influential social movements need the legitimacy and support provided by local groups, but must at the same time think local and act global, because the networks of power act simultaneously at different levels (Castells 2001: 142–143).

The internet played an important role during the years of Indonesian occupation of East Timor. From 1997 an internet domain for Timor (.tp), managed by Connect-Ireland, was available online, hosting entities and organizations that supported the Timorese cause. Another example of the use of the internet during the Indonesian occupation is the information services destined to create awareness about East Timor. Examples of such networks can be found on the Portuguese TimorNet (http://www.uc.pt/Timor), the American ETAN (http://www.etan.org), Mojo Wire (http://motherjones.com/east_timor/), the Australian news service Timor Today (http://www.easttimor.com) or the Indonesian Solidamor (http://www.solidamor.org). Hacking, or more accurately cracking, became another use of the internet in order to protest against Indonesia. Between October 1997 and 2000, a group called 'Portuguese Hackers Against Indonesia' launched inter-mittent attacks against Indonesian networks (McKay 1999). Their most successful hit was achieved in April 1997 when a group called 'toxyn' capped a two-month protest over the Indonesian government's treatment of East Timor by breaking into the Indonesian Military Net-work Homepage and altering the page. In February 1997, the group had started the protest by altering the homepage of the Department of Foreign Affairs, Republic of Indonesia. This altered homepage was online for three hours. Among other things, there was the title 'Welcome to the Foreign Affairs Ministry of the Fascist Republic of Indonesia'. After this first attack, Indonesian hackers countered by breaking into the East Timor site, hosted at Connect-Ireland, and re-registered East Timor top-level domain names.

In the East Timor protests, many of the potential constituencies of the movement were geographically too distant from one another for face-to-face interaction to take place (Smelser 1988, 1989: 722). The actions promoted by the East Timor protest had to act simultaneously in four continents: Asia (East Timor and Indonesia), Oceania (where the closest intervention forces were placed and where the ASEAN meeting was being held), North America (where the USA was the traditional political ally of Indonesia, and the country where the Secur-ity Council of the UN is located), and finally Europe (home of the EU and the place (primarily, but not exclusively, Portugal) where people were promoting a social movement in defence of the human rights of the Timorese). From the moment the main objective of the protesters became the deployment, in the shortest time possible, of a UN peace-keeping force in East Timor, the use of the internet as a resource was widely encouraged and, interestingly, promoted either by the traditional mass media, private telecommunication companies or individuals on the web.

The website 'Guia do Activismo Online' (Silva 2000), a web directory of social protests through the web, displayed in February 2000 a total of 60 actions of protest dedicated to East Timor. Although many didn't display an online counter, it was known that more than 190,000 people used those websites to send emails to, among other decision-makers, Bill Clinton (at the time President of the USA), J.B. Habibie (former President of Indonesia) and the UN Secretary General, Kofi Annan.

Other imaginative uses of the internet during September 1999 included a human chain that intended to multiply the references to East Timor available on the world wide web, the distribution of banners about the lack of freedom of expression in Timor by the Portuguese Journalists Union, or the campaign Free East Timor managed by the Portuguese ISP Netc, which gave one cent for the reconstruction of the territory for each visit to its homepage.

The first actions using the internet through emails and faxes started on 5 September. A web programmer offered help to the TSF radio station and got the fax numbers and email addresses, via the internet, of the political decision-makers at the UN, USA and Indonesia.

Soon after TSF, other media and commercial websites started their protest actions, and so the numbers and email addresses started to circulate in an informal, viral, way through the internet so that soon many other websites were displaying similar texts to be sent to the UN and to the White House. In this process the ISP portals and telecom companies played a fundamental role. More than half of the emails sent were gathered through SAPO – the portal of the leading Portuguese ISP – and Portugal Telecom created a fax gateway and free fax numbers through which people could send faxes (Portugal Telecom 1999) to the White House and Security Council.

This participation of commercial companies (whose main objective is profit) in the protest campaign is one of its most interesting components. One can argue that under a situation of generalized popular discontentment with Indonesia and support of the Maubere people, this kind of action can be looked at as a public relations investment, or that for particular events national identity might still be a decisive element for the decision of private companies. The explanation might also, however, reside in the internet's very own culture (Castells 2001: 61). The companies that supported the protest, both technologically and financially, were new economy companies (Castells

2001: 65), where the internet culture is more widely present, and where the technocratic belief in the progress of humans through technology is more commonly accepted. Those companies being the holders of the technology – the portals or the internet fax-gateways – necessary for the success of the movement's societal goals, it is possible to argue that in the Information Age social movements might include in their ranks not only citizens and NGOs but also some of the new economy companies.

Another example of internet protest actions was the online polls being conducted in their interactive services by global media broadcasters such as CNN and the BBC, as shown in Table 7.1.

The online polls promoted by the BBC constitute one of the most interesting empirical examples gathered in this analysis, because only half of the messages and responses came from Portugal, which gives us an idea of how the movement was evolving from the national to the global level. At the BBC website, one could find messages from British and North American citizens stating their support and underlining the parallels between East Timor and Kosovo and the need for the international community to have a common standard for human rights violations (Viegas and Gomes 1999).

Another example of how a national protest became one of global reach is the analysis of the web pages still available today about East Timor and the number of different languages they are expressed in, as shown by Table 7.2. The origin and number of posts in newsgroups during the month of September 1999 can be analysed similarly (Table 7.2).

Dutton reminds us that the focus of the Information Age should not be 'information' but 'access'. Technology has not made information a new resource, for it has always been a critical resource; instead, it has changed the way we gain access to information, and while doing so the ICTs have also redefined the ways in which we can access other people, services, and technologies themselves (Dutton 2000: 172). The ability to use technologies to access and process information more rapidly and to interconnect people around the world in real-time frames enabled the movement to reach its objectives. During the month of September the East Timor protest slowly faded as events started to move towards the devised movement's societal goals. Interestingly, the enrolment of the international media became generalized only after the first set of images from the protests in the streets of Lisbon arrived at the international news agencies and emails appealing for support started to circulate widely on the internet. The online polls were the confirmation that the problem was finally getting the atten-

Table 7.1 Online polls on the East Timor question

Online polls	Situation	Support	Duration
Send Portuguese soldiers to East Timor? (Virtual Azores)	Finished	84% Yes	12–15/09/99
Send US Troops to East Timor? (MOJO Wire)	Finished	64% Yes	10–15/09/99
Send UN Troops to East Timor? (*Time*)	Finished	65% Yes	8–14/09/99
International forces in East Timor? (*Jakarta Post*)	Finished	94% Yes	9–10/09/99
Naciones Unidas en Timor? (*El Mundo*)	Finished	98% Yes	9–14/09/99
UN peacekeepers to East Timor? (CNN)	Finished	95% Yes	7–10/09/99
Militares Portugueses para Timor? (ID Digital)	Finished	94% Yes	8–15/09/99
Imposto excepcional por Timor? (*Público*)	Ongoing	54% No	Since 08/09/99
East Timor: Time to intervene? (BBC)	Finished	96% Yes	7–09/09/99
Indonesia and East Timor (CNN)	Finished	52% Yes	07/09/99

Situation as of 3 February 2000; (http://members.tripod.com/~Protesto_MC/timor.html)

tion of international public opinion. The battle for media coverage fought by the pro-East Timor movement reached its objectives when the images of the siege on the UN compound in Dili were broadcast worldwide; this showed that the information blackout promoted by Indonesia could only confirm what the people were saying all over the internet: that a violation of human rights was being perpetrated in East Timor.

The outcome

Although the exact number of emails and faxes sent between 5 and 15 September is not known, what we do know about the effect of the protest actions is that they led to the disconnection of several phone lines at the UN building in New York and at the White House. The Indonesian presidential web server was disconnected due to an overload of messages, and the UN and White House servers from 7 September onwards would not accept emails sent from the .pt domain (Viegas 1999).

Table 7.2 Web search for 'Timor', February 2002, and messages exchanged including the word 'Timor'

Language of web pages	Number of web pages	Language of newsgroups	Messages posted
English	600,000	English	27,400
Portuguese	38,800	Portuguese	3,390
Spanish	35,900	Indonesia	982
French	24,900	Italian	786
German	20,000	Dutch	784
Indonesian	19,300	French	534
Italian	18,200	Spanish	429
Dutch	7,410	German	208
Total web pages	1,140,000	Total messages posted	190,000

Sources: (for web pages) Google, (for newsgroups) Dejanews, 1–30 September 1999.

On the other hand, we can also relate these actions to the timing of the shift in the international community's approach to the situation in East Timor. Both Kofi Annan and Bill Clinton recognized publicly the role played by the worldwide awareness campaign in the final outcome of the East Timor people's struggle (Bebiano 1999). On 9 September 1999, the very same day on which the internet online polls of the BBC and CNN showed the widest support for a multi-national force in East Timor, the British Prime Minister Tony Blair and the President of the USA, Bill Clinton, made public their agreement on the need for a multinational force under the mandate of the UN to be dispatched. On 12 September Indonesia formally requested from the Secretary General of the UN the presence of a multinational force in East Timor, and on 16 September the Security Council approved Resolution 1264 mandating the Secretary General to implement the sending of troops and the interim administration of the territory. The Australian-led multinational force arrived in Dili, East Timor, on 20 September 1999. We can argue that it took the pro-East Timor movement 11 days of network actions combined with an integrated management of ICTs and the diplomatic action of the Portuguese state to put pressure on the Security Council in order to achieve a resolution.

The pro-East Timor protest as a networked social movement: bridging across and combining traditional and new media

For many scholars, ICTs are potentially the first true public sphere, not only because they allow for massive and potentially uncensored knowledge to be shared (Ford and Gil 2000: 202–203) but also because they compensate the near monopoly of radio and television given to the older groups such as parties and interest groups (Gibbins and Reimer 1999: 114). Contemporary social movements tend to have in common the assimilation of ICTs as instruments of action and organization. But, although the internet is becoming the central axis of action allowing social movements to act globally, we should question whether ICTs play a purely instrumental role in developing citizenship and political expression or whether, on the other hand, by taking part in the political system, they can go as far as changing its rules (Castells 2001: 137). On the other hand, we should not overlook the integration of traditional mass media by social movements, and the role played by journalists and other social actors – for instance, the new economy companies – in the process.

The movement here depicted developed under the characteristics of the social movements of the Information Age (Castells 2001: 140). Like the December 1999 protests against the WTO (Castells 2001: 141), the East Timor movement was a specific coalition for specific goals, focusing on cultural values (the defence of human rights), acting from the local in an attempt to influence the global (the political decision process at the UN), and using ICTs as a fundamental tool for the success of its actions. The displayed visual symbolism aligned the collective identities of the Portuguese people towards the suffering of the Maubere people and set the preconditions for the eruption, in September 1999, of collective action for the defence of human rights.

Like Castells (2001) and Touraine (1981a), we argue that the novelty in contemporary social movements might be found in the network, but if the network is the prevalent organizational form surfacing from the integration of the internet, the movement's goals can be achieved only when combined strategies of traditional and new media usage are implemented. That is why, though considering the East Timor protest movement as a networked social movement, it is our belief that a social movement can be regarded as truly networked only when it achieves the combined use of the traditional mass media and new media as organizational resources and linkages to reference groups. Table 7.3 summarizes the integration of the different ICTs in the achievement of the pro-East Timor movement's goals.

The analysis of the pro-East Timor movement shows how social movements might themselves be changed due to the interactions they establish with different ICTs. Under the analysis developed here, it was also shown how the social integration of ICTs by the protest movement influenced the role played by specific information mediators, the journalists, and social actors such as the new economy companies.

Table 7.3 Media integration by the pro-East Timor movement

Media	Emergence	Mobilization	Organization and coordination	Protest	Range
Fax	–	–	–	Yes	International
Television	Yes	Yes	–	–	International
Radio	Yes	Yes	Yes	–	National
Newspapers	–	Yes	–	–	National
World wide web	–	Yes	Yes	Yes	International
Email	–	Yes	Yes	Yes	International
Chat	–	Yes	–	–	International
Newsgroups	–	Yes	–	–	International

Analysing the pro-East Timor movement, we can find the novelty of such protest in the fusion between media and movement, especially through the participation of agents seldom directly involved in the organization of such protests (journalists and new economy companies). The way in which traditional and new media were brought together, informing and orienting each other's actions, constitutes another dimension of the novelty associated with this protest, showing how ICTs facilitate traditional forms of protest and become both a tool and a target for collective action.

Looking at the movement from the political opportunity structure and societal context standpoint, it can be observed that the lack of direct diplomatic influence by the Portuguese state on the international level obliged the protesters to take on other repertoires of direct (new media-mediated) and indirect (mass media-mediated) action. They did so using not a clear and rigid organization, but a fluid network-like set of informal ties, which allowed protesters to voice their opinions. Many of these protests had, from the resource mobilization point of view, the grassroots guidance of both the new and the traditional media.

From the above, it can be argued that the pro-East Timor movement represents a clear example of the role played by the new media in social movements' achievement of their goals. The background of newly embraced late modern values and the catalytic power of images and internet communication succeeded where formal and institutional action had failed.

Maybe Russell Dalton has been able to capture the essence of what is new about the contemporary social movements: they have greater discretionary resources, enjoy easier access to the media, have cheaper and faster geographic mobility and cultural interaction, and can call upon the collaboration of different types of movement-linked organizations for rapidly organized issue campaigns (Tarrow 1998: 207–208). Now we must understand also how those elements are combined towards the achievement of their societal goals.

The evidence of the pro-East Timor movement's use of digital media raises new questions in the study of social movements. How can traditional and new media be combined in mobilizing and protesting towards the achievement of the social movement's goals? Can it be that the internet culture, which promotes the technocratic belief in the progress of humans through technology, is transforming social movements by incorporating new economy companies as social actors for collective actions? Are journalists replacing or joining intellectuals in their traditional role of framing and construction of collective identities and leverage of latent social movements?

Note

1 During the years of occupation of the territory, the population suffered systematic violations of human rights, confirmed by international independent organizations and individuals, which led to accusations of genocide being perpetrated by Indonesia against the Timorese people.

The award of the Nobel Prize for Peace in December 1996 to two Timorese, the Catholic bishop Ximenes Belo and the Foreign Minister of the Timorese Resistance Movement, Ramos Horta, marked a turning point in the awareness of the international community towards the situation faced on this part of the Timor island.

At the beginning of May 1999, Indonesian President Suharto was forced out of office by Indonesian student-led demonstrations and replaced by B.J. Habibie. This change in the internal politics of Indonesia, combined with an increase of worldwide public opinion support to Xanana Gusmão, facilitated a breaking of the stalemate in the negotiations between Portugal (the internationally recognized administrative power of the territory), the United Nations and Indonesia. An agreement between the three parties was reached on 6 May 1999, and the date of 8 August was chosen for the implementation of a referendum destined to ask the Timorese people for their views about the future of the territory.

The people were asked to choose between a special autonomy, integrating East Timor into the Republic of Indonesia, or to reject the autonomy leading consequently to separation from the Republic. After outbreaks of violence across the country, the referendum was postponed to 30 August, and on 4 September, the results were finally known: 78.5% of the 410,000 participants rejected the autonomy and the path to independence was open for the territory.

The next 16 days were characterized by fierce violence perpetrated by armed militias against the supporters of independence; violence that led to the killings of 5–7,000 and the displacement of several hundred thousand people. Indonesian armed and police forces gave wide support to the violence of the militias until 20 September, when the United Nations-supported International Peace Keeping Force (INTERFET) arrived at the Timor Capital, Díli. The INTERFET implemented the retreat of the Indonesian army, disarmed the armed militias, and implemented the arrival of a UN transitory administration for the territory.

8   ATTAC(k)ing expertise

Does the internet really democratize knowledge?

Brigitte le Grignou and Charles Patou

During the past years, who hasn't been fooled by those advertisements or articles presenting the internet as a panacea which could both free people and be considered as the origin of a 'new economy' promising sweet hereafter?

(Laurent Jesover, ATTAC-France's webmaster)

This chapter attempts to challenge the potential democratizing function of the internet as used by social movements by examining the case study of the Association for the Taxation of Financial Transactions for the Aid of Citizens (ATTAC[1]). ATTAC, as this chapter will show, is a unique organization, particularly in terms of its membership. Started in France in June 1998, the association claimed during its plenary assembly (in La Rochelle, December 2002) to be able to claim representation via 250 local committees as well as having 30,000 supporters, 28,700 of them being paid-up members. ATTAC was, indeed, surprised by its success. Over 6000 people attended its General Meeting in January 2002: more than double the board's expectations.

ATTAC's influence has spread through French political life, with communities signing up as members of ATTAC; members of parliament and senators have created an 'inter-group' within the French Parliament. Its power was recognized by the President's invitation to Bernard Cassen, the former chairman of the association,[2] to a conference organized by the diplomatic department of the Elysée Palace.

ATTAC has also achieved international growth, with 35 separate movements being created around the world (mostly in Europe but also in Brazil, Japan, Quebec, Senegal, etc.). This internationalization means that ATTAC-France has a team of 500 translators who translate all the data and documents of the website into Spanish, Portuguese, English, etc.

The founding act of the movement was an editorial, 'Disarming markets',[3] published in December 1997 by the director of the monthly magazine *Le Monde Diplomatique*. It firstly prompted an electronic discussion, and then stimulated, in June 1998, the creation of an association of individuals (journalists, academics, lawyers) and corporate bodies such as trade unions, associations and newspapers. Its founding members and its support thus comprise an unusual mix of actors from the intellectual and cultural fields together with members of trade unions and associations, thus producing an interesting bridge between postmodern lifestyle politics and the politics of modernity.

ATTAC shares many features with a new generation of social movements in a globalizing world (della Porta *et al.* 1999), so it can be viewed as in some ways emblematic. Like other social movements in a 'globalizing world', ATTAC is committed to 'supranational arenas' (1999: 16), i.e. transnational targets, focuses and organizations. Like them, it adapts its means and forms of action to contemporary conditions of protest, and contributes to the renewal of 'repertoires of action' (Tilly 1978). It should be understood as a continuous process where new shapes and more mature shapes come together. This way, specific 'arenas of action' and the transnational nature of many of their targets encourage the actors who constitute social movements to utilize the internet, firstly to get organized (instrumental use) and secondly to support their cause (via what is now called 'hacktivism'). Nevertheless, this turning to new technologies does not supersede traditional actions; it is merely an addition to the movements' more traditional repertoires of action. However, the tendency to put the internet at the core of a 'new age' of protest is the result of an enchanting account of protest action (e.g. the struggle against the Multilateral Agreement on Investment (MAI) in 1998). According to Ayres (1999: 133), 'the rather remarkable collapse of the MAI illustrated the changed dynamics of contention in the global age. The failure to ratify the MAI was in response to a successful internet campaign by nongovernmental organizations.' Ayres concludes: 'welcome to contentious politics Internet-style'. We would rather adopt a more realistic view, where the internet is considered as an instrument among others, or to endorse Ollitrault's description of it in relation to environmentalists as being 'an additional step within a dynamics of transnationalization initiated by these movements since the 60s' (1999: 158). So ATTAC, like many contemporary movements, embraces several types of action and uses various repertoires. It combines traditional actions (demonstrations, debates, or leaflets) with dramatic happenings (supporters bathing in the sea to protest against the European Summit in Nice in December 2000). It resorts to transnational forms of action (against international meetings) and to new technologies, not only to build its own organization, mobilize people, and protest, but also to 'hunt' information and acquire the skill of experts.

Like other 'new' social movements, ATTAC's relation to politics is rooted in 'reluctance to any power delegation' (Neveu 1996: 24). This reluctance is expressed through critiques of traditional organizations. It often favours 'rather flexible organizational forms and mobilization means which largely leave the initiative to the basis' (*Mouvements* 1999: 37). This attitude prevails through ATTAC membership and it is illustrated in the loose organizational structure and the emphasis on transparency[4] and democracy within ATTAC. At present, the association pays only six members, and local committees have claimed and obtained a strong autonomy. It is very easy to become a member of ATTAC: all you have to do to receive the newsletter, without paying any contribution, is to be web-connected or to organize, with friends or others activists, a conference: thus you become a *de facto* member (active member). ATTAC's membership provides a good example of a 'distanced engagement' (Ion 1997: Chapter 5) characterized by several short-term activisms instead of long-term activism in one organization. Use of the internet and its huge opportunities of creating and renewing networks (of people, organizations or projects) appears to be a practical illustration of this neo-activism (Granjon 2001). The democratic organization of the association allows or eases this particular kind of involvement. It has to be considered as a main feature of its success and, in a broader sense, as a main reason for the success in several contemporary mobilizations against globalization.

Despite the common features ATTAC shares with other social movements, it should be singled out for its specific projects. Its singularity and (perhaps) force of attraction for would-be activists seem to dwell in its project(s) and its ability to reinterpret those projects in line with local concerns. The initial target of taxing financial transactions (the Tobin tax) has quickly been reshaped into a project to help citizenship, characterized by a material redistribution and, above all, a 'spreading of knowledge' concerning economic mechanisms. Those who forged the foundation platform wished to create an association 'that would allow them to produce and diffuse information to work together' (ATTAC's platform 1998[5]). A bit like the eighteenth-century public sphere actors, they aim to shed 'light' on the secrecy of the decisions taken by international organizations (e.g. World Trade Organization, International Monetary Fund) and to fight against the opacity of many public policies. Also reminding one of the nineteenth-century pedagogues' project, they vow to promote education so as to 'regain control altogether over the future of our world' (ATTAC's platform, 1998). Besides, the movement's supporters and leaders refer to it as a 'people's education movement'[6] or, in the president Bernard Cassen's words, a 'people's education movement oriented towards action'. In other words, the movement aims at producing *counter-expertise* and *counter-experts*.

The features of the association converge to confer a central place on 'knowledge'. This is clearly apparent in ATTAC's genesis – an editorial in *Le Monde Diplomatique* – and when examining its organization: the board honorary chairperson is Ignacio Ramonet, Director of *Le Monde Diplomatique*, and the first chairperson was, until December 2002, Cassen, General Director of the same newspaper. The ATTAC National Committee consists of a board, made up of about a dozen people coming from the press and trade unions, and, at the top of the organizational chart, a Scientific Council comprising approximately 20 academics and researchers.

The importance of knowledge in ATTAC can also be seen by its structure and by the characteristics of its members. Educated categories are over-represented, especially 'teachers' (12.8 per cent) and 'other high-ranking intellectual professions' (6.3 per cent), whereas labourers are under-represented (0.6 per cent) (Trautmann 2001: 63–64). The importance of knowledge as a keystone of ATTAC's foundation stems from the combination of the social logic of membership recruitment, which favours a strong social homogeneity, and the strategy subsequently implemented by the movement. Similarly, the make-up of ATTAC supporters differs from the sociology of the people who back the 'movements of the deprived' (from ID, from housing, from work, etc.). The association aims at helping all citizens, and not just at pointing out the suffering and claims of mobilized victims. Everybody here has to be the actor of their own emancipation, and mobilization happens in the name of reason rather than emotion. So, one can argue that ATTAC 'overcrowds the cognitive sphere' (Patou 2000: 76) and that, among the main repertoires such as quantitative mobilization, the recourse to scandals, and the expert speech (Offerlé 1994: 110), the association has definitely chosen to favour expertise, both as a repertoire of action and as an aim.

Again, the internet, as an endless source of information and a space for debates, would seem to be an accurate vector for this modern pedagogic enterprise (spread of knowledge), its democratic organization and its particular kind of involvement.

On the one hand, the internet should favour the democratic life of the association by easing access to the decision-making process and agenda-setting, in order to achieve the goal of democracy and transparency within the association. However, Trautmann (2001) showed that the internet was not such a powerful tool to raise the level of democracy within the association despite the notions of increased representation associated with it.

On the other hand, the internet is apparently conducive to the second aim of ATTAC: the spread of knowledge. This study will focus particularly on this aspect, which is important in two ways. Firstly, 'adult education' is one of the main goals of ATTAC (perhaps in some senses the only one). Secondly, adult education can be viewed as an aspect, among others, of democracy within the organization. Actually, the use of the internet by ATTAC highlights the strain between two somewhat contradictory goals: the democratic aim of a social movement that seeks to spread knowledge as widely as possible, and the unavoidably restrictive feature of expertise.

We will analyse the mutual links between the expert appraisal favoured by ATTAC and the use of the internet, that is to say not only how the quest for expertise allows, eases and constrains the way it has been used, but also how this quest has been transformed through the use of the internet.

We will focus in particular on three dimensions of this topic:

- how the internet eases the circulation of knowledge in ATTAC
- how the internet modifies (or does not modify) the knowledge gap between grassroots activists and experts
- how the internet shapes the expertise in a particular way.

Our study is based on the electronic tools of the national website of ATTAC France (http://france.attac.org/site), the list of national discussion, *Attack talk*, (http://atlas.attac.org:talk:msg) and *Le Grain de Sable*, an information letter sent twice weekly to almost 60,000 people.[7] In order to understand how these tools are used and internalized, but also to dismiss the 'technological revolution' fantasy, our study will be completed by direct observations made during meetings and interviews with local and national supporters.[8]

The internet: a tool devoted to expertise

Generally speaking, the involvement of most of the contemporary social movements at supranational level can be linked to the expertise repertoire as well as to the internet. Commitment to 'supranational arenas' tends to favour logic of expertise that is implied partly by the complexity and technical nature of the issues, as well as the specialization of the actors involved. Many of these movements are oriented towards the notion of 'expertise', which we will define as the acquisition and diffusion of competencies grounded in a specialized knowledge. In this respect, ATTAC could be considered as an 'epistemic community', i.e. 'a network of professionals with recognized expertise and competence in a particular domain and an authoritative claim to policy-relevant knowledge within that domain or issue-arena' (Haas 1992). One of the ways in which these contemporary movements professionalize is by mobilizing specialists on a permanent or occasional basis. As they make available their often professional competency in a specific field (law, economics, chemistry, etc.), these 'resources people' (Sommier 2001: 55) intend to support a cause. This kind of professionalization, characterized by the important part granted to intellectuals, can be regarded as a key feature of ATTAC. This is why it could be an example of a 'new commitment of the scholars' (Sommier 2001: 57).

ATTAC's scientific council can be seen in many ways as a good illustration of this commitment of the scholars. The scientific council brings 'food for thought' on various action campaigns, and aims to 'nourish the publication of the ATTAC books'. It comprises approximately 15 members, mostly scholars in economics and leaders of unions that also have a high level of economic skills. In 2001, the scientific council was divided into five thematic groups,[9] each producing documents of various sizes from a page of synthesis to a report of 20 pages including references and differing levels of technical difficulty. In its own words, the scientific council is 'placed in the core of ATTAC. Its goal is to produce information easily accessible and to spread it, particularly to ATTAC's local groups'.[10] To some extent, the scientific council seems to achieve its mission.

The relationship between the scientific council and activists is clearly a 'top-down relation', but this does not seem to upset the activists. Actually, many activists acknowledge the role and specificity of the scientific council. They willingly use 'the document of the council as a main source of information and work' for their own actions. Moreover, they clearly accept the asymmetry of knowledge. In the words of one activist, 'the scientific council is to stand security' for their own thoughts.

In that context, the internet is seen by activists as a way to bypass 'the professors of the scientific council'. The internet provides each activist with the same data, documents and arguments and contributes to the process of becoming an expert, that is, it raises new matters of concerns on the agenda. The internet allows each activist to become an expert, to spread knowledge about globalization and to diminish the differences between experts and non-experts.

The important part played by the internet since the beginning of ATTAC is stressed by the webmaster, who underlines that the 'virtual' shape of the movement preceded its physical shape. It is also claimed by grassroots activists that: 'Anyone who wants to be committed to ATTAC has no choice but to be connected to the internet'. The internet is almost a necessity to whoever wishes to support ATTAC. This is also clear to those who are not connected: 'I don't have the internet at home, and I am aware it makes it difficult for me to know what is going on. But well, I can manage.'

Our research highlights the importance given to electronic resources in the supporter's activities, i.e. the research of information, documents, opinions and sources, or even images. As one activist remarked, 'As for me, when I go to the site, I am looking for documents, dates, data, and also images or mottos to design leaflets.' The internet hence appears as a 'documentary goldmine'. Generally, people say it is 'very convenient, full of good documents'. It is regarded as a seminal resource to develop the supporters' critical distance. This is of course the main target of ATTAC and of adult education: in aiming to make information simple and turning the decision receivers into 'active citizens within society' who will eventually attain control for the future of our/their world. As one activist commented, 'Thanks to the internet, one can have access to other pieces of information. You know, all newspapers look alike; they give the same kind of information. So, the internet is an alternate way to get information.'

But, paradoxically, the internet tends also to complicate, and in some cases to forestall, the pedagogic aim of ATTAC. Major problems with the internet actually concern the growing number of documents, interventions and syntheses put online: 'Since anybody can put anything on the Net, you should really be very careful about it. So, never take anything for granted . . . there is much fake information.'

This is so when each day, more and more information is published on the web and more and more people have access to ATTAC's website and discussion list. According to Jesover's chronology (2001), about 20 new documents are put on the website each day. There was one weekly information report in 1998, and this figure went up to five in 2001. It results in what could be called a 'buzz', because not everybody is interested in all the subject matter. One way to cut off this buzz comes from specialization. Indeed, members of ATTAC are very keen to concentrate on just one or two main topics according to their own sensibilities and affiliation to other associations.

Thematic groups provide a good illustration of how the internet strengthens this specialization of competencies. Firstly, these groups are locally based. Then they tend to develop along a thematic line, and are even described by activists as a 'specialization within specialization'. According to some activists, thematic groups facilitate a 'division of work which is possible on the Net, because the internet allows one to level discussions upwards'. Thematic groups also permit the development of synergies and the potential to 'share knowledge mutually' (Jesover 2001: 4). For instance, ATTAC Saint-Malo, which is located near Jersey (an offshore tax haven), has initiated a group on fiscal paradises, and its members work increasingly closely with the other groups from western France on such campaigns.

While the autonomy of local groups and the various origins of the supporters lead to a specialization of competencies, they also widen the range of interests of ATTAC and therefore the nature of its expertise. In 1998, when the association was set up, it focused on claims on the implementation of the Tobin tax. Since then, its targets have kept growing:

> The Tobin tax, the cancellation of debt of the South and Eastern Europe, fighting against the existence of fiscal paradises in Europe and throughout the world, struggling against the rising empowerment of multinational corporations, against the treatment of health, education, and public services as simple market goods, bioethics, the prevailing free-market ideology, the cultural standardization, the worldwide reign of finance . . . Here are the points we tackle altogether with other partners.
>
> (Welcome page, ATTAC-France, October 2001)

One can see that the internet is an efficient tool in terms of the diffusion of protest (Della Porta *et al.* 1999) and the consistency of protest, in order to achieve a 'consensual mobilization' (Ollitrault 2001: 124). It actually brings together, on a single page, issues such as Commander Marcos, 'mad cow disease' and human rights in Tunisia. In this way, the internet makes obvious and visible the link uniting these different subjects of contention. This unity is materialized by the icon 'click here' according to an audiovisual logic replacing articulations through visual transitions. The use of the internet is above all an important element of the unity of ATTAC because it permits a link to be made between hitherto apparently unconnected issues (at least, in so far as those issues can be listed together). Nonetheless, this unity does not delude anyone, since 'the main problem for ATTAC today concerns the unification of the movement and the way to give it a more unified content'.

The internet could then be considered as an efficient tool in keeping with the process of 'frame extension' (Snow *et al.* 1986: 472). It can also be linked to the process of 'frame clouding' (Snow *et al.* 1986: 478), i.e. the loss of any thematic visibility of the movement, which would then look like a hotchpotch of ideas, as a local member once said. So, on the one hand, the internet makes visible the fragmented plurality of its action by listing together subjects and causes. On the other hand, it simultaneously makes homogeneous and coherent a set of analyses, activities and movements which would otherwise be scattered. For ATTAC's supporters, 'everything is connected when it comes to world globalization'.

The knowledge gap

Meyer and Tarrow's remark on the professionalization process could be applied to internet users: 'Professionalization is about drawing boundaries between accredited persons and others' (1998: 15). Furthermore, according to the authors, 'new technologies and forms of social organization have complicated this picture further'. One could apply the hypothesis of a widening of the knowledge gap, verified with regard to television, to internet users also. Just as television can be seen to educate those who are most educated and know how to select and capitalize knowledge, the internet would 'over-inform' a minority of citizens who are already well informed (Hill and Hughes 1998). According to Dahlgren, 'The Internet allows people to do better what they usually do, more than it changes them' (2000: 175). This way, within ATTAC, the frontiers persist between the knowledgeable ones and those deprived of knowledge, the information-rich and the information-poor, between active supporters and people who just pass by. These frontiers even tend to be reinforced by the use of the internet. One can clearly see that the connected supporters make up a minority, belong to the most educated categories, and that the internet users are the most active people within the association.

Jesover, the webmaster, says that in 2001 15 per cent of the supporters were connected, i.e. approximately 4,500 people. As Dahlgren notes, 'the sociological features of the internet users are clearly defined nowadays. There are strong biases in favour of young and rich men, having an important cultural capital' (Dahlgren 2000: 174). Such bias is seen as a potential factor widening the gap between those who get information and those who do not (Loader 1998; Vedel 2000). The professional distribution of connected supporters within ATTAC shows that this population is more privileged from a social point of view and more endowed with cultural capital than the whole body of the adherents. More than 30 per cent of the connected supporters are 'researchers or teachers in high school/university', and 12 per cent belong to the category 'other up-range intellectual professions' (Trautmann 2001: 64).

Finally, we put in perspective the part played by the internet in political commitment. 'The Net makes up a tool, a resource for those who are politically committed, but it does not generally draw in important crowds of new citizens towards the public space' (Hill and Hughes 1998: 177). Other research sheds light on social and cultural factors which favour commitment or otherwise (Gaxie 1978). It appears clear that anyone who wishes to search for information or consult a site committed to a cause, and *a fortiori* to take part in a forum has to comply with certain prerequisites. It implies a special interest and a preliminary commitment, so that the 'issue of proclivity to political commitment is relevant when it comes to the commitment to the Internet, even if it is loose or occasional' (Ollitrault 1999: 167). In this perspective, among internet groups dealing with environmentalist issues, expressed opinions and experts' debates essentially come from educated people, most of them having an academic background. To them, the 'ticket to the Net' is cheap, since it is a professional tool, which they may use every day for free. Trautmann's conclusions about the supporters' activity within ATTAC point to the same conclusion. There is actually a clear link between 'the use of electronic tools and activities committed to "classical" causes' (Trautmann 2001: 25), e.g. distributing leaflets, participating in meetings. As confirmed by our interviews, it shows that the more active the supporters are, the more they actively use the internet. The internet is then likely to reinforce a 'cleavage' between a minority of very active supporters[11] who spend much time and energy on committed (cyber) causes, and the grassroots other members.

The webmaster argues that 'ATTAC is a citizen association, which intervenes on the traditional political stage, rather than as an electronic association. Henceforth, our adult education movement cannot directly get involved in the teaching of the Internet and computer uses' (Jesover 2001: 4). He implements a policy that tends to strengthen the distinction between 'serious practices' and 'entertaining practices', as he tries to discourage occasional web-users from considering 'interactivity as a gimmick':

> 'Our emailing lists do not come with any excerpts of texts available on the Web site. This aims to persuade people to read the document put on line. Besides, there is no forum on the Internet site, so that 'passers-by' are discouraged from quickly glancing at the discussion or making a short statement.
>
> (Jesover 2001: 8)

This 'passer-by' can be described as a new version of Olson's 'free rider' (1978), in so far as his/her activity can consist of paying a subscription, collecting information more or less related to ATTAC's targets, and 'chatting' or holding controversial discussions on the discussion list.

There is actually a clear difference between two discussion lists: *Attac Local* and *Attac Talk*. The former is a working list reserved for local electronic correspondents; it aims to coordinate activities among local committees. The latter is a discussion list open to everybody. This underlying difference is enhanced by the different online protagonists. Firstly, the webmaster regularly insists on the strictly informative character of the first list, different from a 'club-internet discussion-list', he says (Jesover in Trautmann 2001: 19). Secondly, supporters claim their disinterest to *Attac Talk*, which is said to be too 'heavy' and 'congested' (although it could be argued that the congested nature of the site, far from being a negative feature of the internet, is an example of the secondary effects of democratizing access to the internet). Local groups warn visitors: 'be careful, there are a lot of messages every day, many of them being controversial'.[12]

Quasi-expert discussions

Internet-users, like readers (Chartier, 1995) or any users of *machine à communiquer* (Jouët 2000: 490), tend not always to follow prescriptions and instructions for use. Trautmann shows how the people participating on the *Attac Local* list start to take control of the tool as they break through the rules explicitly given by the webmaster. As a result, they reshape a list originally designed to convey information into a 'vector of inner debates'. The *Attac Talk* discussion list is used as a place where a small group shares political feelings rather than economic data.

The study of the discussion list[13] sheds light on contributions, which are located in an intermediary position on account of certain characteristics of their authors, subject matters and style. The authors actually seem to be very active supporters, situated by their pedagogical standpoint between 'real' experts from the scientific council and grassroots supporters keen on learning. The subject matter combines political opinions with economic arguments; the style corresponds to Hert's 'quasi oral speech' (Hert 1999: 213). This discussion list reveals another side of expertise or, to use Hert's expression, a *quasi-expertise*.

Our observations show how selective the list is (although it is open to everybody). There are few speakers, since the debate is *de facto* limited to ten people or so. For example, in October 2000 there were 428 messages, 29 of which came from collective bodies (*Le Grain de Sable*), i.e. approximately 400 messages emanated from about 100 people. Eleven people wrote at least ten messages each, and 162 messages in total. In other words, 11 per cent of the speakers (most of them being men) produced 40 per cent of the messages. The figures for September, November and December are similar: between 325 and 480 messages; between seven and eight per cent of the speakers wrote from 33 to 48 per cent of the messages. Our figures correspond to those given by Trautmann. She mentions 334 messages posted by 94 people in March 2000. She also notices that 76 messages, i.e. about a quarter of the whole, were sent by just four people. She remarks that the proportions are 'constant' in April and May. We found regulars who are on familiar terms with each other, use the other's first name ('hello Roger'), spontaneously respond to each other ('I am not O.K. with that, Michel . . .') and moderate each other ('Come down Benoît'). The few messages from newcomers ('Hi everybody, Let me add that . . .') do not receive any comment or answers.

Trautmann's analysis of the *Attac Local* list also underlines this foreclosing of the speakers. She seems to attribute it to the necessary fragmentation of an excessive level of information on the internet: 'when they are too segmented, debates very rapidly require a high level of technique. Then, speaking becomes the monopoly of a few' (2001: 52). On *Attac Talk* (and maybe in other offline political debates), it seems that the factor of selection is less linked to the technical nature of the debates. It would seem to be related to the feeling of possessing a political competence, according to which one would be allowed to express one's opinion and mood, and is likely to be tied to the 'closure effects of a written exchange' (Hert 1999: 218).

Generally, economic issues are at the core of the discussion. They generate the highest volume of messages, even if they fail to represent more than half of the subjects dealt with. For instance, in October 2001, ten per cent of the messages concern questions like 'what is exactly economics?', 'Lesson of economics', 'symbolical and economic wealth'. The economic issue competes with 'Israel and the Occupied Territories' and many other 'micro-debates' on the reduction of working time, the French Communist Party, the privatization of Thomson, the 'anti-capitalistic revolutionary movement', the independence of the media, etc. In November 2001, a quarter of the messages were devoted to economic issues. Some messages look like a lesson in political economy: 'The Bretton Woods system collapsed on 15 August 1971, when President Nixon decided that dollars could not be exchanged against gold any longer . . .' But in general, they are not really didactic: 'it could happen that the costs induced by the leverage of the tax might not exceed its direct product. In this context, it is clear that the indirect product is defined as the result from the reintroduction of available assets within real economy.' The title 'Professor' is ironically attributed to bash any speaker who is perceived to give lessons and does not abide by the etiquette.

Many figures of speech associate the discourses with narratives rather than scientific demonstrations. In this respect, one can find metaphors ('Everything which can hinder profit, every grain we can add into the gearing system can only accelerate the crash of the system') or allegories ('This system is faithless and lawless'). 'Quasi-oral speech' is a hybrid form, which conjugates written messages and spoken exchanges. It tends to favour a 'slipshod' and informal tone, spontaneous judgements, immediate reactions, controversies, and also 'tactic actions' which aim at imposing a leader through synthesis, quotations or manipulations of messages (Hert 1999: 239ff.). This is illustrated by the often vehement or controversial tone of the list. It quickly evokes suggestions from the webmaster 'for an optional self-moderation' (July 1999) which in turn gives way to counter-propositions to 'moderate the *moderator* instincts'. This results in a debate ironically entitled: 'MODERATO debate – for how long again?????' In October 2000, the discussion started with an exchange entitled 'Will you have some more respect?' It was followed by interventions, the simple titles of which indicated how animated the debate on rules of communication was: 'Excuse me', 'it's not my fucking problem', or 'let us speak, let us stop insulting each other'. Even the economic expertise can be expressed in a tone reminding one of insults more than pedagogy. For instance, here are the first lines of the exchange entitled 'Close to zero in economics':

> What you wish is valuable, but your knowledge in economics is close to zero . . . you just make stupid remarks (when it comes to economics of course. 'cause in politics, everything has some kind of value). If you need someone to teach you economics, I'd be happy to help you.

In January 2000, a vote took place in the European Parliament on a resolution about the Tobin tax, which generated a debate on the net offering an illustration of how the list could be used as a place where opinions and political moods are expressed. The vote in the European Parliament triggered much anger among supporters of the Tobin tax. The resolution did not pass partly because the voices of the three Lutte Ouvrière (Arlette Laguiller's Trotskyist party) representatives and that of the Ligue Communiste Révolutionnaire leader, Alain Krivine, were missing. The online debate took two paths. On the one hand, it became a vehement critique of the political position of the two Trotskyist leaders; on the other hand, it took the shape of a debate on the old and seemingly never-ending question: 'of reform or revolution?' The messages clearly showed that the cyber-supporters had the know-how to use the internet. The first texts were a call to protest via the internet: e.g. 'Go on Arlette! Go on Krivine! This is a real scandal. Does anyone know the e-mail address of those "revolutionaries"? I suggest we should deluge them with protest letters.' Or: 'We should definitely write to them . . . and we don't mind if it can't change anything yet. At least, it'll bring some kind of relief.' They also bear tracks of an anti-capitalist political culture. A specifically political reaction could be viewed in this letter sent to the LO and LCR representatives. It read that

> If I have ever voted for one of your candidates, believe me, it won't happen again. I will always remember how you voted on the 21st when I go to the ballots. You will never see the revolution you've been expecting, 'cause you didn't do anything to start it. And if it ever happens, it won't be thanks to you.

One of the speakers brings his own touch: 'And be quick, because I get old, and you do too!' A message is signed by 'PH G. Liberal since I was born'.

Some, albeit just a few, resort to caricatural arguments, which recall provocative methods used during some public debates. For instance, when it comes to the European representatives who did not vote for the resolution, one could find the following barbed comment: 'their dogmatic attitude reminds me of the Inquisition or the Khmer Rouge!'

However, the debate was quickly re-framed. It became a political analysis starting with some thoughts about the Tobin tax, finally resulting in a questioning of what it meant to be committed to ATTAC: 'I think there is no everlasting solution to inequality and injustice, when we deal with capitalism. From this point of view, I am not satisfied with the TT [Tobin Tax].' One of the answers is 'so what should we do?? . . . A revolution! You didn't knock at the right door. It isn't the aim of this association!'

Conclusion

Following Dahlgren, one can regard the internet as the contemporary form of a public space:

> We can establish some kind of analogy between the Bourgeois living in the end of the XVIIIth century, who used to speak of trade and politics in their clubs and cafés. According to Habermas, a public space emerged through the discursive practices of these élites and the blooming media (press, books and booklets).
>
> (Dahlgren 2000: 182)

Yet one should also consider a few critiques of the standard model of the bourgeois and literate public space, i.e. about the exclusions founding it (Fraser 1997) or about the idealization of a unique model (Baker 1997). So, within ATTAC, electronic tools seem to be required for the democratic promotion of expert actors (either at economics or at activism). But they also contribute to select the actors, and they henceforth maintain and even enlarge the gaps between 'expert' and 'non-expert' contributors. Finally, they facilitate an uninhibited expression, which appears more as an exchange of opinions than an exchange of arguments rooted in reason. The internet is a long way from bringing to ATTAC 'the sweet hereafter'. It appears to date as an instrument that is hardly able to be used to make the adult education project come true. It tends to root in, or at least to maintain, the frontiers between active supporters and non-active supporters. These frontiers replicate more and more the boundaries between experts and amateurs. The internet reinforces in ATTAC an inclination to fragmentation, to the individualization of projects, since it favours a virtual commitment made up of discussions and contests within small circles of specialists. As a grassroots activist put it:

> To me, the Internet tool is pretty delusive, that is to say, people feel they participate in a *network* as soon as they are connected. In actual fact, the tool has never structured anything. The tool is a tool – for something which is already structured . . . But as long as you don't *network* with local groups, the Internet is a big fair devoted to individual projects.

Notes

1 Association pour la Taxation des Transactions Financières pour l'Aide aux Citoyens.
2 Since the general assembly of La Rochelle, on 1 December 2002, the chairperson is Jacques Nikonoff, an academic economist.
3 www.france.attac.org/a644
4 For instance, 27 per cent of the documents available on the website of ATTAC deal with the organization of the association.
5 'Plate-forme de l'Association ATTAC'. ATTAC's Platform, adopted by the Constituent, 3 June 1998. http://www.attac.org/fra/assoc/doc/plate formefr.htm
6 'Mouvement d'éducation populaire'.
7 To be exact, 59,165 (http://attac.org/indexfr/index.html).
8 Fifty questionnaires were administered by telephone to local committees, and about ten supporters and national or local leaders were interviewed in 2000–2001. All the quotations without reference are taken from these interviews.
9 Control of financial transaction; financial criminality; Fonds de pension & Epargne salariale; Employment and finance; sustainable development.
10 http://france.attac.org/a602
11 There were 3582 voters at the Tours general assembly on 3 and 4 November 2001. There were approximately 4500 connected supporters at that time.
12 http://www.local.attac.org/paris11/mailing.htm#archives
13 The study concerns the *Attac Talk* discussion list in the year 2000, and more particularly the last four months of that year, as well as the discussion on the Tobin tax held in the European Parliament in January 2000 (http://attac.org/indexfr/index.html).
14 'Tous les grains de sable qu'on peut mettre dans les rouages de la machine . . .'

Part III

Citizenship, identity and virtual movements

9 The Dutch women's movement online

Internet and the organizational infrastructure of a social movement

Arthur Edwards

Political parties, interest groups, social movement organizations and the media are the main intermediaries that are involved in what Lawson (1988) coined as the 'linkage chain', the chain of connections that runs from the citizens' wishes to political decisions. It has been claimed that one of the effects of the increasing use of information and communication technologies (ICTs) in the public domain, notably the internet, will be that the intermediary roles of these actors will erode, because citizens will be able to bypass them. Such a 'disintermediation' has been welcomed as one of the potential benefits of the internet, as it would allow for a direct, unbiased representation of citizens' demands in political decision-making (cf. Bryan *et al.* 1998). However, disintermediation has also been designated as a threat to democracy, because intermediaries are important sources of judgement and selection, social integration and checks and balances (Shapiro 1999).

Disintermediation in politics has, to date, mainly been discussed with respect to political parties. In various studies it has been established that there is a weakening of the once strong linkages between social class, religion and party identification and that the importance of parties as channels of political participation is steadily declining (Smith 1998). Benjamin (1982) was one of the first authors relating the disintermediation of political parties to ICTs. New technologies such as two-way cable television and direct mail would allow for direct communication between politicians and voters and would therefore contribute to the decline of political parties as mediating institutions.

It seems that social movements are taking over some of the terrain lost by political parties. In the 'market for political activism'

(Richardson 1995), social movements have certain advantages: by concentrating on specific issues, they offer modern citizens the opportunity to be more selective in their choices to invest time and energy in political participation. Nevertheless, it can be argued that the disintermediating potential of the internet will affect interest groups and social movement organizations as well. Davis (1999) presents two scenarios, one of which is that political organizations, as we know them, will fade away:

> Citizens will gather their own political information on the Net, even very specialized information . . . Then they will respond spontaneously and independently, identifying the policy makers they need to reach and crafting their own messages based on their own Internet-based research.
>
> (Davis 1999: 63)

In the same vein, Abramson *et al.* (1988) foresaw that membership-based interest group politics would give way to a politics of 'mobilized categories', characterized by high activism, temporality and low cohesion. Davis' second scenario is the emergence of new cyberspace groups promoting issues that are not addressed by existing organizations. As Hill and Hughes (1998) argue, because of the low costs of going online, small organizations, which address very specific issues or those with extreme points of view, will get better possibilities to reach a wider public.

Empirical research in this field is still rare. Davis (1999) investigated the websites of various interest groups and his main finding was that these groups are rapidly becoming internet-enabled. He concluded that the two scenarios hardly match reality.

In this chapter I examine one particular social movement, the Dutch women's movement. By looking at a social movement as a whole, it is possible to investigate both how existing, 'physical' organizations within the movement are appropriating the internet, and how new 'virtual' organizations are entering the field. I focus on the movement's *organizational infrastructure*, i.e. the entirety of organizations, which make up the movement's basic capacity to fulfil its intermediary roles. The questions to be answered, therefore, are 'how are internet uses reshaping the organizational infrastructure of the Dutch women's movement?' and 'what impact do these changes have on the capacity of the movement to articulate social problems, to mobilize support and to influence the political agenda and political decision-making?'

The women's movement consists of a broad variety of organizations and groups, with both formal, membership-based organizations and informal groups and networks. It combines characteristics of both an instrumental and an identity-directed movement with its typical strategies and action-repertoires (Rucht 1990). In the Netherlands, with its uniquely Dutch political opportunity structure (cf. Kriesi 1996), the women's movement has been embedded and institutionalized in structures of representation, consultation and cooperation. Recently, however, some indications of disintermediation can be observed. Firstly, a part of the women's movement faces an ageing of its membership. The size of the membership is declining.[1] Moreover, the central government is taking a more distant approach towards the 'middle field' of established organizations. This tendency is also visible in relation to the women's movement. The central government tends to develop its policies more autonomously, without prior consultations with the field (Outshoorn 2000).

Conceptual framework and selection of cases

An exploratory study of the uses of the internet within the women's movement was undertaken, examining what these uses are, how they can be explained, and their impact on the intermediary functions of the movement (Edwards 2001).

Figure 9.1 depicts the conceptual model. It is assumed that – within the context of a given political opportunity structure – the internet uses of a movement organization can be explained by the interplay of three sets of variables: (1) organizational characteristics, namely the goal orientation of the organization, the function that the organization fulfils within the movement and its internal structure; (2) the availability of resources; and (3) the organization's perception of opportunities of the internet. These factors bear upon the processes in which organizations develop their internet uses and embed these uses in their ordinary practices ('process of appropriation of the internet'). The internet usage has an impact on the capacity of organizations to manage problem perceptions or frames, to mobilize resources and to establish and maintain relations with their environment. This chapter examines the internet uses of existing 'physical' organizations within the women's movement, as well as 'virtual' organizations that have formed themselves on the internet. For the virtual organizations the scheme has to be read differently, as they are not pre-existing organizations whose characteristics have to be taken account of.

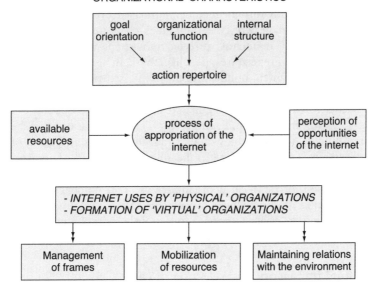

Figure 9.1 Conceptual scheme

Organizational characteristics

As to the organizational characteristics, my focus is on the *function* of the organization within the women's movement. A very useful approach is Kriesi's (1996) categorization of 'movement related organizations'. He uses two criteria: (1) whether the organization depends on the direct participation of its constituency, and (2) whether the organization pursues a political goal (an authorities orientation) or is primarily constituency- or client-oriented. In this way, he distinguishes organizations that are specialized in political mobilization (*social movement organizations* or *SMOs*), in giving service (*supportive organizations*), in self-help or altruism (*movement associations*), and in political representation (notably *parties* and *interest groups*). I take these four categories as constituting the organizational infrastructure of a social movement, as far as 'physical' organizations are concerned.

Internet uses by existing 'physical' organizations

Several authors have pointed to the ways in which the internet can facilitate the performance of social movements (Myers 1994; Hill and Hughes 1998; Davis 1999; Greenberg 1999; introduction to this volume). I distinguish the following *communicative functions* to describe the uses of the internet:[2]

(a) information dissemination and information retrieval
(b) recruitment
(c) mobilization
(d) soliciting opinions, opinion polling
(e) discussion
(f) facilitating contacts between the organization's members
(g) service
(h) networking, communication and coordination with other organizations.

Most of these functions were included in Davis' study (1999) of interest group sites.[3] Information dissemination and retrieval appeared as the most common uses of the internet. The internet was used by most organizations to supplement their offline efforts to provide information to their members and the wider public. About 70 per cent of the sites included a solicitation for membership recruitment.

'Mobilization' comprises (1) mobilization-specific information, such as information about bills under consideration or information about which policy-makers to contact and how to do so, and (2) actual mobilization, both offline and online grassroots lobbying. In Davis' study, about 40 per cent of the sites included information on pending legislation; almost 50 per cent used the site to urge members to participate in group events; 20 per cent of the sites included a solicitation to join email distribution lists for news and action alerts. A striking result of Davis' study was the absence of solicitations of opinions. Most sites provided email addresses, but the internet was not used to solicit opinions on specific issues. According to Davis, such solicitations pose serious problems for group leadership, because they provide opportunities for members as well as others outside the organization 'to take control of the group's agenda'. In line with this, discussion forums were seemingly used as mobilization instruments, but not for opinion formation.

Availability of resources

In terms of relative (transaction) costs, the internet is a cheap medium to reach a wide public (Hill and Hughes 1998). The costs of setting up a simple website are low. Still, for grassroots organizations the initial costs of going online can be difficult to afford, particularly if these costs include the investment in hardware. Davis (1999) found in his research that of the poorer organizations, 50 per cent had no website against only 15 per cent of the richer organizations. Moreover, grass-roots organizations may have difficulties in affording the staff to maintain a website. They are dependent on the know-how of volunteers and their willingness to invest time. Differences in available resources between organizations also affect their further uses of the internet. According to Davis, resource-rich groups are more likely to have websites with more content, an attractive layout and more technical possibilities.

Perception of opportunities of the internet

The internet attracts certain perceptions of what its possibilities are for the functioning of organizations (Snellen 1994). For the Dutch women's movement, the Fourth UN World Conference on Women in Beijing (1995) was a catalyst for the first internet initiatives. During the UN conference a 'mirror conference' was held in Amsterdam, with an internet connection with Beijing. As a result of the success of this facility, the internet was now taken seriously within the Dutch women's movement. According to several interviewees, the internet fits well with the culture of the women's movement, in which communication and international networks have always been important. The internet gave the movement new opportunities to realign itself, notably on international issues. Also, it gave a new dimension to empowerment. The only threshold was 'the technology itself', in particular the masculine images that were surrounding it (cf. Green and Keeble 2001).

Virtual organizations

Thus far, we have discussed internet use by existing organizations. 'Real' or 'physical' organizations function in a physical space, usually with clear boundaries between means and people that belong to the organization or do not, and in which the activities, means and people are ordered within dimensions of time and space. The internet makes new, virtual organization patterns possible that are characterized by place-independent cooperation between persons or organizations. In virtual organizations, a network structure is emerging of information flows and relation patterns (Bekkers 2000). Virtual organizations function within a non-physical cyberspace; the boundaries between organizations, the dividing lines between resources and people that belong to the organizations or not, are waning.[4] From Bekkers (2000) I derive three types of virtual organizations that one can expect to find within the women's movement.

1 Portal organizations: a website functions as a bridge to various other organizations, databases, etc.
2 Platform organizations: a website functions as a shared space for cooperative work and communication.
3 Web organizations, like virtual communities.[5]

Together, physical and virtual organizations can be considered as making up a new organizational infrastructure of a social movement. Building on Rosenkrands' study of websites within the anti-corporate movement (Chapter 3, this volume), and combining his results with Kriesi's (1996) categorization, I reconstruct this new organizational infrastructure as in Table 9.1.

Effects of internet use

To establish the effects of internet use for the political functions that are fulfilled by social movements, I follow van de Donk and Rucht (Introduction, this volume), who group these effects into three categories:

(a) *management of frames.* Social movements have certain perspectives on social problems; they try to disseminate these frames, and to influence the public agenda. They try to create and maintain a collective identity that directs their aims and strategies. The internet can function as a new medium to expose frames and problem definitions and as a space to create shared meaning and identities among the membership and the constituency.

Table 9.1 The organizational infrastructure of a social movement

Organizations in physical space	Organizations in cyberspace
Social movement organizations	Platform sites oriented towards mobilization
Movement associations	Virtual communities
Supportive organizations	Sites oriented towards information provision, information portals
Representative or umbrella organizations	Umbrella platform sites with a lobbying function

(b) *Mobilization of resources*. This approach focuses on the organization's ability to assemble and to use resources. The internet is a powerful tool to build an organization, to collect money, to assemble information and to recruit and mobilize people.

(c) *Maintaining relations with the environment*. The internet can improve the capacity of organizations to maintain networks and to coordinate actions. Moreover, if organizations are online, they can advance their points of view directly to a wide public, bypassing the traditional media.

Initially, the internet uses can be expected to enhance the effectiveness and efficiency of an organization's existing action repertoire. When the organization further develops its internet uses, some innovations might occur, for example in new forms of collective action. Gradually, an organization might undergo a transformation into a new type of organization, including a new action repertoire, organizational structure and ways of maintaining relations with the environment.

Selection of cases

This study follows a broad definition of the women's movement as including all organizations and groups that are directed at improving the position of women or strengthening female gender identities in society.[6]

The findings are based on an in-depth study of 12 physical organizations. In line with Kriesi (1996), these organizations were selected within the four types of 'movement-related organizations' mentioned above: social movement organizations (SMOs), movement associations, representative organizations and supportive organizations.

As to the first two categories, it became apparent that while some organizations specialize in either political mobilization or mutual support and social activities, these activities are often combined.[7] Therefore, the two categories were combined: 'grassroots organizations with an internal or external function'. Six organizations were selected within this category. Three supportive organizations were selected. In the category 'political representation', three umbrella organizations were selected.[8] Apart from this, the cases were almost evenly distributed among the three generations of the women's movement. In its historical development, the women's movement has gone through different 'emancipation waves', in which different demand patterns were put forward (Brouns 1995). In its initial stage (last decades nineteenth century/first decades twentieth century), the women's movement demanded basic political and social rights, such as the right to vote, the right to work and education. The women's organizations that were the offspring of the second feminist wave (1960s and 1970s) thematized the unequal distribution of paid and unpaid labour in society, the participation of women in political decision-making and individual autonomy in issues of life-politics. Within the newest generation of women's organizations, there is more emphasis on diversity on the basis of specific identities, such as ethnicity, sexual orientation or age.

Furthermore, social movements can be distinguished according to certain biographic or social characteristics (such as age, gender, sexual orientation, ethnicity, economic position/income, consumer/client) or by their orientation to a certain problem area (environment, globalization, etc.). Some women's organizations were selected that embody various combinations with one of these characteristics: one organization of elder women, one organization of women on social security, two organizations of black women, migrants or refugees, and one rural organization. Lastly, the cases vary according to factors such as size of membership, number of professional staff, government subsidy, and organizational structure.

As to the virtual organizations, seven cases were included: one mobilization site, three information portals, two virtual communities and one umbrella site with a lobbying function. Apart from the wide field of virtual communities, this choice was less a matter of selection than a reflection of what exists.

The websites of these organizations were inspected twice, in March 2001 and May 2002. This allowed for some observations as to the ways in which these websites have developed. In addition, interviews were held with members of the board of the organizations, and with (other) members or staff engaged in the development of the organizations' internet uses. A short description of the cases is given in the appendix.

Grassroots organizations with an internal and an external function

An estimate of the number of grassroots organizations – at least at the national level – can be inferred from the membership of the three umbrella organizations (see 'Representative organizations' below). The number is about 70. About half of them have their own website. Table 9.2 gives an overview of the communicative functions on the websites of the six organizations that were included in this study.

Table 9.2 Uses of the internet by grassroots organizations

	1	2	3	4	5	6
Information provision	××	××	×	×(×*)	×	×
Recruitment	×	×	×	×	×	×
Mobilization	×	×				
Soliciting opinions	×	×		×*		×
Discussion				×*	×†	
Facilitating internal contacts				×*		
Service						
Networking with other organizations	×	×		×	×†	

×× A particularly large amount of information.
* Present on the members-only section of the website.
† On the common web pages of organizations of rural women.

1 Netherlands Association of Women's Interests, Women's Labour and Equal Citizenship.
2 National Point of Support of Women on Social Security.
3 WOUW ('Wise Old Women') Amsterdam.
4 Netherlands Association of Women with Higher Education (VVAO).
5 Catholic Women's Organization (KVO).
6 Network for Black and Migrant Women with a Higher Education.

The organizations are numbered in order of their focus on external (political) activities. The first two organizations are primarily political organizations (SMOs); the last one functions primarily as a 'movement association'.

Information provision and recruitment are present on the websites of all organizations. This accords with Davis' findings. The two organizations that focus most on their external political functions are also using the website for political mobilization. When the first phase of this study was completed (spring 2001), no site had any opinion-soliciting or discussion feature. One year later, this had changed. With one exception, all websites now have such features, although the opinion-soliciting feature is in most cases no more than an email provision.

The websites of the more external-oriented organizations (cases 1 and 2 in Table 9.2) are the most developed ones. The Association of Women's Interests was one of the first women's organizations that went online (1996). Since 2000 it has gradually expanded its website, mainly with information, both about the main problem area that the association addresses (the man/woman proportion in politics) and about its activities. For example, the section 'Women and politics' gives detailed information on the man/woman proportion in representative bodies on the local, regional, national and European levels. In the period before the municipal elections in March 2002, the association tried to stimulate the nomination and election of more women in municipal councils. The website section on this project facilitated the mobilization of grassroots in local action.

The website of the National Point of Support of Women on Social Security has existed since 1999. In 2001–2002 the website expanded rapidly. Also in this case, it was mainly used as an information outlet relating to the issues the organization addresses and its activities. However, the organization used the interactive possibilities of the internet by asking women to forward their experiences, complaints, remarks and questions about welfare regulations and agencies. This is a clear example of how the internet can facilitate the articulation of citizens' demands and concerns, via a social movement organization.

The website of the Netherlands Association of Women with Higher Education (VVAO), online since 1999, is unusual in that it developed a new website with a members-only section. The public section gives short overviews of the aims, activities and publications of the association, a list of the 33 local branches, two-thirds of which had their own web pages, and contact information including information about how to become a member. The restricted section is more extensive. It contains an electronic list of members, with a search facility to find members with the same interests, a discussion group, a bulletin board, and a possibility to download documents and publications.

In contrast, the website of the Network of Black and Migrant Women with a Higher Education, online since 1998, has not been enlarged but has gradually been reduced, with the section on 'Policy' as well as all the links having been expunged. In 2002, a form was included to forward remarks. Internally, there is a newsletter that is emailed to the members. The development of this website reflects the more inward-looking orientation of this organization, which decided to drop its objective to influence government policies in order to function primarily as a network for its members.

In the website development of grassroots organizations, internal communication purposes go hand in hand with external purposes. The Association of Women's Interests is engaged in a process of improving its internal communication by the use of email and its website. It decided to replace the internal news bulletin by an email provision. The National Point of Support of Women on Social Security aspires to develop a communication network with the local committees. In cases 4 and 6 (Table 9.2), the internal purposes seem to take primacy. These findings seem to suggest that grassroots organizations' uses of the internet pass through different phases. At first, the emphasis is on external information provision. The 'first generation' websites contain basic (static) information about the organization. Then, organizations expand their websites so as to include more information: background information on the problem area that they address, as well as dynamic information about their activities. Subsequently, organizations develop their ambitions further, and these are more focused on using network technology for internal communication purposes. Next, organizations start to develop more advanced interactive functions of the internet in their communication with the environment.

The internal communication orientation could be explained by various motives. Firstly, to enhance the effectiveness and efficiency of the internal communication, e.g. the Association of Women's Interests. Secondly, to create value that is exclusively available for the members. This might have been the dominant motive of the Association of Women with a Higher Education when it decided to create a restricted section. Thirdly, to strengthen the organization's cohesion and its ability to mobilize internal support for political action, as in the case of the National Point of Support. For most organizations, however, this means that the internal communication has to proceed at 'two speeds'. Only a part of the membership is connected to the internet, the figures ranging from 10 per cent (Association of Women's Interests) to 45 per cent (WOUW Amsterdam). In the Association of Women's Interests it was decided that members with email have to 'adopt' members without email. Two organizations (KVO and VVAO) are in a process to connect the local branches. Of the 250 branches of the KVO, approximately 15 per cent are online; of the 33 VVAO branches approximately two-third are online at the time of writing.

As to the effects of internet use, some impact on the ways in which organizations mobilize resources, maintain their relations with the environment and try to manage frames is noticeable. As can be inferred from the interviews, until now the result seems to be largely more effectiveness and efficiency in existing action repertoires. The internet has supported organizations in the dissemination and retrieval of information, at a lower cost than was previously feasible, in the recruitment of members and subscribers and in the management of projects with other organizations, particularly on the international level. It has provided organizations with better possibilities to expose the organization's mission, the issues and problems it addresses. There are also a few examples of innovations. The Association of Women's Interests reported that it is proceeding to a more integrated approach of its magazine and its website. The way in which the new website of the National Point of Support is soliciting women to forward their experiences with welfare regulations and agencies can be seen as an innovation, although this fits more or less within its existing practices. The Catholic Women's Organization (KVO) has found that, since it adopted an online presence, it has more opportunities to exert influence on the policy-making of other organizations.

Representative organizations

Three organizations were studied: the Netherlands Council of Women (NVR), Women's Alliance and TIYE International (the umbrella organization of 12 organizations of black, migrant and refugee women). They are the main umbrella organizations in the Dutch women's movement. The three organizations differ considerably as to their financial and staff resources. Their internet uses, in particular their site development, follow these differences closely. The NVR has been online since 1998. The board of the organization faced many problems, especially as a result of limited personnel and financial resources, in developing and maintaining a website that offers more than static information about the organization. The website of the Women's Alliance, online since 1996, is more developed. It offers a wealth of information about current activities. Much of its documentation (reports, press releases, etc.) can be downloaded. During the course of 2001–2002, its website was fully reorganized. Two interactive features were added, a discussion forum and a provision to forward questions and remarks. TIYE International has been online since spring 2002. Due to a lack of resources, the organization did not succeed in realizing its internet ambitions at an earlier time.

The internet ambitions of the NVR and the Alliance are both directed at strengthening relations with their member organizations. The Alliance intends to build an intranet. With this, it aims to strengthen support of its members for the organization's political work without doing harm to its decisiveness. Network technology enables political umbrella organizations to combine internal support and external effectiveness. The NVR has the same interactive ambitions with the internet, in particular to strengthen its platform function. It also perceives the potentialities of the internet as enabling the organization to enlarge its membership, so as to include networks that do not possess a corporate personality. In this field, the NVR faces increasing disintermediation. The internet ambitions of TIYE International have a more external focus. The TIYE board sees the internet in the first instance as an indispensable instrument in national and international lobbying.

Supportive organizations

Two of the three supportive organizations in the sample, the International Information Centre and Archives for the Women's Movement (IIAV) and E-Quality (an expert organization on gender and ethnic relations) are, according to size of staff, the most prominent supportive organizations at the national level. The Foundation Women's Centre Amsterdam was also included in the research.

The IIAV offers a vast amount of information resources and is nowadays one of the main international actors on information provision for the women's movement. It initiated the European Women Action 2000 website for facilitating global strategies for enhancing the position of women. The website of E-Quality functions mainly as an information outlet, but offers also some interactive facilities in the 'interactive expertise center'. The Women's Centre Amsterdam provides the portal site 'Women's Square'. It edits a digital bulletin board, which also fulfils a mobilizing function.

Service organizations experience a strong incentive to integrate the internet in their daily operations. For the IIAV, information provision is its core business. With its sizeable staff of information specialists, the organization was able to informatize its work effectively. Its ambition to develop the organization to a 'virtual information centre' entails a *transformation* of all aspects of the organization, notably the relationship with the clients. The Women's Centre Amsterdam has seized the potential of the internet to create a new profile of its mission, to facilitate feminist activities. This organization proceeded to offer internet courses for activists of grassroots organizations within the women's movement, established a public terminal and was one of the initiators of the portal site Women's Square. By this *innovation* of its action repertoire, the foundation also succeeded in enhancing its financial autonomy.

Virtual organizations

The organizational infrastructure of the Dutch women's movement has been enlarged by a number of virtual organizations. Firstly, several information portals have been established. Women's Net and Women's Square were both initiated in 1995–1996 after positive reaction to computer network activities during the UN Conference on Women in

Beijing. The portal Women's Net formulated two aims: (1) to enlarge the access to information that is important for women and to make it more widely known, and (2) to stimulate cooperation and to facilitate communication between women's organizations. The network is managed by a steering group on which the IIAV, E-Quality and a provincial Emancipation Office are represented. As the network functioned in practice, it succeeded in serving its first aim. The network has been conducive to the visibility and accessibility of women's organizations and groups. It was less successful in furthering cooperation, mobilization and discussion. As organizations appropriated the internet, they invested their scarce resources in their own internet activities, rather than involving themselves in Women's Net.

The Women's Square has created a profile as a network of women's organizations in Amsterdam. The Square provides links to more than 100 organizations. It also provides a bulletin board on which activities and events are made public, as well as links to ongoing discussions. The Women's Square was an initiative of the Digital City of Amsterdam (DDS) and the Women's Centre Amsterdam. DDS offered a virtual space of 'squares' on which social and political organizations and groups could present themselves on the internet (Francissen and Brants 1998). As the Centre developed its own internet expertise and commercial providers came to offer cheaper arrangements, the balance of costs and benefits of the relationship with the Digital City of Amsterdam became less favourable. The Women's Square is now one of the internet services of the Women's Centre Amsterdam.

In 2000 the website Emancipation.nl was set up by the Joke Smit Foundation, initially with the aim of disseminating publications of and information about the Dutch feminist Joke Smit (1933–1981). Soon, this objective was broadened to cover emancipation issues and policies. Its website expanded very rapidly and is now a huge portal to information resources such as newspaper articles, press releases and publications. It also provides various links to emancipation sites, to records about emancipation themes and to the major government information resources on emancipation. Emancipation.nl entered into cooperation with the IIAV.

A common feature of the three information sites is that they are all set up and managed by supportive organizations. This underlines the importance of supportive organizations within the organizational infrastructure of the Dutch women's movement, and possibly of social movements in general.

A second category of virtual organizations are the *web organizations* or *virtual communities*. Looking at the gender dimension within this field (cf. van Zoonen 2000), two virtual communities were chosen in this study: (1) the Dutch branch of Webgrrrls (Women on the Web.nl), a mailing list for women in computers and (2) Maroc.nl girls, a discussion list that existed within the site of Maroc_nl. Both web organizations can be taken as forming a new type of grassroots organization representing 'cultural politics' (Giddens 1991), in particular those social practices that are oriented towards empowerment and self-construction by individual agents. Women on the Web.nl has been characterized by Van den Boomen (2000) as a combination of cultures of self-help, work, identity and passion. Visitors on Maroc.nl girls discuss topics such as love, careers and Islam. In contrast to the other virtual organizations in the sample, these web organizations have no institutional relationships with the women's movement. The editorial board of Maroc.nl explicitly stated that they do not consider themselves to be linked to the women's movement. Women on the Web.nl has no political aims, nor does it stand for a feminist philosophy. Still, with regard to ICTs, it gives substance to the idea of empowerment, and in its ICT-related activities it contributes to the development of ICT expertise within the women's movement.

A third category is *platform organizations* for mobilization and lobbying. In this subfield it is more difficult to find appropriate cases. In 2002 the Women's Alliance launched the website www. emancipatiepolitiek.nl to further the implementation of the Platform of Action – the recommendations of the UN Conference on Women in Beijing (1995) – on the local level. The site informs policy-makers, political parties and citizens about the themes of the Platform of Action, gives examples of good practice and shows citizens how they can influence municipal policies. In 2000 the IIAV initiated the European and North-American Women Action Network (www. enawa.org) with the aim of empowering NGOs to participate in global strategies to enhance the position of women. It started with the review process of the agreements made at the Beijing Conference. The website provided a platform to search for information, to collaboratively prepare and strategize, to hold critical discussions and to find other organizations for lobbying.

Conclusions

My research centred on how the internet is reshaping the organizational infrastructure of the Dutch women's movement and what impact these changes have on the capacity of the movement to perform its intermediary political functions. Following the conceptual scheme, two sub-questions have to be addressed. Firstly, how existing 'physical' organizations use the internet and how these uses influence their capacity to articulate problems, mobilize resources and maintain relations with their environment. Secondly, which new, 'virtual' organizations have come into being and how they contribute to the movement's organizational capacity.

It was estimated that by early 2002 approximately 40–50 per cent of the grassroots organizations within the movement had their own website. The website development of the six grassroots organizations that were included in this study follows the organizations' main orientation on external (political) or internal (social) activities. The two external-oriented organizations in the sample have the most extensive websites, along with one of the more internal-oriented organizations that developed a new website with a restricted, members-only section. 'Extensive' means that the website offers static and dynamic information about the organization and its activities, background information about the problem area that the organization addresses, and some interactive features.

As to the three representative or 'umbrella' organizations, the differences in the development of their internet uses are great. Inequalities in available resources seem to be of even more importance to the potential of representative organizations to develop websites to meet their ambitions than in the case of grassroots organizations. The internet uses of supportive organizations are the most developed. Furthermore, supportive organizations were also active in initiating several virtual organizations, especially information portals.

The virtual organizations add a new layer to the movement's organizational infrastructure. In this field there is, first of all, a strong presence of information portals. The same holds true for the virtual communities of women. They have the same functions as the movement associations within the movement, such as social encounter and self-help. However, if we take self-identification as a standard, the virtual communities seem to stand outside the institutional women's movement. As a third category, and the most recent addition to the organizational infrastructure, two platform organizations were looked at. They contribute to the mobilizing and lobbying capacity of the movement. Together, these virtual organizations give a picture of what may constitute a new infrastructure for the movement in the virtual domain:

- portal sites with links to organizations, groups and networks
- a common information and knowledge pool

- communities for empowerment, identity-construction and mutual learning
- platform sites for mobilization, lobbying and interactive policy-making.

The conclusion is that the internet is reshaping the organizational infrastructure of the women's movement. The impact is most visible in the movement's increased capacity for mobilizing resources. To a lesser extent, there are also effects in the management of frames. The movement's internet uses are giving more exposure to emancipation and gender issues. However, the interactive functions on the websites of organizations in the physical domain are still in their infancy. This research has yielded only some indications as to the effects on the movement's relations with the environment. Platform sites, for example, may provide new channels for 'interactive' policy-making on emancipation issues. These facilities are, at the time of writing, in an initial phase of their development. The findings lend support to Davis' conclusions (Davis 1999) that interest groups and social movement-related organizations are, although not always 'rapidly', becoming internet-enabled and that the scenarios of disintermediation do not match reality. Furthermore, the finding that several virtual organizations are set up by established supportive organizations even suggests that the existing organizational patterns are being *reinforced* (cf. Danziger *et al.* 1982). However, a qualification has to be made with respect to the virtual communities, as these seem to stand outside the (institutional) women's movement. Further research is needed to reveal whether the virtual communities will prove to be more attractive competitors of the 'traditional' grassroots organizations, or, alternatively, will prompt women to join these organizations. In the latter case, there will be a reintermediation of the (Dutch) women's movement instead of the opposite. As Van Aelst and Walgrave (2001) have argued, although the availability of new communication technologies makes traditional organizations somewhat dispensable for mobilization purposes, a certain institutionalization remains necessary in order to exert a more lasting political influence.

Notes

1 Figures suggest that, in this respect, the Dutch women's movement follows the pattern of 'old' intermediaries such as political parties. In the period 1980–1996, the churches lost 10 per cent of their membership, women's organizations about 25 per cent and political parties about 40 per cent (Sociaal en Cultureel Planbureau, 1998).

2 For the purposes of this chapter, the internet encompasses (a) the world wide web and (b) communication technologies such as email.

3 His sample included 80 interest groups, 41 of them *public* interest groups.

4 The distinction between 'physical' organizations and 'virtual' organizations is an analytical one. By going online, 'physical' organizations gain a virtual existence, whereas many 'virtual' organizations also develop an existence in 'real life'.

5 On the character of virtual communities in comparison with organic communities, see Van Dijk (1996).

6 This means that I do not take 'self-identification' as a criterion for including an organization within the movement. I follow Outshoorn (2000) in this.

7 This concurs with Olson's view that political lobbying can be seen as a by-product of organizations that have the capacity to mobilize a group with 'selective incentives'. These can be social or recreational benefits to its members (Olson, 1965). The combination of these activities may also be taken as resulting from the coexistence of instrumental and identity-directed orientations within the women's movement.

8 Kriesi (1996) takes this category as the outcome of an institutionalization process in which a movement creates its own representatives in institutional politics, namely political parties and interest groups.

Appendix

Grass roots organizations with an internal and an external function

Netherlands Association of Women's Interests, Women's Labour and Equal Citizenship
www.vrouwenbelangen.nl

This organization was founded in 1894 as the Association for Women's Suffrage. After the realization of women's suffrage in 1919, the organization broadened its aim towards equality for men and women in political as well as in socioeconomic and other societal areas. The actual membership is about 800. The association went online in 1996, and was one of the first Dutch women's organizations with a website of its own.

National Point of Support of Women on Social Security
www.bijstandsvrouwen.nl

At the end of the 1970s the first local committees of women on social security were established. In 1984 the national 'point of support' was founded. Broadly, it fulfils a lobbying function towards the national policy-makers, and a coordination and communication function towards the (80–90) local committees. The organization is subsidized by the Department of Public Health, Welfare and Sport. Still, it is primarily dependent on volunteers. The website of the organization has existed since 1999.

WOUW-Amsterdam
www.xs4all.nl/~wouw

WOUW-Amsterdam (Wijze Oude Wijven: 'Wise Old Women'), founded in 1991, aims to increase the influence and the esteem of older women in society. It combines various social as well as political activities. The association has 230 members. It started its internet activities in 1996, following experiences during the UN World Conference on Women in Beijing (1995).

Netherlands Association of Women with Higher Education (VVAO)
www.vvao.nl

The VVAO was founded in 1918, with the aim of strengthening the mutual ties between women with an academic education. Soon the association was also addressing policy issues. The VVAO has about 5000 members, in 33 local branches. Since 1999, it has had its own website.

Catholic Women's Organization (KVO)
www.vrouwen.net/zijactief

The KVO is one of four organizations of Catholic women living in rural areas. It was founded in 1921. With 25,000 members (in 250 local branches), this is the largest organization in our sample. It combines a wide array of social and educational activities with interest representation. The first internet initiatives date from 1998/1999.

Network for Black and Migrant Women with a Higher Education
www.netwerk-zmv.nl

This organization was founded in 1989 with the objectives (1) to further a more positive image of black and migrant women in society, (2) to stimulate mutual contacts and (3) to influence government policies. In the current action repertoire, the last objective has been dropped. The organization has been online since 1998.

Representative organizations

The Netherlands Council of Women (NVR)
www.nederlandsevrouwenraad.nl
The NVR was founded in 1898. The council brings together 54 national women's organizations. It aims to fulfil a platform function, a 'mouthpiece' function and a representation function. The board characterizes the council as a 'classical, rather closed middle field organization'. The organization has two (part-time) staff; it receives some project subsidies from the national government. The NVR has been online since 1998.

Women's Alliance
www.vrouwenalliantie.nl
The alliance is a collection of 45 organizations. It originated from a merger of two organizations, founded in the early 1980s, that addressed issues of economic independence and redistribution of (paid and unpaid) labour. In comparison with the NVR, the Alliance is more directed at exerting influence on policies. The Alliance receives a structural subsidy from the Ministry of Social Affairs and Employment. It has six part-time staff. The organization developed its first website in 1996.

TIYE International
www.tiye-international.org
This is an umbrella organization of 12 organizations of black, migrant and refugee women. It was founded in 1994 with the aim of improving the social participation, participation in political decision-making and economic independence of black, migrant and refugee women. The organization is directed at influencing policy-making at the national, European and global levels, and is almost completely dependent on volunteers. It has been online since 2002.

Supportive organizations

Foundation Women's Centre Amsterdam
www.vrouwenhuis.nl
The Women's Centre Amsterdam provides various facilities to organizations (of women), persons, politics and government to support emancipation processes. These facilities include the renting of rooms and offices, a library and an internet support point. Founded in 1973, the Centre can be seen as an offspring of the second feminist wave.

With three staff members, the degree of professionalization has been kept low. The foundation is subsidized by the city of Amsterdam.

E-Quality
www.e-quality.nl

In 1997 the Ministry of Social Affairs and Employment took the initiative of founding a new institute to support emancipation developments. As a result of this initiative, E-Quality was founded as a merger between four expert organizations in the field of emancipation. E-Quality's goal is 'to improve the quality of society by stimulating equality in gender and ethnic relations'. It wants to be a centre of expert knowledge, thereby to initiate and participate in public discussions and to influence public policy. E-Quality has about 20 staff members and is subsidized by the Ministry of Social Affairs and Employment.

International Information Centre and Archives for the Women's Movement (IIAV)
www.iiav.nl

The IIAV, founded in 1935, is the centre of information provision in the Netherlands on the position of women. Its core tasks are the development and preservation of a specialized scientific library, a documentation centre and an archive. It has a staff of about 35. The centre receives a structural subsidy from the Ministry of Social Affairs and Employment and from the University of Amsterdam.

Virtual organizations

(a) Information portals

Women's Net
www.vrouwen.net

Women's Net was initiated as a resulting of positive reactions to the computer network activities during the UN Beijing Conference in 1995. The network is coupled to Antenna, which was the representative in the Netherlands of the worldwide APC Network (Association for Progressive Communications). Women's Net has two aims: (1) to improve access to information that is important for women and to make it more widely known, and (2) to stimulate cooperation and to facilitate communication between women's organizations. The network is a host for a lot of Dutch women's organizations. Part of its content is only accessible to members. In this closed layer, various foreign networks, newsgroups and online conferences can be found. The Women's Net has a steering group in which the IIAV, E-Quality and a provincial Emancipation Office are represented.

Women's Square
www.vrouwenplein.nl
This initiative was launched in 1996 by the Women's Centre Amsterdam in cooperation with the Digital City of Amsterdam (DDS). DDS offered a virtual space of 'squares' on which social and political organizations and groups could present themselves on the internet. The squares were interconnected so as to form a huge portal for Amsterdam 'civil society'. Since 2000 the Women's Square has been a service of the Women's Centre Amsterdam.

Emancipation.nl
www.emancipatie.nl
This website was set up in 2000 by the Joke Smit Foundation to disseminate publications of and information about the Dutch feminist Joke Smit (1933–1981). Soon, this objective was broadened to cover emancipation processes as well as emancipation policies. This website expanded very rapidly to several hundred pages.

(b) Platform organizations

European and North-American Women Action Network
www.enawa.org
This network was an initiative of the IIAV with the aim of empowering NGOs to participate in global strategies to enhance the position of women. It started with the review process of the results of agreements made at the Beijing Conference. The review congress took place in 2000 in New York.

Emancipatiepolitiek.nl
www.emancipatiepolitiek.nl
This site was set up by the Women's Alliance in 2002 to further the implementation of the Platform of Action – the recommendations of the UN Conference on Women in Beijing (1995) – on the local level. The site informs policy-makers, political parties and citizens about the themes of the Platform, and shows citizens how they can influence municipal policies.

(c) Web organizations

Women on the Web.nl
www.womenontheweb.nl
This website is the successor of the Dutch branch of Webgrrls. It is a virtual meeting place for women interested in computer technology, as well as for other business purposes and informal contacts. About 4000 women participate in the mailing lists of the network. It is also possible to become a member in the 'classical' sense (with membership dues); there are about 500 members.

Maroc.nl girls.
www.maroc.nl
This discussion list formed part of the site of Maroc_nl. This website was established by the foundation Maroc_nl, which aims at improving the access to digital communication functions for (ethnic) minorities in the Netherlands. Topics have to do with, for instance, intimate personal relationships, careers and Islam.

10 Dis@bled people, ICTs and a new age of activism

A Portuguese accessibility special interest group study

Rita Cheta

The relationship between disability social movements (DSMs)[1] and new technologies is crucial to understanding the problems of DSM identity politics, its framing, transformation and evolution. Identity politics and framing analyses (discussed below) are interlinked within a social constructionist approach. We see identity politics as a mode of political activism typically, though not exclusively, initiated by groups excluded from traditional mainstream politics. Such marginalized groups generate a self-designated identity that is substantiated by both the individual and collective identities of its constituents. Social movement organizations (SMOs) lay claim to certain rights drawn from the inseparability of politics and collective and individual actors (Duyvendak 1995; Gergen 1995).

With the concept of framing, social movement (SM) theory problematizes the 'values', 'issues' and 'interests' that provide an entire SM common pattern of perception, interpretation and a sense of direction in action. Rather than assuming that SMOs pursue interests that are given, the values and preferences of collective actors are seen as resulting from a process that develops over time and which may seek to achieve goals such as challenging the dominant codes of society (Melucci 1989), broadening the arena of the political (Gamson 1996), (re)presenting the views of a particular constituency to a wide audience (Edwards and Hulme 1992), and raising the consciousness of the latent members of the social movement (Campbell and Oliver 1996).

An analysis of the Portuguese Accessibility Special Interest Group (GUIA) as a case study demonstrates the uniqueness of this disability SMO. At the level of information and communication technologies (ICTs), it shows the possibilities of reframing the master frame on disability and technologies. It is also a good example of a communicative means of protest. The goal here is to study these two principal dimensions, framing for change and mobilizing for change, as discussed below, at several levels:

- to understand how GUIA contributed to redefining/challenging outdated frames on disability and new technologies
- to identify the framing processes that underlie GUIA's actions
- to analyse how GUIA has launched a new ethos and new *modus operandi* with repercussions at the national, European and international levels, during its short timespan
- to illustrate some of the most striking GUIA initiatives, such as the popularity achieved with the first electronic petition to improve internet accessibility launched in Portugal and Europe and GUIA's online protests for multiple accessibility to ICT.

Through this case study, we present a dual strategy that characterizes a new ethos and style of mobilization of GUIA within the DSMs: the definition of the ICT accessibility principle as a core value of framing identity, and the mobilization and management of ICTs as means of protest.

Methodology

Methodologically, the study relies on interviews with the GUIA co-ordinator[2] and representatives of other Portuguese and international DSMs with Portuguese affiliates. The results allow contextualization of the emergence and development of DSM, and the identification of the main 'master frames' that emerge from the relationship between disability and technology (from 'medical–rehabilitative technologies' to 'empowering technologies' and 'enabling technologies') so that they correspond to different aspects of identity politics.

A content analysis of GUIA's website (www.acessibilidade.net) is also used. The site offers access to a large archive of this DSM's campaigns and activities during its two-year existence from December 1998 to January 2001. It includes all GUIA newsgroup and mailing list messages, coverage of all events and campaigns, conferences, legislative documents, e-books, e-guides, online training kits and software tools on accessibility; some new media services testers, online assessment reports and recommendations on accessibility to ICT and new media, and other materials.

Development of the disability social movement in Europe and in Portugal

The development of the international disability social movements

For the disability social movements (DSMs), the technological issue was associated with the dynamic of reconceptualization of its identity politics during the second half of the twentieth century. In the 1950s and 1960s, based on a medical and rehabilitative perspective, the normalization of people with disabilities (PWDs) was proposed through 'politics of care or rehabilitation' (an approach based on welfare aimed at individual intervention composed within medical criteria of impairments) that favoured the development of what we may call 'care technologies' (assistive technologies that aim to compensate individuals' personal impairments or handicaps). The disability movement supported the sectoral development of new technologies aimed at finding adaptive solutions for different impairments. It also favoured the organization of its redistribution through a delivery system of assistive technologies based on an eligibility principle as defined by medical and bureaucratic powers (WHO 1980; Hutton 1995; Johnson and Moxon 1998).

Disability was produced as a particular social fact, as an individual problem requiring medical treatment to gain access to a process of bodily and intellectual normalization. Old age has become a similar construction under the capitalist mode of (re)production that emphasizes the value of ableism,[3] scrutinized by both medical professionalism and labour market exclusion. Capitalist work, medicine, and bureaucracy have played an important role in shaping the construction of disability – as the incomplete and imperfect self, as a dual object of pity–charity and of expert management – in modern times (Oliver 1990, 1999; Hughes 1999).

The transition to late modernity has led to demands for the inclusion of those previously excluded, in the sense that the shift in the mode of historicity in western societies corresponds to a shift in the central struggle of those societies (Touraine 1981b). Consequently, the interpretation of disability as an individual medical problem, addressed to a politics of care managed within the context of social welfare rights, came under attack, and attempts to construct a notion of disability in a social and political form commensurate with integration rather than rehabilitation, and empowerment rather than normalization, have been appearing in the sociopolitical agenda. An alternative approach to disability issues – the sociopolitical model of disability – was produced from within a new sector of the disability social movement led by disabled academics,[4] who have been supporters of the *Disabled People's International* movement, and became prominent during the United Nations Decade of Disabled People (1983–92).

During the 1980s, this sociopolitical perspective displaced the locus of transformation from internal variables of the individual (impairments) to external variables (living environments, social representations of disability, cultural attitudes, etc.). Correspondingly, the development of 'empowering or emancipatory technologies' is fostered within rights-based initiatives, which act at a situational level in the transformation of 'disabling environments' (i.e. the contexts of daily interaction such as school, work, housing), and at a more structural level in the changing of modern social institutions that reproduce the 'ideology of disablement' (medicine, state, law, education, mass media). This renewal of the agenda results from the reconceptualization of the 'disability dominant' notion into a framework of 'politics of civil rights' and 'collective empowerment', based on principles of 'equal opportunities'.

Disability is a sociological notion that addresses the disabled people's power (and powerlessness) experiences and attempts to focus on those aspects of disabled people's lives which 'can' and 'should' be changed in order to reverse the unequal distribution of power and its benefits and opportunities in society (Barnes and Oliver 1991). From this approach, the memory of disability is reconstructed and its categorizations are contested as social constructions of modernity and its dominant institutions (medicine, bureaucratic state, law, school education, mass media). The notion of disability is then redefined and operationalized in order to develop specific programmes and politics for the defence of disabled people's civil rights, and it is incorporated into the 'master frame' of the emancipatory politics of the disability movement. Traditionally, 'disabled' defines internal (physically–bodily) and individual features of people with disabilities, which address themselves as objects of rehabilitative care provided by the organizations of the welfare state. 'Disability' defines an external imposition of a powerless status on disabled people, which is socially and politically changeable. Therefore, people with disabilities are more likely to be seen as subjects of social transformation than as objects of welfarism (Oliver 1993; Oliver and Barnes 1998).

Some major aspects are highlighted by this emancipatory politics, such as the citizenship rights of disabled people; the right of disabled people to be involved in the design and production of their own welfare going beyond the ideology of care; a need for a political mobilization of disabled people (and their constituency as a political pressure group) in reaction to the commitment between the development of social policies that tend to reproduce the power structures of realpolitik; publicizing the social and environmental barriers to the achievement of self-reliance and full equality of opportunities by disabled people; and resistance to discrimination perpetuated by the bureaucratic system of social compensations for PWDs, among others (Barnes and Oliver 1991; Davis 1996; Finkelstein 1992; Fitzgerald 1997; Geiecker 1995; Johnson and Moxon 1998; Thornton 1993). By raising and contesting the legitimacy of the processes of medicalization and bureaucratization of disability (and the exclusionary practices faced by disabled people in school, employment and housing) and by asking for alternatives, this new approach serves to challenge the normative structure of society.

Since the mid-1990s, in a context of maturity of the sociopolitical perspective, a political pragmatism has emerged interested in re-examining the very construct of 'disability'. It is at the core of the framing process of the disability movement which re-vindicates the universalism of ICT use in the transition to the information mode of (re)production, which in turn no longer depends on conditioned access resulting from an eligibility system, but on a lifestyle choice in a universal accessibility context. In the information-network society, the aim is to act at the level of institutional change through media and technology, which play an increasingly important role in social organization. Moreover, as it claims to drive an action-based philosophy and change-related action, and to channel it directly to public debate and public opinion, it is in itself a direct challenge to the dominant structures and systems that are, in turn, indifferent to communicative action and debate (Finkelstein and Stuart 1996; Roe 1991; Sapey 2000; Thornton 1993). The disability movement may have currently gained a transitional status characterized by both engagement in the conflict over distribution of assistive technologies that the welfare state can provide (typical from the 1960s and 1970s) and, simultaneously, struggling in new conflicts over the new media and ICT market that arose in several domains (e.g. social integration, cultural reproduction, socialization, consumerism) during the 1980s and 1990s as a response to structural changes which engendered new problems and issues for disabled people.

The development of the Portuguese disability social movement and GUIA's context of emergence

The Portuguese disability movement[5] first developed and spread during the political democratization process after the democratic revolution in 1974. Concerned parents and professionals involved in rehabilitation and special education formed a network of grassroots associations to develop a political agenda. The aim was to publicise PWD needs and demands in terms of qualified services that would break the cycle of exclusion and isolation of PWDs in the domains of health, education, professional training and employment. Simultaneously, the Portuguese SMOs started supplying some services to fill the void left by the state. In the early 1980s, the disabled movement mainly developed to provide 'care' and 'cure' services through an articulated system that brought together SMOs by sector and the national state. Their policies were designed to plan, manage and run expertise services for PWD in health, education and training supported by welfare clusters.

As a result, Portuguese disability welfarism was, and still is, organized on differing levels of responsibility, funding and service types. These include a plethora of national and regional co-ordinating SMOs and local action-oriented SMOs relying strongly on state funding for project eligibility. As a consequence of this bureaucratization/institutionalization process, the Portuguese disabled movement became strongly institutionalized. It is a movement constituted by dozens of SMOs 'for' and 'of' disabled people which are hierarchical, fragmented and sectorialised (by types of impairment), professionalized, service-provision-oriented and government-dependent.

Critics of the development of the disability social movement in Portugal and new generations of related SMOs may be divided into several groups. Some lambaste the absence of autonomy and of a real 'emancipatory politics'. Others contest the hybrid model that appears to confuse representative democracy with participatory democracy (whereby it is not clear where governmental politics end and other social actors' action begins) because of the absorption of disability SMOs into the *status quo* of welfarism. There are also criticisms of the incapacity of a transformation inspired by the sociopolitical model drawn from the international disability movement that would turn 'the disabled movement' into a 'disability movement'. However, advocates of DSMs also exist. Some praise the role of SMOs in the initial definition of the national rehabilitation system. Others support the existing model, which reflects the social and political context of the emergence of this social movement and its possible trajectories of survival and development. Lastly there are those who compromise within a matrix of 'legitimized politics', which simultaneously generates renewal from the centre and incorporates the 'willingness for change' protest that occurs at its threshold.

GUIA is a very small and flexible SMO without an associational or sectoral base. It started as an informal, online, activist network that had no physical address but existed merely in cyberspace. Its main goal was to improve ICT accessibility for all citizens. Its activity focused on negotiating between ICT enterprises and the political–legislative camp to bridge the divide between the private and public sectors. It lobbied for the inclusion of PWD and the wider public in general, relevant decision-making. It also advocated consumer rights in an information society that was, increasingly, undermined by a market mentality. It strategically articulated the dialogue between the private sector's production interests and the government's regulatory obligations to protect ICT use by its citizens. As it is led by experts and strategically oriented toward parliamentary lobbying, we could categorize GUIA as one of what Campbell and Oliver (1996) define as old social movements that tend to campaign on single issues. However, the literature on new social movements clarifies some other facets/ forms of action, which are also evident in relation to GUIA.

New social movements are recognized to be oriented philosophically and in terms of action to 'alleged innovation in their non-productivist analysis of society' (Burgmann 1993: 5), 'to tap the failure of NGOs to make the right linkage between their work and the wider systems and structures of which they form a small part' (Edwards and Hulme 1992: 13); to be actively involved in the construction of a reflexive democracy rather than a reflective democracy, based on a model of participatory rather than representative democracy (Humphrey 1999); to seek change in cultural, symbolic and political domains, at times collectively but also sometimes by the way of self-change (Melucci 1989). Also, from an organizational point of view, new social movements tend to be flexible, informal and virtual.

If we focus on the criteria presented by Campbell and Oliver (1996) to evaluate a new social movement aimed at disability rights, the following stand out: the extent of consciousness-raising and empowerment of people with disabilities, the promotion of disability rights from human and civil rights perspectives, reframing the core values; the extent to which disability issues are raised beyond the national scale, and new fields of embededness of discussion and action; the experiencing of new means of protest and mobilization.

Models of SMOs: social movements, identity politics and framing analysis

In order to elucidate GUIA's role in the symbolic construction, mainte-nance and negotiation of a collective identity and framing relying on technology and new media, in which ICTs play a role, some theoretical remarks on social movements, identity politics and framing are now given.

Framing for change: how ICTs penetrate to the very heart of dis-ability politics, aiming to negotiate the reinterpretation of a core ideological problem – the relationship between disability and new tech-nologies in late modernity, its dimensions, causes and potential frame-works of action. Which framing processes underline the changes? (Snow *et al.* 1986; Snow and Benford 1988; Melucci 1989; Gamson 1996; Tarrow 1998; Crossley 2001).

Mobilizing for change: which roles do ICTs play in the mobilization of encounters, discussion and publicity of the disability social move-ment? To what extent are ICTs central for a new style of communica-tional protest launched by the DSMs (Tilly 1978; Klandermans 1989; Shakespeare 1993; Gamson 1996; Tarrow 1998)?

Framing analysis develops an approach that reflects the 'problems and issues' around which movements tend to mobilize. The notions of frame and framing clearly point out questions of meaning, culture and interpretation on the agenda of SMOs. Since 'frames' are constitu-tive aspects of the subjectivity of social agents from which those agents cannot detach themselves (Crossley 1996), they act like an ethos. A central concern of the collective action of the disability movement, globally, has been the attempt to change the way in which PWDs are perceived, and the frames applied to them. 'Disability politics' defines the framework of action of the DSM by changing the technological framing in the context of the information society. Disability politics aims at the transformation of disabilities into abilities, of needs into rights and into lifestyles, on the grounds that actions need to be set up concerning the disabled people's interests and should be conducted by themselves rather than by the welfare state (Campbell and Oliver 1996; Johnson and Moxon 1998). This involves a politics of identity that concerns questions of recognition, representation and dominance of certain cultural codes in institutionalized contexts or fields of fram-ing, such as the media, political, medical, and academic fields.

Therefore, questions of who represents the disability movement, who defines its core values, in what contexts and so on, have signi-ficant implications. Hence, movements may experience a different balance of opportunities and constraints in the various fields in which they engage, and they will most certainly find that they are required to play a different game in each of these fields (Crossley 2001). Indeed, the media game is quite different from the legal game, which is dissimilar from the parliamentary game and the academic game; and we need to be aware of this if we are to analyse struggles that traverse these domains. This leads us to the assumption that 'the aim of new movements is to bring about changes within these particular fields. In the more traditional and formal, political and legal fields' (Crossley 2001: 158); we would say that both the market and the new media should be added as significant fields or contexts of framing in late modernity.

Drawing from the GUIA case study, we would argue that this SMO acted on at least at four levels, according to a framing analysis.

First, it dislocated the question of new technologies, through the problem of 'accessibility' of ICTs as a core problem of framing for the disability movement and the concept of 'disability' itself. Second, it reviewed the dominant disability–technology dichotomy that is inseparable from the process and structures of modern society. Third, it shifted the locus of discussion/protest from the logic of asymmetrical distribution underlying the disability policy promoted by the welfare state, to inscribe it in the fields of creativity and pre-production at the level of ICT and new media R&D and at the level of the regulation of the ICT market from the supply side. Fourth, given the strategic character of intervening at a regulatory level, GUIA placed its action towards negotiating between the political–legislative camps and the research and development and marketing of ICT. Instead of unilaterally negotiating in the public or private sector (as is normally the case with traditional SMOs), it invented methods of action and mobilizational support to intervene at strategic moments and on specific issues where sectoral issues intertwined.[6]

In this manner, GUIA acts as a centre for change-oriented resources and as an incubator of sociopolitical experiences within a participatory matrix. GUIA ensures that PWDs and other potential users are neither forgotten nor excluded from influencing decisions made by the dominant forces in the ICT and new media market. It participates in discussions regarding development and regulation and creates a parallel avenue for experimentation, testing, participation, advertising, and reviewing what would otherwise remain exclusively mainstream interests. As a result, it has become a major player which cannot be ignored.

Cooper's work (1999) is relevant here, when one considers that if the political power of disabled people may be most easily seen in traditional SMOs running 'old politics' oriented toward debating issues with governmental policy-makers, a greater cultural power may be with individuals and smaller groups working almost without funding, inspired by consciousness-raising and sociopolitical approaches, armed with anti-discriminatory legislation, and engaged in change-oriented and participatory initiatives for the new politics agenda on disability. For these groups, of which GUIA is an example, strategies focusing on politics and media attention are crucial.

Along with the visible media and legislative protests, there is an aim to seek sociocultural alternatives by promoting the emergence of a project identity, which in turn may challenge 'disablism' as a production of modernity, 'disability' as a product of a hierarchy of able-bodily identities, and the 'politics of disablement' as the politics of a 'dominant identity' and resistant 'habitus'. By challenging both the collective interpretative resources and the daily lives of disabled people, it has been promoting the emergence of a new project identity which is aimed 'at the transformation of society as a whole in the continuity with the values of communal resistance to dominant interests enacted by global flows of capital, power and information' (Castells 1997: 357).

We suggest that GUIA engaged in a new project identity. First, it showed that the time was ripe to overcome directly the interests of the established groups and challenge their interpretation of master frames on disability and technologies. Second, it demonstrated the existence of cultural, political and media opportunities that should be achieved as the costs of inactivity increased enormously. Third, it suggested that there were rewards to be obtained from action for those disability SMOs, groups and individuals that participated in protest activities through a more flexible and creative style of mobilization. Consequently, GUIA may constitute a 'pioneer' of a new ethos and *modus operandi* and may have partially reinvented the field of the disability social movements in Portugal and in the wider European Union.

We suggest that the most recent changes in the DSM framing tend to dislocate the core problem for disabled people from access towards accessibility to technologies in general, and ICTs in particular. Instead, we assume that this dislocation of focus is not independent of the redefinition of the very notions of 'disability' and 'disabled people' in the present societal context (e.g. population ageing that will raise the number of PWDs with acquired age longevity-related handicaps; the crisis of the welfare state; the emergence of the informational-network society and the worsening of the info rich/info poor gap). We question the meaning and configurations of the change led by the GUIA at two main levels of analysis: first, at the level of its politics of identity (see Table 10.1); second, at the level of its communications *modus operandi* (see Table 10.2).

Case study analysis

Framing for change: reframing from 'care politics' to 'lifestyle politics', and from 'eligibility' towards 'access' and 'accessibility' core values

We argue that three master frames on disability and technologies exist: 'care or rehabilitative technologies', 'empowering technologies' and 'enabling technologies' (see Table 10.1). These master frames differentiate the varied ethos of protest that coexists and conflicts in the midst of DSMs. They express different ways in which disability and disabled people's identities and interests can be framed. In the most traditional aspect, the implementation of 'care politics' favoured the development of 'rehabilitative technologies' guided by medical expertise and state bureaucracy, the main agents of eligibility processes and the normalization of PWDs.

From the sociopolitical perspective, the implementation of an 'emancipatory politics' gave primacy to the development of 'empowering or emancipatory technologies' able to transform PWD living environments into collective systems that assure equality and opportunity of access. Law, schools, and academia were the main areas where equality of opportunity was implemented.

In contrast to the conflictual nature of these two aspects, a more recent feature initiates a new politics on disability linking 'enabling technologies' with consumer and lifestyle politics, and if ICTs' reclamation as a potential means of transformation is not merely to constitute a novelty, then reframing based on consumers' rights to participate fully in the information society combining with a broader identity project illustrates such a linkage.

Among most disability SMOs, a strong resistance to the *interiorization* of new (or partly new) frames seems to occur predominantly, in the (still dominant) medical–rehabilitative approach and in the emancipatory sociopolitical approach. However, the findings of GUIA's experience suggest the emergence of a new ethos.

Table 10.1 Framing for change

	Master frames		
	Care, rehabilitative technologies	Empowering technologies	Enabling technologies
Identity politics/framing of protest	Care or normalization politics **Needs/eligibility principle**	Emancipatory politics Access/opportunities principle	**New politics on disability; consumer politics; lifestyle politics** Accessibility principle
Focus of protest	Social welfare users' rights (better conditions and facilities to meet needs and financial compensations)	Civil rights; minority groups' rights; Disability rights ('equal opportunities')	Consumers' rights Advocacy by theme-oriented issues (design for all on all media, from TV to ICT; accessibility on internet; on digital TV; third-generation mobile communications)
Contexts or **fields** of framing	Medicine Bureaucratic state Welfare state Capitalist mode of production	Political Academia Law School	Market (ICT and new media markets) Media (mainly internet and new media) R&D

Audience of protest	Individuals, laypersons Corporations, enterprises and other potential funders (non-technological market) Experts and professionals on medical rehabilitation and assistive technologies	Political field Academia (fields of education, social sciences, political science)	Internet users (PWDs or not) Experts and professionals on disability (worldwide networks) ICT researchers and professionals ICT corporations (multinational and transnational), ICT market Parliament (EU level, national level)
Scale of protest	National, regional sectoral	National EU International	National EU International Global
Aims of protest	Legal frameworks (general) Organizational needs Funding for assistive technologies Vocational training Rehabilitative care Segregational support environments	Legal frameworks (specific fields) Enclaves and integrative environments – housing, education, professional, employment, recreational, transport subsystems Independent living centres	R&D on accessibility of ICT and new media (disability sensitive) Communicational networks and inclusive environments – training, learning, working, sociability, living, public administration

If GUIA seems to adopt the master frame that refers to the newest structures of meaning in the disability movement ('enabling technologies'), it also seems to perform a task of communicatively 'frame bridging' its own perspective with the other actors' perspective. Both are insiders and outsiders of the disability movement, thereby moving a step forward to explore the deeper dynamics of persuasion and 'framing alignment' negotiation. In fact, GUIA shifted the thematic agenda from 'care–rehabilitative technologies' to 'empowering' and 'enabling technologies'. It became clear that a wider discourse about citizenship was emerging because the protests and campaigning did not express views or point out priorities about the rehabilitative care system and the related social services and policies. Once the 'care-and-welfare users' politics' had been addressed, should disabled people's claims be considered 'citizen politics' or 'consumer politics'? To overcome the ideology of normalization and care may not signify a solution to the problems of care. It may, instead, open the discussion of a new type of identity politics.

We must accept the hypothesis that GUIA's protest activities may not have generated a new master frame. Instead, they may have had a significant effect only in challenging and changing certain basic dispositions and strategies of some social agents, making them more available for future persuasion and actions ('frame bridging'). The process by which agents are persuaded to adopt new or partly new frames can be seen in the attempt by GUIA to bridge with the interpretative schemata of its potential constituents through the convergence in the enunciation of master frames ('frame aligning').

A good illustration of this frame alignment results from GUIA's enunciation of a new category, namely 'citizens with special needs', which has been created in order to manage the problem of disability–ICTs accessibility. That category fuses both sub-frames (social and medical) within the disability movement under the notion of PWDs with the political frame of elderly people that as a social group is said to have similar special needs to PWDs regarding accessibility to technologies issues. A range of possibilities for framing negotiation is likely to arise between the distinct master frame and its representatives.

GUIA has also attempted to amplify beliefs about the causes of discriminatory ICT research, design and social policies that rule technological services delivery systems, and the possibilities of solving those problems ('frame amplification').

One outcome of the frame amplification dimension was the firm pressure that GUIA put on the enforcement of the 'design for all principle' on ICT research and development. The universalism of the 'design for all' principle on ICT and all new media constitutes an alternative value to the 'minority rights framework' which underlines the segmentation that takes place in the assistive technology R&D, marketing, distribution and consumption. It may contribute to a repositioning of the core value of 'equal opportunities'. This construct of 'equal opportunities', whether it means that treatment and distribution of social compensations is equalized (with the PWD perceived as a welfare user) or that opportunity is to be equalized (with the PWD perceived as a consumer) (Michailakis 1997; Rosenberg 1995), is a crucial framing question which guides GUIA's calls for 'equality', 'liberation' and 'design for all' principles (on the supply side) and against 'subtle discrimination' by the market and administrative delivery systems (on the demand side).

In addition to the latter, another major concern has been to shift successfully the 'access' principle to the 'accessibility' problem, which represents a significant 'management of frames'. It comprises the challenge of administrative and professional notions of 'physical barriers' and 'virtual barriers' as elements to be challenged. Thus, GUIA made explicit two levels of understanding of the accessibility principle/ claim. First, accessibility characterizes the flexibility of information and interaction regarding the respective vehicle of ICT, which refers to the interconnection of users–environment–situation. Second, it is a more structural and institutional level of understanding which looks for new opportunities for citizens with special needs through the information society, such as new concepts of care, independent living, and new contexts of communication, learning, working, consumption, and sociability. Implicit in both is a notion of 'abilities' that claims 'enabling technologies', both as external (interaction tool) and internal (skills) features.

Consequently, GUIA created a counter-image of the disabled people/ new technologies relationship which goes beyond the conventional sector of assistive technologies which are medically and professionally driven and also of the mass media examples of misframing (Pilgrim *et al.* 1997). It also goes beyond the double principle of action 'care'– 'cure' underpinning provider professionalism based on the model of welfarism, which according to the sociopolitical approach of disability made PWDs 'patients–recipients', not 'active citizens'. The reform of the welfare state as a site of struggle is replaced by the market and R&D. The 'right of consumerism', which emphasizes the right of individual consumers to make decisions and choices according to new lifestyles, is combined with the right to participate and influence R&D, as consumer–tester groups. As a result, disabled people also seek direct consumer power through engagement with new contexts of framing.

Intervention in the shaping of the new media's role in society is foreseen as an issue of major importance. It may determine who owns, accesses, produces and controls information, images, persuasion, debate, propaganda, and other kinds of communicative action. GUIA influenced the legislative agenda of ICT and new media R&D and market segmentation in Portugal based on accessibility issues (namely on the internet, universal mobile telecommunication system (UMTS) and terrestrial digital television).

GUIA not only created the agenda but also stimulated online debates that reunited expert and lay knowledge on the grounds of disability and accessibility to new media and ICT (the public, the private and the movement sectors) at an international level. It encouraged the participation of all those interested (leaving open GUIA's membership criteria) in ICT development, design and market segmentation, policy formulation and implementation as integral parts of citizen rights and responsibilities. According to Humphrey (1999: 178), it constituted an experience of participatory and reflexive democracy that underestimated the questions of representativeness and internal organization of the group in favour of critical dialogues oriented toward the content and objectives of action. Although the GUIA members tend to highlight their successful experience of conducting the first electronic petition on web accessibility in Europe, we would argue that they tend to overestimate that event. In fact, one can only understand the depth of GUIA's new profile when analysing its articulation with the communicative *modus operandi* (its mobilizing for change strategies). We now look more extensively at content analysis of the GUIA's website, www.acessibilidade.net, to highlight the new profile.

Mobilizing for change: setting up a virtual modus operandi *through the internet*

Acts of communication presuppose certain rights of expression on the part of agents and take place within a context where speakers enjoy unequal degrees of legitimacy and privilege (Bourdieu 1992). Whose voice is privileged? Who gets to say what on behalf of whom? What means of communication are used for protest? And what effects are reached? These are questions that address the asymmetries in the power game, in which more flexible and informal SMOs (such as GUIA) may emerge in the intermediate areas not filled by more institutionalized SMOs of the disability movement and by the medical monopoly itself as the traditionally legitimated expertise system. So, along with the bridging and amplification of frames, did GUIA create transitional areas of communication previously unlikely or non-existent? And did GUIA innovate in mobilizing for protest?

Although some authors do not distinguish between the terms 'mobilizing' and 'organizing' SM, there are some differences that may have consequences at the analytical level of operationalization. Mobilizing refers to the process by which inspirational leaders or other persuaders can get large numbers of people to join an SM or engage in a particular SM action; organizing refers to a more sustained process whereby people come to understand an SM's goals deeply and empower themselves to continued action on behalf of those goals. We will mainly emphasize the importance of new forms of mobilizing DSMs on the internet, although organizing is also present in the analysis.

Goals, strategies and tactics to mobilize for change are influenced by the reframing of DSM master frames, type of DSM organization and its communicational means of protest. We call these three variables a DSMO 'communicative *modus operandi*' (see Table 10.2).

Drawing from a detailed content analysis of GUIA's website – www.acessibilidade.net – some findings may clarify particular aspects of its communicative *modus operandi*. First of all, GUIA used the internet as its main means of protest and mobilization. In fact, GUIA was born through an online mobilization that launched the first initiative of electronic democracy in Portugal legally recognized as such. While conducting the first European electronic petition for accessibility on the internet, GUIA pressured the alteration of the law of right for petition and recognition of signatures collected electronically in Portugal, to facilitate actions of mobilization through the internet. It did so through its electronic petition that collected (exclusively online) the signatures of the subscribers, which were sent by email to the national parliament and EU Council, for further recognition, approval and implementation. GUIA accompanied the rhythm of the legislative agenda, launching both proactive and reactive campaigns and sending proposals to be approved in due time, which after being approved were presented online as 'fair results' of their protest. Emphasis on the legislative/legal framework is analysed by several authors that conducted empirical studies related to the disability movement (Michailakis 1997; Crossley 1996; Cooper 1999; Jayassooria 1999).

In addition to the virtual *modus operandi*, GUIA also set up a more traditional means of protest. In fact, GUIA has constructed a strategy

Table 10.2 Mobilizing for change

	Master frames		
	Care technologies	Empowering technologies	Enabling technologies
Means of protest by type of media	Annual funding campaigns Annual sales campaigns Interviews with representatives on TV, radio, press Outdoors TV spots Concerts, sport events, etc.	TV programmes on disability issues (disabled people on the media) Events performed by PWDs (Paralympics, independent living centres, etc.) Alternative press (by DSMO) Civic/concerned marketing Conferences for experts Forums for lay people 'Open house' of disabled people, schools, training centres, living centres, etc.	TV, press ICT and telecommunication fairs and events ICT tools developed and managed by disabled people Public presentations and showcases on innovative projects Showcases on best practice Internet, websites Electronic petition Videoconferencing Newsgroups (both expert and expert–lay people)

Type of SMO organization		
Institutionalized	Self-help groups	Mailing lists (lay–expert people)
Professionalized	Development of specific applications	Websites (set up by every SMO)
Sectoralized	Intra-networks	Electronic handbooks and self-help guides
Formal membership	Technological application to specific environments (experimental tools applied to several fields, from education and training to housing)	Electronic delivery of best practice and tools
Sector-oriented		Telework
		Electronic activism
	Professionalized and self-help groups	Flexible
	Fragmented	Informal
	Management of sheltered environments	Virtual
	Situation-oriented	Theme-oriented

of message anticipation in the mass media, as well as the organization and treatment of information in its website for journalistic self-service. Although GUIA had to work through mass media to broadcast its views and sentiment tapping, its leadership was aware that mass media do not represent the interests of DSMs. For this reason GUIA created its own website, an unmediated media centre which produced and delivered its own messages, organized dossiers for mass media professionals and also for the public in general, and stored mass media coverage. Therefore, it tried to adjust the timing of the mass media field with the timing of the parliamentary field (where official legislative documents are created). It simultaneously speeded up the rhythm of the actions in its own online channel of communication, which led on the one hand to the preparation of proposals that were non-official but certified by specialists, and on the other hand to raising general support at the level of public opinion for its campaigns for accessibility on ICTs and new media. This rigorous management of resources and networking resulted in a maximization of results in terms of public opinion mobilization, political influencing and ICT R&D and market involvement/engagement. It also contributed to reducing action–reaction timings.

GUIA existed predominantly through its website; perhaps for this reason the site was named from that very mobilized thematic, the accessibility issue (www.acessibilidade.net). Constituted by an informal and flexible human structure, with only two coordinators[7] and five PWDs that participate in it occasionally, its existence materialized in the dynamization of campaigns and supporters, in discussions made through mailing lists and discussion groups, which have produced recommendations, directives and action proposals that followed the success of the first electronic petition.[8]

In terms of internal communication, GUIA innovated at the level of interaction between the DSM establishment in Portugal (which can be characterized as fragmented, sectoral and institutional) and the network of informal support and mobilization around a common objective transversal to the sectoral interests specific to DSMOs. It is important to highlight that the 'political pragmatism' style of GUIA revealed not only the ability of negotiation in the ambit of the national and international disability movement dynamics, but also the ability to read into the structural changes that determine its acting (framing and mobilizing) when power and influence on the information society are increasingly gravitating to transnational markets and bodies. Additionally, it constituted an example that demonstrated to disabled people an alternative model of mobilization to the one connected to

DSMOs; simultaneously it demonstrated to DSMOs the opportunity and the interest of online campaigning, discussion and participation in the information society.

At the level of external mobilization, GUIA stood out from the traditionally institutionalized mode of action and from an old politics profile conducted by disability-related SMOs in Portugal. It mobilized public opinion to act as a protest and pressure group directly over the actors in the political field (parliament, government, EU Council) and in the market (telecommunications and ICT corporations, regulatory bodies, experts and professionals), in support for citizens with special needs to challenge and take control of the forces which construct disablement. GUIA also stimulated unlikely interactions among actors that normally act in different fields: DSMOs and the ICTs and telecommunication sectors in the field of entrepreneurial innovation, market and consumption. GUIA's *savoir-faire* in the democratic game within the disability movement, and with the political establishment, market, R&D, academia, mass media and general public, was decisive to its successful experience. Indeed, GUIA persuaded many relevant social agents (such as several DSMOs, government, parliament, EU Commission, ICT professionals and researchers, ICT corporations, regulatory bodies, international and national academic and business experts), as well as individuals in the general public, that their already existing values logically required them to subscribe to this particular campaign for internet accessibility (and, later, accessibility to UMTS and terrestrial digital TV, etc.).

However, it is mistaken to limit the action of GUIA to its successful electronic petition on accessibility to the internet. Drawing on our main findings concerning GUIA's protest actions, it can be stated that its predominant online feature was a series of events, produced in interaction with allies, bystanders and opponents located in various fields, that came into being as various communication arrangements (electronic petition, online forum, mailing lists, online newsgroups, video-conferencing, web broadcasts, campaigning reports and documents, press releases, campaign symbols, protest posting, calendar of events). Moreover, GUIA's campaigns and actions were heavily dependent on the internet and, thereby, were widely discussed and supported on the internet. Becoming wired was not a goal in itself, but a means to achieve major goals such as: reach the public debate and gain attention and support; participate in the decision-making process; negotiate legislation and policy design; present a convergent mobilization of a wide set of DSMO profiles; ask for support from expert and peer groups at the international level; activate dialogue and partnerships across public–private sectors, expert–lay knowledge, national–EU–international levels; and aim for multidimensional achievements in legal, market, civic, political, and persuasive dimensions.

In this sense, 'be born for campaigning on the internet' may enclose a complex generative mode of existence; simultaneously a way to learn, get involved and influence the intermediary and the more diffuse areas of the power game. It may be argued that GUIA never intended to play this power game outside the system in the first place; indeed, the struggles entailed the use of parts of the system while other parts were strategically and skilfully attacked. For instance, it lobbied in order to achieve both goals at the parliamentary and EU levels, and thereby contributed to the significant process of legislative production and recommendation for actions concerning accessibility to ICT issues for disabled people.[9] But it also speeded up the legal process of validity of electronic petitions when it created the first electronic petition officially recognized in Europe.[10] Furthermore, GUIA's website – www.acessibilidade.net – has constituted a model for best practice in the application of WAI[11] rules, and has imposed public debate and its regulation on websites of public administration and public corporations at national and European levels. This began as an initiative to establish its presence and assertiveness in an international plan, with objectives distributed on a national, European and international scale.

Related to this, it is important to mention that it is one of the few websites of Portuguese SMOs that is in both Portuguese and English; that has created and managed mailing lists and newsgroups on the international scale for both lay–expert and exclusively expert individuals and groups; and that has projected a non-fragmented and sectoralised image (by type of impairment) of the Portuguese disability movement. In addition, several experimental tools and testing, training and public discussion environments have been successfully created and managed online during its two years of existence. These include, *inter alia*: the 'electronic petition for Internet accessibility'; training courses on WAI rules; launching of e-books and e-guides on accessibility legislation and training; electronic delivery of best practices and tools; promoting of the voluntary self-labelling 'accessibility award' for accessible websites; PWD consumers panel for assessing new ICT solutions and implementations; expert–lay observatories on accessibility to ICT and new media; and the 'Solidarity Web' that aimed to join together all related disability SMOs in a virtual space, regardless of their traditional or new ethos, national or international locus of action. Two goals were targeted: on the one hand, to search and explore constructions of meaning most likely to come into a DSM shared agenda on ICT and new media; on the other hand, to stimulate new means of communication for internal and external mobilization, and the emergence of some transitional areas of communication not occupied by more institutionalized disability SMOs and traditional institutions. The number of grassroots DSMOs operating online and on a transnational basis is increasing rapidly, mobilizing participants from around the globe in enabling disabled people. However, the expected mushrooming of ICT e-tools and e-contents and also the development of virtual communities that would promote non-disabling environments, informal networks of testing and sharing materials, para-market sites, incubator sites for accessibility solutions, etc., is developing at a slower pace. At present these are only at the beginning of their potential development.

Lastly, it is worth mentioning that GUIA's dissolution in January 2001 was an act of communication itself: the general announcement to the press of a mission completed; the constitution of an online archive that prolongs its memory; and the decision to maintain its 'leading' mailing list (acessibilidade@egroups.com) attached to a recent but largely legitimized entity (CANTIC, an academic research centre on accessibility to ICT) to which the coordinator of GUIA belongs.

Conclusions

When examining the two-year experience of GUIA, one may wrongly assume it to be a single-issue politics group which was born to set up a new grievance in a period of latency (Melucci 1989, 1996) 'where' and 'when' opportunities were relatively open, and that consequently died when its protest became institutionalized and the value of its framing partly incorporated into the *status quo*. In fact, GUIA dis-solved after the release of the 'Accessibility Software Guidelines 1.0' and the pre-official formation of ANASOFT (National Alliance for the Software Accessibility)[12] with representatives of R&D, business, the ICT industry, government, and the Solidarity Web, and the recycling and further actions from the European Disability Forum that have furthered the manifesto on the information society and disabled people. However, according to Tarrow (1998), a more complex expla-nation may follow in which 'exhaustion' plays its part in a very small, flexible and informal SMO, as well as 'a process of institutionalization' undergone since the struggle itself has altered the institutional context.

The transformation of disability politics was pursued by GUIA as the political and social context around DSMs changed, partly due to moderate political reforms inside the welfare system, the development of the new technological domains, changes in people's minds and forms of protest, and also while power, decision-making and regulation of people's lifestyles were increasingly gravitating towards transnational networks, markets and bodies.

On the one hand, GUIA's framing for change contributed to overcoming the understanding that defines disability as a physical defect inherent in bodies, and going beyond the understanding of disability as a way of interpreting and socializing bodily differences among individuals and groups. The latter has undoubtedly been important to the understanding of PWDs as active agents that could further politicize the field of disability by themselves. But GUIA seeks to move forward in showing how PWDs, as their own advocates, become transformative agents in the field of ICT and new media development, regulation and daily/common use.

Most likely, the point is not to eradicate traditional frames and vocabularies of action. Rather, GUIA seems to have participated in the generation of a new style of cross-framing/reframing, a new consciousness, a new vocabulary of action and a range of practices. This expanding and fertilization of disability politics has acted in the intertwining of the two more democratic DSM frameworks of action: emancipatory politics/empowering new technologies and new politics on disability/ enabling new technologies.

On the other hand, GUIA's mobilizing for change has adopted a new style of mobilization through the internet. This *modus operandi* has probably been one of GUIA's most successful achievements, and a model for other DSMOs. GUIA linked grassroots organizations with international and transnational, formal and informal networks of discussion and participation on the internet. It has made an effort to deinstitutionalize and decentralize the *modus operandi* of the more traditional DSMOs. Identity politics mobilizing has become more diffuse as it has become increasingly less reserved for the arena of politics (e.g. campaigning, voting for representatives, office holding, programme and project funding) held by more traditional DSMOs. Identity politics practices are moving into the arena of daily life (e.g. in business, in consumption, in sociability, in schools, in work, in housing, in daily communicating, in R&D and market testing).

Interlinked with the transformation of disability politics in both disabling and enabling new technologies and new media, and ICT in particular, GUIA has experimented with ever-broadening and innovating forms of collaboration among actors inside and outside the DSM. As a result, a more diffused and defused collective action seems to emerge. Diffused action in terms of its expansion and cross-fertilization of means, fields and actors involved into continuing practices that may replace traditional practices of specific groups in particular places and dates. Also, defused action in terms of reducing its alienation and isolation posture by adopting and promoting a more subtle intermingling of identities and practices.

In short, if emancipatory politics and consumption–lifestyles politics converge in the generation of a new ethos and in the process of enabling technologies fostered by GUIA's multiple protest initiatives for accessibility to ICT and new media in Portugal and the EU, some more practical questions related with DSMO mobilization may remain open in the near future.

Notes

1 The adoption of the concept of **'disability movement'** instead of **'disabled people movement'** follows the approach of British social science studies on impairments and disabilities, and related activism, since the early 1980s. M. Oliver and C. Barnes have been two of the best known representatives of this field of 'disability studies', related to journals such as *Handicap, Disability and Society* and *Disability and Society*.

2 Francisco Godinho, an engineer in rehabilitation and ICT, a professor at UTAD university and researcher at CANTIC in Portugal; ex-adviser of the President of the Portuguese Republic on science and technology, and an electronic activist.

3 Ableism defines a set of principles overvalued within the capitalist society, such as work, productivity and efficiency.

4 Among others, Colin Barnes and Vic Finkelstein, researchers at the Disability Research Unit for the British Council of Disabled People (within the Department of Sociology and Social Policy of the University of Leeds), which has recently developed to a more broadly based interdisciplinary Centre for Disability Studies at the same university. Also Mike Oliver, professor of Disability Studies at the University of Greenwich.

5 There are only a few analyses of the Portuguese DSMs. One is UNICS/ UNIDE (1998) *Diagnóstico do Sistema Nacional de Reabilitação e Integração de Pessoas com Deficiência*, Relatório de Investigação, ISCTE, Lisbon.

6 It organized online forums for experts, free market tests for new products and services, experimental tests for PWD volunteers as focus or test groups, forums on dates when legislative bodies (Portuguese as well as European) were scheduled to deal with ICT regulation, mailing lists to present new proposals or alternatives, kits/modules for online training on WAI regulations for users and webmasters, troubleshooting and personalized online training, online software access WAI centre and promotion of commercial lines making compatible software solutions available, creation of a parallel online market, online petitions to lower access costs and taxes on ICT and new media solutions, electronic petitions to

regulate ICT production (especially regarding 'design for all' and WAI), diffusion of its positions to the mass media and the creation of its own media centre.

7 A researcher in rehabilitation engineering and ex-adviser of the minister of science and technology, and a computing professional who set up the first Portuguese activism website in 1998.

8 http://br.egroups.com/group/acessibilidade,   http://groups.yahoo.com/group/eeurope-pwd/, accessibility@egroups.com.

9 Decision to approve the eEurope initiative Action Plan, which includes a specific initiative on eAccessibility (http://europa.eu.int/information_society/eeurope/index_en.htm), and output of an international expert forum on the internet, the International Accessibility Board Meeting, can be found at http://group.yahoo.com/group/eeurope-pwd/, http://www.acessibilidades.net/doc/acessibilidade/forum/inter_forum.html.   For public contests on accessibility to internet, digital broadcasting, terrestrial TV and UMTS, see http://www.acessibilidade.net/umts/debate_nac.html, http://www.acessibilidade.net/umts/guia_acess01.html, http://www.acessibilidade.tv/menu/guia_acesstv10.html,   http://www.aacs.pt/bd/Deliberacoes/20010328a.htm.

10 http://www.acessibilidade.net/petition/government_resolution.html, http://www.acessibilidade.net/petition/parliament_report.html, http://www.mct.pt/legislacao/despachos/cneinter.htm.

11 WAI – Web Accessibility on Internet. GUIA's campaigning on WAI has drawn on the experience of the USA, Canada, Australia and Brazil, which began in 1996. No European DSMO had a similar initiative before GUIA, although some were lobbying for the 'European manifesto on the information society and disabled people' launched by the European Disability Forum (1999).

12 http://br.egroups.com/group/anasoft.

11 The Queer Sisters and its electronic bulletin board

A study of the internet for social movement mobilization

Joyce Y.M. Nip

Social movement organizations have employed the internet to a high degree. Hundreds of social movement organizations network with each other by email lists. Many also have websites and electronic bulletin boards or other conferencing spaces on the internet where users can interact directly with each other. For social movements, which typically have limited membership and financial resources, 'the Internet is revolutionizing the rule of the game' (Leizerov 2000: 462). The Zapatista movement in Southern Mexico, which first clashed with the Mexican government in 1993 and which Manuel Castells called 'the first informational guerrilla movement' (1997: 79), owed much of its success to its communication strategy (Castells 1997; see below). In the campaign against antipersonnel landmines in the 1990s, 'the global web of electronic media, including telecommunications, fax machines, and especially the internet and the world wide web, have played an unprecedented role in facilitating a global network of concerned supporters around the issue' (Price 1998: 625; see below). Almost everyone directly involved in the campaign against the Multilateral Agreement on Investment, the antecedent of the anti-WTO globalization campaign, agreed that the internet was vital to the success of the campaign (Deibert 2000; see below).

Little is known about the different ways in which the internet may help social movement mobilization, but studies have highlighted two functions of the net: first, it helps communication in information dissemination, formal networking, and action coordination; second, it helps in building a collective identity among participants and potential participants of the movement. This study seeks to examine the identity-building capacity of the internet in social movements.

Use of the internet by social movements

Diani (2000), who is one of the few who explore the overall impact of computer-mediated communication on social movements, conjectures that the main contribution of computer-mediated communication to social movements is the facilitation of communication among existing sympathizers. Diani (2000) is uncertain as to whether computer-mediated communication would help build new identities, as he concludes that the contribution of computer-mediated communication seems to be mainly instrumental rather than symbolic. Prior to Diani (2000), Myers (1994) also tried to understand the overall impact of computer networks on social movements. Arriving at a different conclusion, Myers (1994) held that direct interactions among participants in computer conferencing did facilitate the development of a collective identity. Most studies that relate social movements to the internet focus on the net's instrumental functions of communication, which include information dissemination, formal networking, and action co-ordination. In the Zapatista movement, the internet, together with tele-communications and videos, played a major role in disseminating information from the Zapatistas to the rest of the world instantly (Castells 1997; Froehling 1997). The internet also organized a world-wide network of solidarity groups, which helped to produce an international public opinion movement that deterred the Mexican government from using large-scale repression (Castells 1997; Froehling 1997). In the campaign for economic sanctions against Burma, Danitz and Strobel (1999) stated that the internet served best as a tool of information. The activists interviewed agreed that the internet could not replace human contact in lobbying and other campaign activities but it did make face-to-face group meetings less necessary (Danitz and Strobel 1999).

At the local level, email and a listserv greatly facilitated the formation and administration of the Telecommunications Policy roundtable in Boston (Klein 2000). Bonchek (1995) analysed seven transnational, national and local social movement cases and concluded that the internet reduced the transaction cost of group organization and therefore helped group formation, group efficiency, member recruitment and member retention. On the other hand, some studies have found that new communities were formed on the internet in social movement campaigns, and seem to support the view that computer networking helps identity-building. Downing (1989), studying PeaceNet, found that computer networks, apart from serving information and coordination functions, act as forums for developing agendas for political action. Price (1998) reported that in the campaign against anti-personnel landmines, the network on the internet created a space for virtual communities to debate politics, on top of breaking open access to the policy process and creating communities of experts outside of government. In the campaign against the Multilateral Agreement on Investment, the internet helped in three main ways: (1) communicating information swiftly among members who lobbied against the Multilateral Agreement on Investment (with several electronic mailing lists), (2) publicizing information about the agreement to those outside the lobby, and (3) providing easy-to-take protest action options (Deibert 2000). Deibert (2000: 265) concludes that the role of the internet went beyond facilitating activism already in place; rather it helped create 'a new formation on the world political landscape'.

The success of other transnational campaigns that have used the internet also seems to suggest that the net helps build identity. It is common in these campaigns that sympathizers are mobilized to take action where few offline organizational forms exist. The campaign against Lotus Development Corporation's plan of introducing a direct mail marketing database (MarketPlace: Households) for Macintosh computers in 1990 was conducted mainly on the internet. Gurak (1999) reported the use of newsgroups, emails, and a specifically formed discussion group on the internet in the campaign. As a result of the 'internet-based protest' (Gurak 1999: 243), Lotus never released the product.

Similarly, the petition against the US government's proposed use of an encryption chip in telephone handsets for security checks was conducted on the internet. An internet-based petition drive organized by privacy advocates in 1994 collected 47,000 signatures and defeated the proposal for the time (Gurak 1999). The campaign against Intel's introduction in 1999 of the Pentium III processor, which carried an electronic personal serial number (PSN) that allowed websites to verify the identity of those who used the sites, was also headquartered and executed almost exclusively on the internet (Leizerov 2000). Three privacy advocacy groups declared a boycott of Intel and created a website to headquarter the campaign. The site provided information about the campaign, was linked to many sympathetic news reports and had a questions and answers page on the support section. In 2000 Intel eventually announced that it would stop using the PSN in its next generation of computer processors (Leizerov 2000).

Collective action in itself is an indication that the actors involved have achieved a certain extent of collective identity (Melucci 1995c), while at the same time being a process of building a collective identity (Calhoun 1991; Melucci 1995c). In this perspective, the fact that the internet succeeded in mobilizing action in the above cases suggests that a collective identity is shared among the actors. Scott (1990: 126) argues that 'It is only by focusing on the process of group formation within informal networks that we can understand how social collective action is at all possible'. The forums for debating issues, as found in some of the studies cited above, seem to embody the very process of group formation.

However, available research relating the internet to social movements is mainly case studies that report the use of specific internet spaces in certain transnational social movement campaigns. It is uncertain to what extent the internet may help identity-building in social movement organizations or social movements in general.

Identity-building in social movements

The two dominant paradigms for the study of social movements are the 'resource-mobilization' paradigm and the 'identity-oriented' paradigm (Cohen 1985). However, some theorists take the view that the emphasis on collective action between groups of opposed interests in the 'resource-mobilization' paradigm is not sustainable without an understanding of the formation of 'groupness' (Cohen 1985; Melucci 1995c). The key to understanding is to be found in the process of identity formation (Cohen 1985), which is crucial to social movements of all types (Calhoun 1991; Taylor and Whittier 1992).

A collective identity is not something static; rather it is 'the process through which a collective becomes a collective' (Melucci 1995c: 43). Reviewing previous work, Taylor and Whittier (1992) identified three elements of collective identity in social movements. First, individuals share a sense of 'we' or solidarity when they define some shared characteristics as salient and important. Second, individuals harbour a consciousness comprising shared interpretive frameworks that include political consciousness, relational networks and the goals, means, and environment of action of the movement. Third, a culture of direct opposition to the dominant order exists.

Collective identity formation and maintenance require a network of active relationships between the actors, which necessitates the direct participation of the individual actor in interactions (Pizzorno 1985). Traditionally the face-to-face setting is where these interactions take place for interpreting grievances and debating opportunities (Mueller 1992). Now the internet allows direct interactions through a medium.

Some are sceptical (e.g. Diani 2000; Tarrow 1998) that computer-mediated communication can develop the collective trust essential to social movements. Can the interactive spaces on the internet be the settings for the formation of collective identities in social movements?

Various authors have pointed out the crucial role of organization in identity-building in social movements. Gamson (1992) stated that solidarity processes focused on how people related to social movement carriers. McAdam *et al.* (1996a) contended that even if system-critical framings could emerge in the context of little or no organization, the absence of any real mobilizing structure would prevent their spread to the number of people required for collective action. In the spaces on the internet, what role does organization play in the building of collective identities?

This chapter seeks to examine the identity-building capacity of the internet in social movements by examining a women's group in Hong Kong, the Queer Sisters, and the bulletin board it created on the world wide web. Specifically this chapter asks: (1) Do participants on the electronic bulletin board develop a collective identity among themselves? (2) If yes, does the identity extend to the offline organization? (3) If yes, does the identity help action mobilization of the offline organization? (4) What role does the offline organization play in affecting the development of a collective identity on the bulletin board? On the basis of the findings to these questions, the chapter discusses the potential of the internet in identity-building in social movements.

The Queer Sisters and its electronic bulletin board

Formed in 1995, the Queer Sisters is the oldest queer/lesbian group in Hong Kong. It proclaims itself a human rights organization fighting for the sexual rights of women. It does not have a membership system and is run by volunteers. A small group of self-proclaimed organizers make decisions for the group.[1] Its monthly gatherings normally draw 20 to 50 people.

Queer Sisters created its website (http://www.qs.org.hk) in November 1997, to which a bulletin board was added in October 1998. The bulletin board was accessible to anyone without registration or subscription by clicking the icon 'chat room' on the home page or by bookmarking the board's address. Anyone can post a message by filling in a pre-formatted form posted on the board or post a reply to a message by clicking on the link built in the message without pre-censorship. Most postings on the board are in Chinese (modern standard form or the Cantonese dialect); some are in English. The board's system administrator, one of the Queer Sisters organizers, has the technical power to delete messages or replies on the bulletin board. Another organizer monitors the content of the board as quasi-moderator.

An indication of the size of the bulletin board participation came from a survey posted by Queer Sisters on its homepage, asking what new features people would like on the site. In six weeks from mid-May to the end of June 2000, over 1000 respondents were recorded.[2]

The Queer Sisters is what some social movement theorists call a new social movement organization. Unlike the working-class movement, which was equated to 'social movement' in the nineteenth century, new social movements – including the student, antiwar, women's, and environmental movements since the 1960s – target the social domain of civil society rather than the economy or state. They are concerned about the democratization of structures of everyday life and work for the creation of new life spaces (Cohen 1985; Johnston *et al.* 1994; Offe 1985).

The Queer Sisters' bulletin board is a good site for studying identity-building in social movements. Identity-building is not only essential for the women's movement, of which the Queer Sisters is part in Hong Kong, it is central to any organization formed around queerness. Heavily influenced by postmodernism and post-structuralism (Esterberg 1996), queer theory challenges the notion that sexual identity is an unchanging sexual inclination of a person (Esterberg 1996; Gamson 1996; Stein 1997). Like other queer groups, Queer Sisters faces the contradictory task of consolidating a sense of identity among supporters and advocating the destruction of a stable identity (Gamson 1996).

Sedgwick (1994) claims that the year 1992 was the moment of Queer. Esterberg (1996) argues that the term 'queer' became more common in 1994. The Queer Sisters was formed in 1995 in Hong Kong by three ethnic Chinese women, one of whom grew up in the United States, and another who completed her university education there. The 'academic' background of the group also brings it into tension with the less political participants of the bulletin board.

Data and methods

With agreement from the Queer Sisters organizers, I announced at the monthly gathering of the Queer Sisters on 29 August 1999 that I would study the use of the internet by the group. I then participated on the Queer Sisters bulletin board as an unobtrusive observer between 1 September 1999 and 1 October 2000. This provided the background for my content analysis of all the 603 messages posted during 1–28 September 1999 and 1–28 July 2000.[3] On 1 August 2000, I posted identical messages in Chinese and English on the bulletin board to invite all participants to fill in my questionnaire, the Chinese and English versions of which were lodged on two websites and accessible by clicking on the links given in my messages. Response to the questionnaire was monitored; invitation messages were posted from time to time. I closed the survey on 13 September 2000 when response dropped to very low. One hundred and two valid responses were received.

Individual interviews with 11 willing bulletin board participants were conducted after the survey until the data yielded were saturated. Interviews with five Queer Sisters organizers and three volunteers were also arranged.

I used the following 10-category scheme for content analysis:[4] information, relational, task, expression, sharing, advice, discussion, management, intrusion, and others. I classified the messages twice, and reclassified those where discrepancy arose.

Identity formation on the bulletin board

In this section, I shall look at the Queer Sisters bulletin board to see if its participants bear a collective identity among themselves, and, if yes, whether the collective identity extends to the offline Queer Sisters group. My discussion focuses on the three elements of collective identities in social movements, namely a sense of 'we', a consciousness, and an oppositional culture.

A sense of 'we'

The existence of a sense of 'we' among board participants is obvious both in the survey and interviews with participants, as well as my observation of the board. The sense of solidarity extends to the offline Queer Sisters group. Seventy-six per cent ($n = 77$) of survey respondents reported sharing a sense of belonging to the bulletin board (Table 11.1). Board participants, be they active posters or not, talked about the bulletin board as a space for 'us' lesbians. An infrequent poster described how she felt when she found the bulletin board on a web search: 'I was very happy, very excited. I felt I had discovered a place that I belonged to' (author's interview, 28 October 2000). She said she could get support from and discuss with 'her kind' when lesbian issues got into the news media so she 'did not feel being

Table 11.1 Survey findings on sense of belonging of 101 bulletin board participants

	per cent	n
Share sense of belonging to board	76	77
Participation in board increased sense of belonging to les/queer community	70	70
Participation in board increased sense of belonging to QS	61	61

alone'. Another rare poster described the bulletin board as 'like a home for the lesbian circle' (author's interview, 24 November 2000). An active poster said the board gave her 'family warmth' (author's interview, 21 November 2000). Another said, 'I feel being very close to the QS board. I go there to chat with my friends every night' (author's interview, 27 November 2000).

Even some of those who disagreed with the fun orientation of the active posters shared a sense of solidarity with them. A board participant said although she was not interested in most of what was talked about on the board, she was glad that the board maintained its activity by attracting lesbians of all interests (author's interview, 28 October 2000). Another said she found the others too young and had little she could share with them, but still sensed being in a group with them (author's interview, 19 October 2000).

The sense of being a group was clearly manifested in responses made to postings considered to be intruding into the board. On 10 October 1999 the following intrusion message was posted: 'ching chang ping pong pussy smells like ding dong!!!!!!!!!!!!!!!!!!!!!!!!!!!!!!!!!!'. In response, three replies were posted:

> Could someone please remove this racist, sexist and anti-lesbigay message? I don't think we need to tolerate ppl like this.

> I trusted that this is a disgusting message, nevertheless, mind me stupid, I never know what it means. So I guess if people don't understand that fxxk fag could not take the pleasure out of such offensive writing.

> Dear ah Q [a well-known fictional character in Chinese literature who imagined that everything would be fine if he did not attend

to it], I CAN understand the sentence and I don't feel comfortable with it. And trust me, the bastard is taking immense pleasure from it. Can ppl be more considerate? Can they see that what they don't understand could be understood by, and offend, others?

The number of responses to the intruding message was small only because many board participants took the view that the intruder would obtain greater pleasure if more responded. Two board participants said that intrusion messages were those they disliked the most. A rare poster described them as 'words posted by outsiders who insulted us', but she thought that the messages should be allowed to stay on the board so participants were reminded 'how others saw us' (author's interview, 20 November 2000). A frequent poster said she was disgusted by 'those messages that attacked tongzhis[5] and that polluted the board' (author's interview, 27 November 2000). She said such messages made her unhappy and she sometimes replied to rebuke them. One of the Queer Sisters organizers, who also said she disliked intrusion messages the most on the board, said the group decided not to delete them because they thought participants needed to face the reality of hate and discrimination. The organizer also realized that 'opposition and insulting voices built solidarity' (author's interview, 3 November 2000). The participants' responses clearly showed the perception of a boundary between 'them' and 'us'.

There is no doubt that the first element of a collective identity in social movements, namely a sense of 'we', existed among participants on the Queer Sisters bulletin board. The question is which collective the sense relates to: Is it the bulletin board alone, is it the Queer Sisters group, or is it the lesbian/queer community in general?

The survey found that 70 per cent ($n = 70$) of respondents considered that their participation on the bulletin board had increased their sense of belonging to the lesbian/queer community (Table 11.1). While it is true that at least some participants' identification with the lesbian/queer community might pre-date their participation on the board, the fact that their sense of identification had increased shows that the bulletin board served as the venue for the maintenance and reinforcement of that identification.

Sixty-one per cent ($n = 61$) reported that their participation on the board had increased their sense of belonging to the Queer Sisters group (Table 11.1). As 75 per cent[6] ($n = 76$) of board respondents first learned of the bulletin board through online channels unrelated to the Queer Sisters (Table 11.2), it could be assumed that most participants did not start with any sense of identification with the group.

Table 11.2 Survey findings on channels through which 101 participants learned of board

	per cent	*n*
Through people known online	36	36
Through website hyperlinks	20	20
Searched from web	20	20
Through offline QS channels	6	6
Through people known offline in QS	4	4
Through people known in offline les/queer community	9	9
Others	6	6

The increase in the sense of belonging to the Queer Sisters is the result of identity-building through active interactions and relationship formation on the bulletin board. Indeed, 62 per cent ($n = 63$) of survey respondents visited the board (almost) every day; another 15 per cent ($n = 15$) visited it two to three times a week. Ninety-four per cent ($n = 95$) had posted messages or replies, with every message usually drawing around five replies. Over half (52 per cent, $n = 53$) had made friends on the board (Table 11.3).

Thus the sense of 'we' was shared among participants of the bulletin board not only as a bulletin board collective, but also as the offline Queer Sisters group and the lesbian/queer community. Multiple identifications like this are natural; the challenge for social movements is how to make the identification with the social movement more salient than others. The multiple identifications reveal that the participants on the bulletin board defined different boundaries of their collective in their various ongoing interactions with each other and with 'outsiders' (Phelan 1993; Taylor and Whittier 1992). In intrusion messages that attacked lesbianism, participants were addressed as a lesbian collec-

Table 11.3 Survey findings of active interactions on the bulletin board

	per cent	*n*
Visited board every day	62	63
Visited board two to three times per week	15	15
Had posted messages or replies	94	95
Made friends on board	52	53

tive; participants' sense of being a lesbian collective was reinforced. When groups based outside Hong Kong wrote on the board to ask for information or publicize their activities, which happened from time to time, participants were addressed as one bulletin board collective and so their sense of being a bulletin board collective was strengthened.

Interestingly, my interviews with the board participants, as reported above, seem to suggest that being lesbian is a more salient shared characteristic than being queer. This reflects the failure of the Queer Sisters in building a consciousness of queerness among the board participants, something that is discussed further in the next section.

Consciousness

The sources of data did not show that participants of the Queer Sisters bulletin board harboured a collective consciousness, the second element of a collective identity in social movements. Nor did they show that the bulletin board shared the same interpretative frameworks regarding the values and aspirations of the Queer Sisters group.

Content analysis found that 34 per cent ($n = 207$) of the sampled messages on the bulletin board were relational messages; 23 per cent ($n = 141$) were sharing messages and 16 per cent ($n = 94$) were expression messages (Table 11.4). The online survey[7] also found that sharing (65 per cent, $n = 66$) and mutual support (64 per cent, $n = 65$) were what most participants said they obtained from the bulletin board.

Relational messages are those used by the poster to address particular board participants for interpersonal liaison. They normally bear the

Table 11.4 Content analysis results

Category	per cent	n
Relational	34	207
Sharing	23	141
Expression	16	94
Information	13	78
Task	4	23
Discussion	3	20
Advice	2	13
Management	0	2
Intrusion	0	1
Others	4	24
Total		603

names of both the poster and addressee(s). Where only one of the names is given, the method of address must give sufficient information about the corresponding parties. Occasionally, no name of either the poster or addressee is given, but if the message draws an expected reply, then it is still counted as a relational message. Sharing messages are those that carry the feelings or views of the poster, typically not addressed to anybody, and that draw replies. Expression messages also carry the personal feelings or views of the poster and are not addressed to anybody, but do not draw replies. The distinction between sharing and expression messages is made on the basis of whether the messages serve the function of sharing or not for the poster of the initial messages, but obviously posters of expression messages are likely to have the intention of sharing with other bulletin board participants.

Consciousness is developed in a process in which groups re-evaluate themselves, their subjective experiences, their opportunities, and their shared interests (Taylor and Whittier 1992). However, observation of the posting on the bulletin board suggested that the relational messages were posted mainly for lovers and friends. While they strengthened the bond between the parties involved, these relational messages served little purpose of building a collective consciousness on the bulletin board. Some relational messages, like this one posted on 2 October 1999, which were meant to solicit friends, might help to reinforce the sense of 'we' among bulletin board participants by addressing them as one collective, but again could not help develop a collective consciousness:

> icq: xxxxxxxx
> I am a 25 years old TB,[8] live in Hong Kong.
> I have a kind heart and sense of humor.
> I am also a sporty person.
> I like to make some les[bian] friends.
> Please feel free to add me.

Sharing messages, typically like the following two, revolved around feelings and views on various aspects of life, and often on romantic love:

> 9 Sep 1999
> I looked in the sky and there I saw a star shining so bright above
> I closed my eyes and wished upon that I would find true love
> Someone who needed me

Someone to share my life
For a love that would be true
I would wait forever . . .
[name]

17 Jul 2000
A few more days and I'll be one year older!!!
I remember when I was young,
I always wanted to grow up
So that I would be independent and be free from mom and dad's
nagging!!!
So that I would be dating and earning money. I was so naïve!!!
Now I am grown up
I don't want to grow old
I want to be 4 or 5 years younger . . .
[name] [author's translation from Cantonese]

Only very occasionally did sharing messages – such as this one
posted on 8 July 2000 – touch on lesbian experiences and offer opportunities for raising the consciousness of a lesbian identity:

> Mom said: Your younger brothers will have their own families. Of
> course they will stop contributing to the family expenses once they
> move out. So I expect you to pay the mortgage for buying a home
> for your dad and me.
> I love them and I am most willing to take care of them. But why is
> it a matter of course that they will have their own families but not
> me?
> They know for sure that I have an intimate girl friend, whom they
> have met. I am 25. Should I not have my own family? Does it have
> to be a man and a woman to make a family?
> [name]

The message drew seven replies, which raised issues including equality between men and women in family responsibilities, social tolerance/
discrimination of lesbians, and strategies for handling the situation.

More than sharing messages, expression messages focused mainly
on romantic love. Categories that might help cultivate a collective
consciousness recorded far fewer messages. Only 3 per cent ($n = 20$)
of the messages centred on discussion (Table 11.4). Thirteen per cent
($n = 78$) of the messages were informational, but further analysis

found that most of them ($n = 47$, 8 per cent of total) were posted by individual participants asking or giving information about lesbian-related leisure activities only.

The personal concerns of the bulletin board were in sharp contrast to the political orientation of the Queer Sisters. To fight for the sex rights of women, the Queer Sisters campaigned with other women's and gay groups and granted press interviews from time to time. They also hosted a radio talk programme broadcast biweekly on a commercial website, and organized essay competitions every four months. On top of that, the group provided telephone counselling one evening a week and organized barbecues, dinner parties, boat launches, and dance parties several times a year as a service.

Core organizers of the Queer Sisters were critical of the abundance of personal emotions related to romantic love displayed on the bulletin board, as one core organizer commented: 'They [participants on the board] are very young, very shallow, and would not look further than their immediate lives' (author's interview, 3 November 2000). One bulletin board participant referred to the call by the Queer Sisters for board participants to phone candidates of the Legislative Council elections during the campaign period as being too political for her. But she did harbour a sense of belonging to the bulletin board and the Queer Sisters (author's interview, 16 October 2000).

The Queer Sisters group believed that the sex rights of women were best accommodated in the fluid sexual orientation of queerness, a value that was again not shared by the bulletin board, as revealed in a debate that erupted on the board in September 1999. After the Queer Sisters' quasi-moderator, in reply to a query, defined the group's main target audience as tongzhis – which the group defined as 'non-heterosexuals of multi-dimensional sexuality' – this posting came on 12 September:

> Why the hell is 'tongzhi' not the same as lesbian?
> Why the hell 'the choice of wording is consistent with the ideals of the Queer Sisters'? . . .
> In organizing an activity you talk about political incorrectness even in picking a word . . . You spend your whole life pondering about the publicity flyer, and leave 15 per cent of your time for organizing it . . .
> [author's translation from Cantonese]

On 14 September came this reply from a queer:

I can see QS is/has become an organization which only serves the narrowly-defined communities, namely LESBIANS. So where the hell are those QUEERS? I have no intention to speak against LESBIANS. I likED this website, i likED this chat room, because i thought it was the only organization in Hong Kong [that] had its own stance which I stand up with and which provided us, as women, as queers or as whatever you dare to be (no matter what gender(s) you fxxk) to talk OPENLY about gender and sexuality . . .
[capitals are the poster's emphasis]

Amid the series of discussion messages and replies was this reply posted on 17 September that indicated the extent of disagreement from the 'queer' value of the Queer Sisters among some board participants:

I'm glad that some serious discussion has surfaced in QS . . . But sometimes the human brain is like a silted-up river or an ancient closet. No matter how much others try, the stubborn old silt or garbage can't be cleared . . .
The perspective on sexual inclination of the Queer Sisters has enlightened me. It liberated my thinking from labels found in the closet . . .
The arguments in recent days have troubled me a lot. This is my last posting for this argument.
[author's translation from Chinese].

Discussion on the issue disappeared from the bulletin board afterwards, but it showed that the Queer Sisters' value relating to queerness was not shared by at least some of the bulletin board participants.

Although participants of the bulletin board shared a sense of 'we' among themselves, they did not manifest a collective consciousness of their position. And although board participants shared a sense of 'we' with the Queer Sisters, they did not share the group's interpretative frameworks regarding political action and queerness.

An oppositional culture

Individuals develop a collective sense among themselves when some shared characteristic becomes salient and is defined as important (Taylor and Whittier 1992). For participants on the Queer Sisters bulletin board, the basis of their collective sense was the identification with lesbianism/queerness, which in itself was a culture opposed to society's dominant mode of male–female relationships. The abundant expression of romantic love (between women), as in the following message posted obviously for a lover on 31 August 1999, was an act that both revealed and reinforced such opposition:

> Although these few weeks you have been busy with your work with no time left for me, and we have little time to meet, I do not mind. I would only support you silently.
> Listening to Kenny G's music while going over the love letters and caring cards between us gives me a special feelings – some sweet, some romantic, some funny, and some moving. In these years I deeply feel your love for me – true, frank, and whole-hearted.
> I feel being very lucky and happy. Thank you.
> No matter what comes ahead, I will stay with you.
> [name]
> [author's translation from Chinese]

When some participant encountered problems related to her sexual orientation, as in the following message posted on 30 August 1999, the supportive responses from other participants formed part of a process of cultural opposition while helping to build/reinforce the participant's sexual identity.

> If your other half does not accept herself as being lesbian – she cares a lot about how others see her – what would you do?
> In fact I have considered staying with her for the rest of my years, but if she can't accept it, what can I do?
> . . . Hope someone can answer me.
> [name]
> [author's translation from Cantonese]

One of the six replies drawn by the message suggested that the poster adopt a queer orientation:

> Don't let your identity tie you down. You love a girl today does not mean you have to wear a sexual identity . . . Just respect your feelings; don't worry about your sexual identity.
> [name]
> [author's translation from Chinese]

Sometimes posters shared their observation or reflection about their own community, implicitly acknowledging each other's identification with an alternative sexual inclination:

16 Jul 2000
I had dinner in Causeway Bay last night and I saw many les. As soon as I got off the bus, I saw a pair who were holding hands. Then I saw some others on the way to Chuen Cheung Kui [name of a restaurant]. In the restaurant was a table of them next to mine. When I left, I saw some others waiting for tables. Suddenly I felt like on another planet. The feeling was: 'Wow, the world has changed.'
[name]
[author's translation from Cantonese]

The culture of opposition to the dominant mode of heterosexual relationships remained at the level of mutual recognition and reinforcement on the bulletin board. Because of the seeming lack of collective consciousness among board participants, the culture of oppositional sexual orientation did not manifest itself as a collective fight to gain recognition from outside their culture.

Implications of identity on the bulletin board for mobilization

The above discussion shows that participants on the Queer Sisters bulletin board on the world wide web fell short of sharing a collective identity in social movements. Participants shared a sense of 'we', which was extended to the Queer Sisters. They exhibited an oppositional culture, but that might not be formed on the basis of queerness as cherished by the Queer Sisters. A collective consciousness seemed to be absent on the bulletin board.

What does this mean for action mobilization by the Queer Sisters? My findings suggest that the process of identity-building on the bulletin board did seem to help increase participation in the offline Queer Sisters group. Among those whose sense of belonging to the Queer Sisters group had increased as a result of participating on the bulletin board, participation in the offline group was 43 per cent ($n = 26$), higher than the 34 per cent ($n = 34$) among board participants in general. Yet whether or not the participants had a sense of belonging to the bulletin board, the percentage of participation in the Queer Sisters group was similar (Table 11.5). This suggests that different

Table 11.5 Survey findings on sense of belonging and participation

	per cent	n	Total
Board participants with increased sense of belonging to QS participating in offline QS	43	26	61
All board participants' participation in offline QS	34	34	101
Participants with sense of belonging to board participating in offline QS	35	27	77

logic governs participation online and offline. Online participants might not wish to take part in offline activities because of resource constraints or other disincentives.

A big difference exists, however, between participating in offline activities organized by the Queer Sisters and being mobilized into offline collective action, the latter involving risks of repression and real costs to the participants. The Queer Sisters were observed to try mobilizing bulletin board participants a number of times, but only for online collective action. An example was the campaign for the Legislative Council elections in September 2000.

A message was first posted on 6 June 2000, and re-posted on 8 June 2000, stating that an alliance of gay and lesbian groups had been formed and volunteers were being recruited for the campaign. On 15 August, a message that gave a schedule of candidate appearances on live forums organized by an online newspaper urged board participants to write in the online forum to press for gay and lesbian rights. Between 3 September and the voting day, 10 September, the Queer Sisters posted eight messages to mobilize board participants. The last of the three messages posted on the voting day ran with the subject heading: 'Only two-and-a-half hours left; go and vote quickly!'

On another occasion, board participants were mobilized to defend their own interests. A message posted by the Queer Sisters on 22 August 2000 called on board participants to launch a one-person-one-email campaign to demand that a pornographic site de-link the Queer Sisters site after hyperlinking it without permission. Continued hyperlinking was likely to bring unwelcome visitors who might disrupt the board.

No data was available about the success of the mobilization attempts, except that the pornographic site later did de-link the Queer Sisters site. Yet the absence of a collective consciousness on the bulletin board made one wonder how successfully the bulletin board could be mobilized for offline collective action by the Queer Sisters.

Role of the Queer Sisters in identity-building on the bulletin board

The absence of a collective consciousness among participants of the Queer Sisters bulletin board may not have resulted from the limitations of the internet in identity-building. I would argue that in fact it was more the result of the way the bulletin board was administered.

Gamson (1992) identified from previous social movement literature two characteristics of social movement carriers that promoted solidarity: first, the use of pre-existing social relationships; and second, the organizational forms that support and sustain the personal needs of participants and embody the movement's collective identity.

On the Queer Sisters bulletin board, pre-existing social relationships were given complete freedom to operate. The bulletin board was accessible to any web user without software installation, subscription or registration. Forty-nine per cent ($n = 49$) of the survey respondents first learned of the bulletin board through people they knew, either online or offline (Table 11.2). In fact the quasi-moderator of the bulletin board reported that a group of seven friends previously conversing on another bulletin board migrated to the Queer Sisters board at one point (author's interview, 26 July 2001).

In terms of organizational forms, what the bulletin board offered for the personal needs of the board participants was a public participatory environment for liaison, expression, sharing, advice and discussion. Given the frustration and discrimination arising from the participants' sexual inclination, the provision of a sharing space alone was an effective organizational form of support.

Some social movement scholars (e.g. Diani 2000; Tarrow 1998) are sceptical that online interactions could develop the collective trust essential to social movements. In the case of the Queer Sisters bulletin board, online interactions led to other opportunities of communication, which together did result in a certain degree of trust among networks of board participants. As reported above, over half (52 per cent, $n = 53$) of participants on the Queer Sisters bulletin board had made friends through first conversing with them on the board. Almost all (96 per cent, $n = 51$) of the friendships formed on the board had extended to other communication channels, including face-to-face meetings (55 per cent, $n = 28$). The fact that participants agreed to meet face-to-face with each other offline indicates that a certain degree of trust had been established between the parties involved. A participant who described herself as shy and introverted said she would arrange to meet face-to-face the friends she made on the board only after they had achieved some understanding of each other. And she was able to maintain the seven or eight friendships made that way (author's interview, 20 November 2000). The relationships formed on the board were not necessarily romantic; many were social in nature. Some of these relationships were maintained on a one-to-one basis, and some among a number of people.

Some of the friends who met offline continued to use the board for liaison although some migrated off the board to more private channels of communication. I estimated from the content of the postings that 64 per cent ($n = 133$) of the sampled relational messages were posted between people who had met each other face-to-face. Given that only 19 per cent ($n = 19$) of board participants first learned of the board through offline contacts (Table 11.2), it was likely that a substantial portion of the face-to-face encounters were results of friendships extended from the bulletin board. The quasi-moderator of the bulletin board played a role in using the pre-existing friendships. By monitoring the board postings, she was able to identify newcomers to the board, whom she would approach (by posting a message) and introduce herself socially. The social contact so established should help rally the networks of relationships for fostering a sense of solidarity with the Queer Sisters.

The building of a collective consciousness – or framing – involves conscious strategic efforts by groups of people to instil shared understandings of the world and of themselves among constituents to legitimize and motivate collective action (McAdam *et al.* 1996a; Snow and McAdam 2000). The Queer Sisters organizers, however, had not tried building a collective consciousness on the bulletin board because of considerations of their resources and aims of the organization. Previous organizers who tried to arouse concern for public issues by posting lesbian-related news did not draw much response (author's interviews, 29 August 1999, 12 July 2000). The present organizers decided that their limited time would be better used in organizing activities (author's interview, 10 November 2000). Only five of the seven organizers of the Queer Sisters visited the bulletin board, and then only infrequently, except for Eunice, who acted as the quasi-moderator.

Various authors have pointed out that successful framing requires argumentative power (empirical credibility) (Snow *et al.* 1986) and sound analysis of the situation (empirical validity) (Gamson 1992).

But the Queer Sisters organizers were concerned that they might not be sufficiently equipped with a theoretical analysis of queer issues to use the bulletin board as a venue for building a collective consciousness (author's interview, 10 November 2000).

The Queer Sisters considered the bulletin board more as a service provided for the lesbian/queer community than as a venue for consciousness raising. They adopted the policy of allowing free expression without censorship, considering that consistent with the group's aims to fight for a space for women to develop (author's interviews, 18 May, 10 November 2000). Observation of the board and interviews with the quasi-moderator revealed that she perceived her role as smoothing over tension that might disrupt the friendly atmosphere of the bulletin board, but not as an enforcer of the values of the Queer Sisters group (author's interview, 21 September 1999). The system administrator of the bulletin board, who was another organizer of the Queer Sisters, had the technical power to delete messages but such power was exercised only in the very early stage when the board was set up.

Running alongside the debate over queerness/lesbianism reported above was a debate about the political orientation of the Queer Sisters. One of the replies to the 12 September reply, excerpted above, simply stated: 'PC sucks!' In turn it drew this response on 14 September that supported the political position of the Queer Sisters:

> I don't think PC sucks . . .
> Individual consumption habits (personal) have serious impact on a global scale, and it's therefore important to tie up personal and political. Personal issues like motherhood or reproduction (and even our sexual preferences) are impacted by global social structures and are thus political in nature . . .
> This is also why the matter of female sexuality . . . is deserving of public attention and political analysis. Following from this, it was also argued that personal behaviour has political impact outside of the self, and can therefore be understood (and judged) in political terms. And thus, in my opinion . . . spending 85 per cent of time to have a deep and critical reflection and discretion about what to do for QS is definitely ESSENTIAL . . .
> [name]

That week could have been a perfect occasion for the Queer Sisters to raise the political and queer consciousness among board participants, but it did not try to do so. It just replied to questions in the name of the quasi-moderator and restated what the group fought for. It did not rebuke the lesbians, nor did it defend itself from attacks by the lesbians. It did not try discrediting the apolitical position of the posters either.

System-critical attribution is an essential component of collective action frames that social movement organizations and actors could offer (McAdam *et al.* 1996b; Snow and Benford 1992). Occasions where messages touching on the personal experiences of being lesbian were posted again provided good opportunities for the Queer Sisters to suggest system attribution, but the Queer Sisters failed to take the chance to cultivate a collective consciousness. To the 8 July 2000 message, cited above, came a reply from the bulletin board quasi-moderator. Instead of focusing on the discrimination against lesbian relationships, the quasi-moderator dwelt on the equality between men and women in supporting their parents.

The Queer Sisters did not respond to the 30 August 1999 message, also cited above. It was two other participants who suggested that the poster adopt a fluid (queer) conception of her sexual inclination. Instead of using the bulletin board to build a collective consciousness, the Queer Sisters adopted the strategy of recruiting potential supporters from the board to its offline activities. The quasi-moderator of the board would identify posters from her monitoring who needed support or who revealed a political awareness, and then encourage them to join the group's monthly gatherings. The Queer Sisters organizers said the group's website and the bulletin board had become the primary grounds where the Queer Sisters recruited their volunteer helpers (author's interview, 3 November 2000).

The disadvantage of the group's policy of administering the bulletin board is that the group gave up the opportunity of an official voice to shape the interpretative frames of the bulletin board participants. The policy, however, is consistent with the group's aims and understandable given their resource limitations. The fact that the bulletin board was openly accessible brought many visitors who might not be sympathetic with the queer value or political orientation of the group. Had the Queer Sisters introduced a screening policy for the bulletin board – say by adding a registration that required visitors to state they agreed with the aims and objectives of the Queer Sisters – the board would have kept participants who were more likely to be interested in the wider political issues and had a queer (not lesbian) orientation. Faced with a more like-minded aggregate, consciousness raising should be easier to achieve on the board.

Conclusion

In this study, the participants on the Queer Sisters bulletin board developed a sense of solidarity with the Queer Sisters and shared a culture of opposition to the dominant order, but they fell short of harbouring a collective consciousness. Nor did they share with the Queer Sisters interpretative frames about the need for political action or queerness as the value to cherish.

I have argued that the apparent absence of a collective consciousness on the Queer Sisters bulletin board is the result of the way the board was administered. Compared to previous social movement studies where an identity seemed to be formed online, this case study differs in two ways, which may also explain the absence of a collective identity on the bulletin board. First, the constituents of the Queer Sisters' project of identity-building were less homogeneous. Second, the Queer Sisters were a subcultural movement organization that faced a dilemma in identity-building.

Past studies of social movements that investigate the role of the internet predominantly focus on transnational campaigns. The anti-Multilateral Agreement on Investment campaign, for example, is an international alliance of transnational and national nongovernmental organizations and activists, rather than a social movement existing solely in cyberspace (Deibert 2000). Much offline lobbying and campaigning was conducted outside the internet. In the campaign against antipersonnel landmines, for example, nongovernmental organizations participated, either independently or as part of states' official delegations, in conferences organized under the auspices of the United Nations (Price 1998). Even in the campaigns against Lotus' introduction of MarketPlace and Intel's introduction of the Pentium III processor – cases where few offline organizational forms existed – privacy advocacy groups initiated the campaigns (Gurak 1999; Leizerov 2000). Offline activities also took place in the Intel case, where Intel officials had meetings with representatives of the privacy groups (Leizerov 2000).

Being a network of pre-existing organizations meant that the campaigns started with a network of supporters of the organizations who were imbued with a sense of collective identity to the organizations. The task of identity-building for these campaigns is to define the issue in terms of an accepted value. Leizerov (2000) reported that the privacy groups faced a difficult challenge of categorizing the Intel issue in their audience's minds as a true danger to privacy. Price (1998) suggested that the effort to delegitimize antipersonnel landmines hinged on the grafting of moral opprobrium from other delegitimized practices of warfare.

The case of the Queer Sisters is very different. The bulletin board on the world wide web was openly accessible to all; only 10 per cent ($n = 10$) of visitors to the board first learned of the board through off-line channels related to the Queer Sisters (Table 11.2). Although the home page of the Queer Sisters did introduce the group's aims and goals, visitors with a lesbian inclination would still find themselves accommodated within the fluid sexual values advocated by the group. Neither the Queer Sisters homepage nor the bulletin board suggested any expectation for board participants to be politically aware of their social conditions. Thus the Queer Sisters were faced with an aggregate of people whose values and aspirations might differ substantially. This made the project of collective identity-building much more difficult.

A number of authors (e.g. Cohen 1985; Pizzorno 1978) have proposed a distinction between strategy-oriented and identity-oriented social movements. Koopmans (1992, cited in Kriesi et al. 1995) has further proposed to distinguish identity-oriented movements into subcultural and counter-cultural movements. Calling strategy-oriented movements instrumental movements, Kriesi et al. (1995) stated that subcultural movements are predominantly internally oriented and identity-based, whereas instrumental movements have an external orientation. According to this categorization, the Queer Sisters would be a subcultural social movement organization, as the homosexual movement and the women's movement are cited as examples of sub-cultural movements (Kriesi et al. 1995). The social movement cases in previous studies of the internet are instrumental movements.

Subcultural movements mobilize far less than instrumental movements. For their participants, the process of identity construction is the predominant motivation for their action (Kriesi et al. 1995). This explains why the Queer Sisters set up the bulletin board not so much as a vehicle of consciousness raising but as a space for expression and sharing. The purposeful and expressive disclosure to others of one's subjective feelings, desires, and experiences for the purpose of gaining recognition and influence is itself collective action (Pizzorno 1978). However, it is uncertain to what extent the expression and sharing on the Queer Sisters bulletin board qualified as collective action in that sense, as coming out anonymously online is much easier than coming out to someone directly offline (Tsang 2000).

Seeing the Queer Sisters as a subcultural movement organization would lead us to expect that even if a collective identity is built on the bulletin board, the collective identity may not contribute to collective mobilization for instrumental goals. Yet it does not explain why a collective consciousness failed to emerge on the bulletin board. The answer, I think, lies in what Gamson (1996) called the 'queer dilemma'. Queer politics – upholding the inessential, fluid, multifaceted character of sexuality – tends to take on the deconstruction of identity as the goal (Gamson 1996). This seems to testify the Queer Sisters' accommodation of the lesbian orientation and explain the lack of a conscious effort to build a queer identity on the bulletin board.

Although this study of the electronic bulletin board set up by the Queer Sisters group in Hong Kong did not find that online interactions succeeded in fostering a collective consciousness among the online participants, such absence is explained mainly by the way the board was administered. Compared to transnational social movement campaigns, the project of identity-building for the Queer Sisters is more difficult. The aims of the group add a further dimension of difficulty to identity-building. However, the potential of the internet in building identities for social movements is revealed in the successful development of a sense of solidarity among the bulletin board participants with the Queer Sisters group. Bulletin board participants were also found to share an oppositional culture to the dominant order. A certain degree of trust, which is considered essential for developing collective identities in social movements, was developed on the bulletin board, although not solely through online interactions. Future studies of how the internet may help identity-building in social movements needs to focus on the role of the organizers in the dynamics of interactions. The implication of the online–offline divide – of identity built online for offline mobilization – is another dimension that calls for further investigation.

Notes

1 The number of organizers and volunteer helpers varies as some leave and others are invited to join. In September 1999 there were four organizers and nine volunteers (author's interview, 21 September 2000), and in December 2000 there were seven organizers and 18 helpers (statistics provided by Queer Sisters' core organizer, 28 December 2000).
2 The record was automatically provided by the free software available from the 'Pollit.com web service' site (www.pollit.com), which was used in the survey.
3 The sampling strategy was used considering the nature of text produced in online groups. The fluidity of participation in online groups means that

those who are most active in posting messages may differ from time to time. Online groups also evolve, as participants inject new interests and concerns to their interactions with other participants. The absence of gate-keeping, as in news organizations, further means that the content produced by an online group may differ substantially from time to time (Nip 2001). Taking reference from McLaughlin *et al.* (1997), who used four blocks of 200 contiguous messages each, this study used two blocks of contiguous messages in two four-week periods. The first block of messages was drawn immediately after my announcement at the Queer Sisters monthly gathering of my study; the second right before the beginning of my web-based survey.

4 Taking reference from previous studies (Correll 1995; Kollock and Smith 1996; McLaughlin *et al.* 1995; Myers 1987; Rheingold 1996; Wellman and Gulia 1999), an initial classification scheme was devised and used to categorize the messages. It was then adjusted to the present form.

5 'Tongzhi' is a transcription from the Chinese term for 'comrade', which communists often use to refer to people who share the same ideals and commitments. The term 'tongzhi' was invented/appropriated by members of the gay community in Hong Kong before the 1997 political changeover to Communist China to refer to members of the community. The meaning of the term has since expanded to include at least lesbians as well.

6 The percentage is calculated by adding the first three rounded-up percentages shown in Table 11.2.

7 Respondents could give multiple responses to this question.

8 TB stands for 'tom boy', the equivalent of 'butch'.

12 Politics and identity in cyberspace

A case study of Australian Women in Agriculture online

Barbara Pini, Kerry Brown and Josephine Previte

In a front-page story entitled 'Confessions of an IT junkie' published in an edition of *The Buzz*, a quarterly magazine of the farm women's group Australian Women in Agriculture (AWiA), rural woman Judy Brewer (2001: 1) says that 'going online has changed my life'. She writes that technology is essential to her business work and an increasingly important element of her social life, particularly given that, as well as having two young children, she lives 60 kilometres from the nearest shop and 200 kilometres from a town-centre.

In this chapter we explore Brewer's (2001) reflections about the impact of new communication technologies on rural women's lives, and particularly the extent to which these technologies have facilitated the political agendas of women in rural Australia. The focus for this analysis is the discussion list of AWiA, which was established in 1998 to support the political and social activities of network members. Using interviews with twenty members of the discussion list, we argue that AWiA women have engaged the technology to constitute new identities for themselves, far removed from the traditional construction of women on farms as 'farmers' wives' or 'farm wives'. These are the identities of 'political activist', 'business manager' and 'community leader'. In tracing this evolutionary process we further highlight the way in which the women's use of technology has reshaped and shifted notions of 'public' and 'private'. To begin, we turn to the literature from rural sociology which provides a context for understanding the way in which technology has been taken up by AWiA.

Farm women and their emerging political identities

American academic Carolyn Sachs (1996: 134), who has made a substantial contribution to feminist rural sociology, has argued that the widespread use of the nomenclature 'farm wife' raises critical questions for investigation. These, she suggests, are:

> Who are farm wives and what do they do? How do they perceive of themselves? In the larger context, what changes are occurring in women's definition of themselves? What is the relation between the state and farm women?
>
> (Sachs 1996: 134)

Of these questions, the first, that of 'what women do on farms', is the one that has, until recently, received the greatest attention from rural social scientists (see, for example, Sachs 1983; Whatmore 1991; Alston 1995). A central outcome of this research has been the realization that the nature of women's work on farms, characterized by pluri-activity and the connection between the reproductive and productive spheres, blurred the traditional definitions of what constituted 'work'.

Sachs' (1996) second thematic question – that of how farm women 'perceive of themselves' – has also generated attention from rural sociological scholars. As a means of addressing this issue, some writers have turned their attention to the discourses of agrarianism and rurality in the narratives of farm women themselves. These discourses, which highlight the moral superiority of rural/farm life and the traditional division of household labour, constitute an identity for 'farm women' that has typically limited their role to the domestic and household sphere (e.g. Fink 1992; Little 1987, 1997). Liepins (1996), in contrast, turns her attention to the media to explore the formation of gendered agricultural identities. She finds, however, a similar marginal position for the subject 'farm wife' in this discursive site in that representations of women are 'almost entirely absent' or limited to their roles as 'wives, mothers and homemakers devoted to home, community service and ancillary support work on the farm' (Liepins 1996: 5).

It is in studying how farm women 'perceive of themselves' that feminist rural sociologists have necessarily engaged Sachs' (1996) third question, that of how farm women's self-definition is changing. It seems that just as the theoretical spotlight was being placed on the nature of farm women's identities, substantial changes began occurring in how these identities were being constituted. This is, perhaps, because the cultural turn within rural sociology coincided with a decade of rural and farm women's political activism across Australia, New Zealand, Canada and Europe. Motivated by the crisis in agriculture, inspired by the impact of the urban women's movement and frustrated by men's numerical dominance of established agri-political groups, rural women formed groups to provide new spaces and places for uniting and addressing their concerns. In order to analyse the changes occurring in farm women's self-perceptions as a result of their involvement in these groups, Mackenzie (1994) and Liepins (1995) undertook discourse analysis of the networks' media. This process revealed the way in which the new farm women groups were contributing to a reconstitution of the identities of 'farm women' and 'farmer'. An important feature of these identities was – and remains today – a role for farm women in the public sphere of agriculture as political activists, as business managers and as industry leaders.

In a recent paper, Fincher and Panelli (2001) contribute to the scholarship on farm women's shifting identities, while simultaneously addressing Sachs' (1996) final question, that of the relationship between farm women and the state. The focus for their analysis is how the political actors of the Australian Women in Agriculture movement are utilizing the state to advance their agendas. To undertake this analysis they draw on what Cox (1997: 21) refers to as 'spaces of engagement' for political change. These arenas are distinguished from the 'spaces of dependence' that are the place-specific and material spaces in which political actors operate. They are, in contrast, often contingent and dependent on the construction of networks (often beyond the immediate physical space).

Fincher and Panelli (2001) identify two ways in which the Women in Agriculture movement in Australia has generated 'spaces of engagement'. The first has been by positioning themselves within specific geographical locations. For Women in Agriculture members this has meant strategically positioning themselves within discourses of 'rurality'. This strategy, the authors suggest, both facilitated the development of a cohesive group identity and fostered a sense of legitimacy in dealing with the state. The second has been to engage strategically both with private and with public space for their activism. To argue this case, the authors demonstrate the way in which the private space has been used by women to develop the skills, knowledge and expertise utilized in the public space. For example, lobbying politicians, holding conferences and submitting press releases, undertaken by AWiA members, are organized and supported through such private sphere activities as face-to-face and telephone conversations between women and home-based meetings.

In this chapter we take up the arguments made by Fincher and Panelli (2001: 13). Our purpose, however, is to address one area of space which the authors do not consider in their analysis of activist women's use of space – that is, the use of cyberspace. This is a particularly important space in which to examine political engagement for a group such as AWiA, because their 600-member constituency is dispersed across the country. This is because technology has the capacity to address the limitations to group identity and political action that may exist when there is a lack of physical connectivity among members. A further reason why cyberspace is an important space in which to examine farm women's activism is that this space offers the potential to disrupt existing power and social relations (Loader 1997). Groups utilizing information and communication technology may challenge dominant political interests and agendas through forging alliances and undertaking activities that do not rely on formalized face-to-face or structured institutional interactions in specific geographic locations.

While Fincher and Panelli (2001) took as their focus for analysis a range of farm and rural women's groups in Australia (as well as an urban-based group), we focus specifically on the organization, AWiA. The group, formed in 1992, has the following objectives:

- uniting and raising the profile of women in agriculture
- addressing rural and agricultural inequities
- working to ensure the survival of agriculture for future generations
- securing local, regional and international recognition
- achieving the status of a political and economic force (AWiA 2002).

In order to understand the extent to which cyberspace may offer a new space for AWiA members to meet these political goals, it is necessary to examine how members conceptualize technology. The following section provides a conceptual framework for undertaking this task.

Gender and the social construction of technology

Social-shaping or social constructivist approaches to technology (MacKenzie and Wajcman 1999) offer a compelling perspective for looking at gender and the internet. This is principally because constructivists' observations of 'technology' recognize not only the built device itself, but also the practices and knowledge related to it and the social arrangements that form around the device, which in turn imbue practices and knowledge (Mackenzie and Wajcman 1999).

The analysis and technological discussion undertaken in this chapter departs from dominant approaches towards technology that typically study the effects or impact of technology on society. Rather, it explores how the social shaping of technology by rural women has facilitated the social process of women's engagement in online activism. In this chapter we apply the specific model of SCOT (Social Construction of Technology) because it has several advantages in analysing users as agents of technological change (Pinch and Bijker 1984). SCOT's conceptual framework focuses on three interrelated components: interpretative flexibility, relevant social groups and closure and stabilization of the artefact.

The focus on 'interpretative flexibility' in the SCOT framework 'underscores artefacts and, in particular, their working as subject to radically different interpretations, that are coextensive with social groups' (Kline and Pinch 1999: 114). The SCOT framework emphasizes that technological studies need to draw attention to technological benefits which are human-centred, usable, equitable, appropriate and responsive to everyday culture and practice (Williams and Edge 1996). This study of AWiA is thus about the usability of the internet for rural women's activism, and the intergroup negotiations between relevant social groups involved online as they work to make their organization a 'political and economic force' (AWiA 2002).

In SCOT 'relevant social groups' which play a role in the development of a technological artefact are defined as those groups that share a meaning of the artefact (Klein and Kleinman 2002). Within AWiA a number of social groups participate in constructing AWiA online. For example, different types of farming women (graziers, horticulturalists, fish farmers, etc.), rural consultants, researchers and bureaucrats participate in the list and collectively construct meanings about rural and agricultural concerns. However, as discussed later in this chapter, these multiple groups embody a specific interpretation of the AWiA list and thus negotiation continues over the design of AWiA's content and communication style. Evidently, different social groups in AWiA associate different meanings with the internet, leading to interpretative flexibility over the discussion list. Interpretative flexibility will cease at some stage and stabilization will occur. At this stage, AWiA has stabilized because there are fewer conflicts and the artefact (discussion list) no longer poses a problem to any relevant social group, and the multigroup process on AWiA has achieved closure. In the SCOT framework, closure by definition occurs when unresolved problems are redefined so that they no longer pose problems to social groups (Klein and Kleinman 2002).

The SCOT approach has two major limitations. Firstly, SCOT says little about the social structure and power relationships within which technical development takes place (Russell 1986). A related concern is the neglect of the reciprocal relationship between technology and social groups. In agreement with Kline and Pinch (1996: 767) we believe 'it is important to show not only how social groups shape technology, but also how the identities of social groups are reconstituted in the process'. Another major concern with the SCOT approach is the absence of a focus on gender and, importantly, the lack of attention to the historical nature of gendered power, which has been of concern to feminists studying technology (e.g. Wajcman 1991; Cockburn and Ormrod 1993). Mindful of this omission, this chapter places gender at the centre of its inquiry. Thus, our study of women's use of technology shifts attention away from the artefacts (internet and computers) and instead privileges the work women undertake online and their processes while online. In this sense, our interest is not in the technology itself, but rather on what Jackson *et al.* (2002: 238) call the possibility to 'envision new or alternative modes of engagement'. Before beginning to explore data on this subject, the following section provides a brief overview of the research methodology used for the study.

Methodology

This chapter is based on twenty semi-structured interviews undertaken with members of Australian Women in Agriculture during their Annual General Meeting in Melbourne in 2001.

A key advantage of this process was its flexibility. Given the differing levels of engagement with technology and opinions about technology held by members, a semi-structured approach was useful in that it allowed us to contextualize approaches to address the views of particular individuals (Cohen and Manion 1989). The interview was also valuable in that it is a method which gives emphasis to the meanings and interpretations of participants and thus provides the means of valuing the voice and experience of women (Limerick *et al.* 1996). Interviews were transcribed and coded thematically for analysis using the software program NUD*IST VIVO (Qualitative Solutions and Research 1999).

As well as drawing on interview data, the chapter also uses documentary evidence in the form of past editions of the organizational monthly publication, *The Buzz*, to provide a more comprehensive understanding of the research questions (Yin 1994). This magazine is useful in elucidating the research question, particularly as a selection of letters on the chat line are published monthly. We thus had an edited, but still important, retrospective picture (Sarantakos 1993) of the topics that have been discussed electronically, as well as the nature and tone of the online discussion.

It is recognized that the use of new technologies by members of AWiA may be undertaken for a range of purposes and by different individuals or subsets within the group and between these individuals and subsets and outside members. The organization itself is made up of women involved in a range of farm-related activities. Some are on farms while others are in government, academia, extension agencies and rural-based commercial enterprises. Currently, the organization has no demographic data on the make-up of its discussion list which could have provided further insights into the data. For the purposes of this chapter we have looked separately at the use of technology, by and for board work by the executive of the organization and the use of technology, by and for the general membership of the group on the AWiA chat line, Australian Women in Agriculture Online. These are discussed below.

The technosocial landscape of AWiA

In this section we will discuss the way in which the technosocial conventions of the AWiA email list have emerged and have come to be stabilized. Members have a historical reliance on technology for conducting the business of the organization. Before internet technology, members had utilized faxes, phone and the pen (mail). The last of these was particularly problematic given that some board members on isolated properties obtain mail only once a week or, in periods of flood or fire, are cut off from mail access for days or weeks. The technologies of phone or fax are also problematic, as is the use of the internet for rural people in Australia who rely on the Digital Radio Concentrator System (DRCS), as it is notoriously unreliable and users are often without lines for days or weeks (Simpson *et al.* 2001).

Members agreed there were advantages in the use of new communication technologies for board members; however, there were also some tensions. Of these, the most commonly mentioned was that there was a difference of opinion as to the degree of informal discussion which should be engaged in a board email. Some saw the issue as the need for board members to restrict any non-business references in board emails. One member commented, for example, that the problem facing the board was that some members could not 'get to the point'. Others believed that informal discussion between board members was important, but that strategies needed to be developed to ensure that this was done using other media such as the telephone. As one interviewee commented:

> The problem with the technology is that people like to chat to each other. How to separate out the chat from the business is difficult. We have had to really work on that to combine both . . . encourage people to ring each other and talk between meetings or email each other for chats as well as for business.

As well as using email for sharing information and networking, AWiA board members also use the technology for communicating with members. That is, they asked for feedback on submissions they had received or for issues they would like raised if a member was involved in a lobbying trip or was a representative on an industry/ government committee. Another purpose of the discussion group for board members was supporting and encouraging membership activities. One executive member summed up this role:

> I try and encourage what's going on. If someone posts something saying that they are having a gathering, I'd write and say, 'Great. Good on you.' So I try and not just contribute by saying something but also by supporting what others are doing and saying.

What the members of the AWiA board do not use the technology for is direct lobbying. One commented, 'We use technology for information gathering to do the lobbying, but typically, the lobbying we do is face-to-face.' This 'face-to-face' lobbying involved annual trips to the national capital, Canberra, where members meet with various politicians and industry leaders. Asked why there was not greater use of new technologies for lobbying politicians, board members argued that they believed there was greater potential to influence people when meeting them in person. These women are thus interpreting technology for a range of political ends including developing their political skills and knowledge, and sharing information between group members. At the same time, they construct technology as being less powerful politically compared with direct personal interaction.

Australian Women in Agriculture Online

The discussion list AWiA was established in 1998 and currently has 206 members. No demographic data on list members is held by the organization and thus it is not possible to present a profile of participants. However, interviews with members as well as an examination of messages indicate that, like the broader membership of AWiA, list members are a mix of women living in rural Australia, government officers working in agricultural agencies, agricultural consultants and rural researchers.

The reasons for only a third of the AWiA membership being involved in the discussion list had not been investigated by the organization, but it was a subject that was of great interest to members of the executive. When asked why she thought some members had not signed up to be part of this group, one current leader and farm woman observed:

> Maybe it is cost. In lots of areas it is still expensive, especially where there aren't local service providers. Maybe it is that they think they're going to get inundated with emails. Maybe they haven't even got a computer yet or haven't had training. I just don't know.

To explain why some AWiA women do not participate in the online list we should think beyond the purely functional role of access as being grounded in infrastructure and technology training towards a conceptualization of geographies of access (Scott *et al.* 1999). Dutton (cited in Scott *et al.* 1999) argues that we cannot think about internet-based technology which simply adds to people's existing capacities and resources. Instead, we must ask other questions. These questions are: To what are women gaining access and how is access to internet-based technologies substituting other activities in women's lives? Some perspective on these questions was provided by three of the 20 members interviewed who are not part of the discussion list. All three of these women are farm women living in different parts of rural Australia. One commented on the fact that her paid work demanded time on the computer, and therefore she did not want to engage in using technology in her leisure and private life. She explained this functional view:

> I use the email as a tool. I find it very time-consuming when time is precious. I spend so much of my life at the computer now, that to

have to email people as well would be a chore. I very rarely send a chatty message. It's just not my thing. I'd rather talk on the phone. I find it impersonal. There's no intimacy about it. People say it's so quick. Yes, it's quick, but it's not intimate.

While the second woman agreed with the participant quoted above, saying that she did not like the impersonality of technology, a third said she was simply too busy. She referred to the fact that often involvement in off-farm paid work, on-farm work and volunteer work meant that something like being part of a discussion group was a 'luxury' she could not afford.

For the remaining seventeen participants interviewed, participation in the AWiA discussion list was critical to receiving up-to-date information and being in a position to provide input into policy. This attitude was summed up by the participant who replied to a question about the significance of the discussion list saying, 'We finally have a voice'. She provided a range of examples to demonstrate what this meant. In one example she referred to a posting by an Australian Broadcasting Commission reporter who said they would be interviewing the Prime Minister the next day and asked members if they had any particular questions they would like addressed. This participant's example along with those provided by others demonstrates the way in which cyberspace provides the opportunity for women activists to subvert what Scott *et al.* have called the 'geographies of public and private' (1999: 550). They are participating in the public world of agri-politics in which they have traditionally been marginalized – and doing so from the private world of their home computers.

It had been the original intention that all members of AWiA would be a part of the online group. Thus, when members joined the organization they were immediately connected to the discussion list. This did not continue, however, beyond 2000, when some members who had been connected complained about the number of emails they were receiving and the content of the emails. This reflects an ongoing tension in the discussion list. It was a tension one board member characterized in terms of the 'different groups' that she said made up the membership of AWiA. One group, she said, were the 'bureaucrats and consultants' who wanted to use the list for distributing information. The second group were those she categorized as the 'broad base of membership' who were interested in obtaining information but also in informal discussion and networking. The participation of actors from different communities of practice, such as bureaucracy, academia, and agri-commerical enterprises provides AWiA with the opportunity to meet its political goals. However, as other research has noted, simultaneous membership of more than one community can create tensions for individuals as we involve ourselves in many potential actions (Becker, cited in Star 1991: 50).

At this stage of the research, we have not undertaken interviews with members from the full range of occupational groups represented on the list or undertaken a detailed analysis of postings according to occupational categories. However, it is possible and likely that the different occupational identities of members will inform their construction of the list. Importantly, members are not anonymous on the list, and typically when postings are made, signatories reveal their occupational position and geographic location. Given the different discursive powers of occupational identities (politician, Minister's adviser, journalist, farm woman), some postings may be seen to be more privileged or legitimate than others. This may be the case with those that have been vocal about how the list should be utilized. This was evident when a list member, whose occupation was not specifically known but who signed herself as 'Dr', wrote to the list saying:

> Is it possible to partially remove me from the email list? I would like to continue to get the outgoing emails from you BUT NOT the returning comments, etc.

Another member, from a farm in the south-western part of the state of Queensland, replied saying that while she did not want to risk 'adding to the gabble', she too would 'like to receive the minimum'.

Quite a different response was elicited in two replies from women in country Victoria and New South Wales:

> Having seen people come and go from the AWiA list I am intrigued to see talk about gabble . . . my understanding was that this forum wasn't just for information dissemination but to hear each other's voices. I sometimes feel it's clutter . . . not gabble and so I only open my AWiA mail (which I prize!) when I have time to read (not hear unfortunately) . . . As rural women this is a valuable way of feeling part of another community. Please consider carefully any changes . . . I like it the way it is!!!
>
> Let's not forget that only a short time ago, access to this amount of information, and opinions, and discussion, could only be dreamed about. Now we can access women from different skills,

backgrounds, farming concerns – all at the click of one email.
I think it's fabulous.

In an interview, the list moderator at the time recalled the debate,
as well as the way in which some members who had been actively
involved in 'chatting' seemed to 'jump off and never speak again'
rather than, she said, 'be assertive enough to say that this is what
we want it for so you get off'. Another member concurred with this
perspective, reflecting on the changes in the list since the tensions had
erupted:

> People wanted to chat about the weather and the kids and that
> was okay. But then a certain percentage of the membership
> wasn't happy with that at all so they started saying things like,
> 'We don't want to hear that it's good drying weather.' So I think
> it's been very quiet in the last couple of years.

An examination of the emails posted during the month of April 2002
attests to the dominance of instrumental communication on the list.
Of the total forty-one posted messages, one focused solely on personal
issues as a new list member introduced herself. The remainder either
provided or sought information. This demonstrates the stabilizing of
technology within AWiA.

At the same time, members maintained that there is still a place
for chat. Many found this aspect of the discussion list particularly
important. One commented:

> Maybe someone will say that we had a meeting today and who
> hosted it and what was discussed and things. And then they'll
> say at the bottom that 'My daughter had my first grandchild
> today'. At the bottom you get that human aspect which really
> makes it more special. You can really picture people.

A range of emails published in previous editions of *The Buzz* attest
to the prevalence of this particular type of discourse, of which the
following is illustrative:

> If you want to get a political skills handbook Joan Kirner and
> Moira Rayner have not long put out *The Women's Power Hand-
> book*. It is a very basic commonsense read about political activism
> in easy to understand language. Published by Viking Press. Had

some great rain this weekend, sorry to hear Moora has copped a flood.

This mention of 'the weather' in an email on the discussion list is common according to interviews with members. Asked why they believed this topic is so prevalent, members pointed to the importance of the weather to farmers and anyone involved with agriculture.

The construction of technology by AWiA members

The technology constructionist approach we have adopted in this chapter to examine the extent to which cyberspace offers women a new space for political engagement focuses attention on the human-centred processes manifest in the technology of the discussion list. The data reveals that the construction of the AWiA members cannot be separated from their own gendered identities. There is, as Cockburn and Ormrod (1993) demonstrate in tracing the life of the microwave oven through design and manufacturing to its point of purchase, a relational and lived process by which technology and gender are 'made'. Thus, the AWiA members' construction of the technology as a 'business tool' has been influenced by their own gendered identities as 'women activists'. The aims and objectives of the AWiA are broad-ranging and reconstruct women in agriculture from a position of assisting on the family farm or 'farm wife' to a political force in their own right in the agri-political sphere. The objectives to raise the profile and political status of agricultural women alongside those of structural adjustment, viability and equity concerns in relation to the agricultural industry signal an intent to engage politically at the highest levels. Adopting a 'business' approach to using the technology demonstrates AWiA members' reconstituted identities as they shift from 'farmer's wife' to 'political activist'.

To understand why the women of AWiA have constructed discussion list technology as being for 'business' rather than 'leisure', it is also necessary to examine the broader gendered context in which their subject positions are constituted. The first contextual factor is that for women, leisure is typically highly circumscribed by gendered power relations (Green *et al.* 1990; Wearing 1998). In their review of the still limited literature on the subject of gender, leisure and ICTs, Green and Adam (1998: 302) make the salient point that because of 'the constraints on women's time, especially their leisure or "uncommitted time", the use of ICTs for leisure purposes is likely to be limited for most women and heavily dependent upon the possibility of combining such activities with the work of child minding or house-work'. This may be particularly pertinent for the farming women who were the subject of this study. This is a group of women who are likely to be responsible for all domestic labour and a number of other on-farm tasks, undertake off-farm paid work and be involved in a number of voluntary and community activities (Alston 1995; Sachs 1996). Thus, these are women for whom time is critical. There is the added factor that the already limited time availability of the women will have been further eroded by their online activity. This was certainly the experience of the participants in Scott's (2001: 416) study, one of whom found responding to the excessive numbers of emails that are possible due to the speed and efficiency of technology 'a bit like housework'. Given this context, it is understandable that the technology used by AWiA members has been largely constructed in ways which give primacy to it as a tool for efficient business use. In this sense the lives of the women have shaped the technology of the discussion list.

The construction of the discussion list by AWiA members as primarily instrumental may shift and change over time. Wajcman (1991: 103) has argued that 'many domestic technologies were initially developed for business use' but have been subsequently reconstructed. Frissen (1995) has illustrated this phenomenon in terms of the telephone, which was first seen as an instrument of 'business' rather than of social interaction: women have, over time, established a dimension of 'sociability' in relation to its usage. It may be that in this period in the early adoption of the internet as a medium of communication, 'business' transactions are given more prominence, but this will change. It is certainly the case that the telephone is constructed by AWiA members as being for both personal and business use. While it is often used for undertaking the business of AWiA, there is no suggestion that a conversation about 'business' on the telephone precludes including some personal opening or closure. Indeed, during the three-day AWiA General Meeting during which time the interviews reported in this chapter were conducted, we noted that it was common and seemingly acceptable for there to be a blurring of conversational/personal and formal/business discourses within AWiA. The more stringent discursive boundaries that have been established by AWiA members in the positioning of the computer technology as purely for (or at least primarily for) 'business' may also come to resemble the conventions associated with telephone or meeting technologies as it becomes more integrated into the women's lives.

A new space for political engagement?

This research has demonstrated that information and communication technology not only has overwhelmingly improved communication between members but also has linked the group into the political process in more effective ways. Through the sharing of knowledge fostered by new technologies, rural women have had opportunities for input into the processes of policy-making and access to government representatives and decision-making forums which were previously unavailable to them. A further outcome of the technology is that it has facilitated the women's identity transformation as they become 'women in agriculture' who are embracing activism to give their organization 'the status of a political and economic force'.

However, there are, to use the terminology of Cox (1997), 'spaces of engagement' available electronically that are not being exploited by AWiA and that could facilitate the organization's meeting its political goals. The technology could be further utilized as a means of collectivizing and empowering members. It could also be used to assist the development of a shared identity as 'women in Australian agriculture', as well as providing opportunities for negotiating the differences and diversities of women involved in farming.

Clearly, there has been some tension among group members because they have viewed the technology as differently located – as a white good, a brown good or a mixture of both. This tension was played out on the list as members voiced their preference for instrumental talk, for social talk, or for a combination of the two. Power dynamics were revealed through these tensions. That is, while stabilization of the techno-social conventions on AWiA has benefited some members, this has not been the case for those who have left the list. Star (1991: 43) points out that 'a network is only stable for some, and that is for those who are members of the community of practice who form/use/ maintain it'. Thus, those 'non-standard' members no longer have their voices heard on the AWiA discussion list. This means that these women no longer are participating in cyberspace as a political 'space for engagement'. It may be that the women who left the list had limited political aspirations. However, their participation in the list may have actually politicized them. This is because involvement in a discussion list such as AWiA Online has been demonstrated to increase women's confidence in using new technologies, sharing points of view, accessing information and resources and expressing one's ideas (Lennie *et al.* 1999). What is interesting is that the importance of a 'private' space in which women may be supported to debate ideas, network and develop skills and knowledge that can be utilized in the 'public' space has been well recognized by AWiA (Fincher and Panelli 2001), but in the online environment this has not been well acknowledged, or, indeed, acknowledged at all. To realize the potential of new communication and information technologies, however, group members need to reconsider the limited way in which they have constituted technology. Such a reconstruction will include relational discourses in defining technology and not only transactional and functional discourses. This is not to suggest that attempting to create a space for open debate and discussion will, by definition, lead to such debate and discussion occurring. However, it is possible that groups such as AWiA can seek to develop online spaces which support inclusive and open debate and discussion.

Conclusion

The incorporation of technology into the political processes of AWiA is relatively new. Given the shifting nature of technology construction and identities, future research on the use of technology by AWiA members will be important to provide greater insight into the potential of new ICTs for political activism. In turn, this will raise new questions about how cyberspace is expanding and reconstituting traditional political engagement. Further exploration is also required to learn more about non-users of the discussion list. This would focus our attention on those women who do not use new communication technologies at all and the extent to which they are being marginalized by increased online political activity. What will be of use about such work is that it will highlight difference and diversity among women. Studies of gender, technology and communication have often claimed that there are essential differences between women as a group and men as a group (e.g. Pew Internet and American Life Project 2000; Reeder 1996). We would argue, however, that instead of examining gender as an independent variable in research on ICTs there is more significance in examining differences across subject positions and seeking to understand why such differences exist. In this chapter we have taken a gender perspective in exploring the technology use of the list participants. However, our focus has been on the participants not simply as women, but as rural and farm women. We have drawn attention to the salience of this latter identity in determining how AWiA members have constructed technology in their lives. There are, of course, a range of other subject positions these women inhabit which will also influence their construction of technology. Thus, to understand fully the relationship of gender and technology in these women's lives, we will need to incorporate into future analysis an understanding of these different subjectivities.

Bibliography

Abramson, J.B., Arterton, F.C. and Orren, G.R. (1988) *The electronic commonwealth. The impact of new technologies upon democratic politics*, New York: Basic Books.

Advice A/S analysis report, (2002) *Dyreaktivisters aktionsformer og netværksdannelse på internettet*, Copenhagen: Advice A/S.

Aelst, P. Van (2000) 'The battle of Seattle. Over Internationale Democratie op straat', *Internationale Spectator* 54: 76–79.

Aelst, P. Van and Walgrave, S. (2001a) 'Nieuwe spelers op het middenveld. Over sociale bewegingen in de 21ste eeuw', *Bestuurskunde* 10, 1: 28–37.

Aelst, P. Van and Walgrave, S. (2001b) 'Who is that (wo)man in the street? From the normalisation of protest to the normalisation of the protester', *European Journal of Political research*, 39: 461–486.

Aggy, K. and Andrew, S. (2002) 'Renegotiating the terrain – autonomous social movements', http://www.melbourne.indymedia.org/front.php3?article_id=26875andgroup=webcast, accessed 26 May 2002.

Agre, P. (2002) 'Real-time politics: the internet and the political process', *The Information Society* 18: 311–331.

Alberoni, F. (1984) *Movement and Institution* (originally published in 1977), New York: Columbia University Press.

Alston, M. (1995) *Women on the land: the hidden heart of rural Australia*, Kensington: UNSW Press.

Andersen, G.J. and Tobiasen, M. (2001) *Politisk forbrug og politiske forbrugere: globalizering og politik i hverdagslivet*, Aarhus: Magtudredningen.

Andrade, C. (1999) 'Tragédia obrigou a tomar partido', *Diário de Notícias*, 29 September.

Argyle, K. (1996) 'Life after death', in Shields, R. (ed.) *Cultures of internet: virtual spaces, real histories, living bodies*, London: Sage.

Arnison, M. (2002) 'Open publishing is the same as free software', http://www.cat.org.au/maffew/cat/openpub.html, accessed 1 March 2002.

Arquilla, J. and Ronfeldt, D. (1996) *The advent of netwar*, Santa Monica: RAND.

Arquilla J. and Ronfeldt, D. (2001) 'The advent of netwar (revisited)', in Arquilla, J. and Ronfeldt, D. (eds) *Networks and netwars: the future of terror, crime, and militancy*, Santa Monica: RAND.

Arrighi, G. (2002) 'Lineages of empire', *Dissonance* 1, http://pages.akbild.ac.at/aesthetik/dissonance%20Kopie/arrighi.html, accessed 1 March 2003.

Arrighi, G., Wallerstein, I. and Hopkins, T. (1989) *Anti-systemic movements*. London: Verso.

Aufheben (2002) '"Anti-capitalism" as ideology . . . and as movement?', *Aufheben* 10.

AWiA (2002) *Annual report*, Melbourne: AWiA.

Ayres, J.M. (1999) 'From the streets to the internet: the cyber-diffusion of contention', *Annals of the American Academy of Political and Social Science* 566: 132–143.

Ayres, J.M. (2001) 'Transnational political processes and contention against the global economy', *Mobilization* 6: 55–68.

Baker, K.M. (1997) 'Defining the public sphere in eighteenth-century France: variations on a theme by Habermas', in Cahloun, C. (ed.) *Habermas and the public sphere*, Cambridge, MA: MIT Press.

Barnes, C. and Oliver, M. (1991) 'Discrimination, disability and welfare: from needs to rights', in Bynoe, J., Oliver, M. and Barnes, C. (eds) *Equal rights for disabled people*, London: Institute for Public Policy Research.

Barnett, S. (1997) 'New media, old problems. New technology and the political process', *European Journal of Communication*, 12: 193–218.

Barton, L. (1993) 'The struggles for citizenship: the case of disabled people', *Disability, Handicap and Society* 8: 3.

Baxi, U. (2000) 'Human rights – suffering between movements and markets', in Cohen, R. and Rai, S. (eds) *Global social movements*, London: Athlone Press.

Bebiano, (1999) 'Rui Um Clamor Digital', *Vida Mundial*, 1st October 1999.

Beck, U. (1997) *Risikosamfundet: På vej mod en ny modernitet*. Copenhagen: Hans Reitzels Forlag A/S, first published 1986.

Beck, U. (2000) *What is globalization?*, Cambridge: Polity Press.

Becker, H. (1960) 'Notes on the concept of commitment', *American Journal of Sociology* 66: 32–40.

Bekkers, V.J.J.M. (1998) *Grenzeloze overheid: over informatisering en grensveranderingen in het openbaar bestuur*, Alphen aan den Rijn: Samsom.

Bekkers, V.J.J.M. (2000) *Voorbij de virtuele organizatie?*, The Hague: Elsevier.

Benjamin, G. (1982) 'Innovations in telecommunications and politics', in Benjamin, G. (ed.) *The communications revolution in politics*, New York: Proceedings of the Academy of Political Science.

Benjamin, W. (1969) *Illuminations*, New York: Schocken Books.

Bennett, W.L. (1996) *News: the politics of illusion*, White Plains, NY: Longman.

Bennett, W.L. (1998) 'The uncivic culture: communication, identity, and the rise of lifestyle politics', Ithiel de Sola Pool Lecture, American Political Science Association, *Political Science and Politics* **31**, 4: 41–61.

Bennett, W. L. (2003a) 'New media power: the internet and global activism', in Couldry, N. and Curran, J. (eds) *Contesting Media Power*, New York: Rowman and Littlefield.

Bennett, W.L. (2003b) *News: the politics of illusion* (5th edn) New York: Longman.

Bennett, W.L. (2003c) 'Branded political communication: lifestyle politics, logo campaigns, and the rise of global citizenship', in Micheletti, M., Follesdal, A. and Stolle, D. (eds) *The politics behind products: using the market as a site for ethics and action*, New Brunswick, NJ: Transaction Books.

Beresford, P. and Holden, C. (2000) 'We have choices: globalization and welfare user movements', *Disability and Society* **15**, 7: 973–989.

Besser, H. (1995) 'From internet to information superhighway', in Brook, J. and Boal, I. (eds) *Resisting the virtual: the culture and politics of information*, San Francisco: City Life.

Bieber, C. (1999) *Politische Projekte im Internet. Online-Kommunikation und politische Öffentlichkeit*, Frankfurt-on-Main: Campus.

Bimber, B. (1998) 'The internet and political mobilization. Research note on the 1996 Election Season', *Social Science Computer Review*, **16**: 391–401.

Blumer, H. (1951) 'Social movements', in Lee, A.M. (ed.) *New outlines of the principles of sociology*, New York: Barnes and Noble.

Bogumil, J. and Lange, H.J. (1991) *Computer in Parteien und Verbänden*, Opladen: Westdeutscher Verlag.

Bonchek, M.S. (1995) *Grassroots in cyberspace: recruiting members on the internet*, Paper presented at the 53rd annual meeting of the Midwest Political Science Association, Chicago, 6–8 April. Available at http://www-marketing.com/virtuelle_gemeinschaft/text/bonch95a.htm.

Boomen, M. van den (2000) *Leven op het Net. De sociale betekenis van virtuele gemeenschappen*, Amsterdam: Instituut voor Publiek en Politiek.

Borgida, G. and Sullivan, J.L. (eds) (1999) *Minnesota symposium on political psychology*, New York: Cambridge University Press.

Borio, G., Pozzi, F. and Roggero, G. (2001) 'Intervista a Sergio Bologna – 21 Febbraio 2001', on the CD accompanying *Futuro anteriore: Dai Quaderni Rossi ai movimenti globali: ricchezze e limiti dell'operaismo italiano*, Rome: Derive Approdi.

Bourdieu, P. (1992) *The logic of practice*, Stanford, CA: Stanford University Press.

Braun, E. (1992) 'Augsteins Spiegelbild' (originally published in 1972), in Redaktion diskus, *Küss den Boden der Freiheit. Texte der Neuen Linken*, Frankfurt-on-Main: Edition ID-Archiv.

Braverman, H. (1975) *Labor and monopoly capital*, New York: Monthly Review Press.

Brewer, J. (2001) 'Confessions of an IT junkie', *The Buzz* **43**: 1.

Brophy, E. (2002) 'The outlaw "net": opposition to ICANN's new internet order', *Computers and Society* **32**, 4, December.

Brouns, M. (1995) 'Feminisme en wetenschap', in Brouns, M., Verloo, M. and Grünell, M. (eds) *Vrouwenstudies in de jaren negentig*, Bussum: Countinho.

Bryan, C., Tsagarousianou, R. and Tambini, D. (1998) 'Electronic democracy and the civic networking movement in context', in Tsagarousianou, R., Tambini, D. and Bryan, C. (eds) *Cyberdemocracy, technology cities and civic networks*, London: Routledge.

Buchstein, H. (1997) 'Bytes that bite: the internet and deliberative democracy', *Constellations* **4**, 2: 248–263.

Buechler, S.M. (1993) 'Beyond resource mobilization? Emerging trends in social movement theory', *The Sociological Quarterly* **34**, 2: 217–235.

Buechler, S.M. (2000) *Social movements in advanced capitalism: the political economy and cultural construction of social activism*, New York: Oxford University Press.

Bullert, B.J. (2000) *Strategic public relations, sweatshops, and the making of a global movement*, Working Paper 2000–14, Joan Shorenstein Center on the Press, Politics, and Public Policy, Harvard University.

Burgmann, V. (1993) *Power and protest*, St Leonards: Allen and Unwin.

Calhoun, C. (1991) 'The problem of identity in collective action', in Huber, J. (ed.) *Macro–micro linkages in sociology*, pp. 51–75.

Calhoun, C. (1995) '"New social movements" of the early nineteenth century', in Traugott, M. (ed.) *Repertoires and cycles of collective action*, Durham, NC and London: Duke University Press.

Calhoun, C. (1998) 'Community without propinquity revisited: communications technology and the transformation of the urban public sphere', *Sociological Inquiry* **68**, 3: 373–397.

Callon, M. (1986) 'Some elements of a sociology of translation: domestication of the scallops and the fishermen of St Brieue Bay', in Law, J. (ed.) *Power, action and belief*, London: Routledge & Kegan Paul.

Campbell, J. and Oliver, M. (1996) *Disability politics. Understanding our past, changing our future*, London: Routledge.

Canadian Security Intelligence Service (2000) *Anti-globalization: a spreading phenomenon*, Report 2000/08, online. Available at http://www.csis-scrs. gc.ca/eng/miscdocs/200008_e.html.

Capek, S.M. (1993) 'The "environmental justice" frame: a conceptual discussion and an application', *Social Problems: Official Journal of the Society for the Study of Social Problems*, **40**, 1: 5–24.

Cardoso, G. (1999) 'As causas das questões ou o estado àbeira de sociedade de informação', *Sociologia – Problemas e Práticas*, **30**: 111–144.

Casarini, L. (2003) 'Throughout Italy: the multitude against the empire', *Rebeldía* **5**, http://amsterdam.nettime.org/Lists-Archives/nettime-l-0304/ msg00100.html, accessed 25 April 2003.

Castells, M. (1996) *The rise of the network society*, Oxford: Blackwell.

Castells, M. (1997). *The power of identity*, Oxford: Blackwell.

Castells, M. (2000a) *Internet y la Sociedad Red*, available at http://www. uoc.es/web/esp/articles/castells/castellsmain.html, accessed 28 February 2002.

Castells, M. (2000b) *The rise of the network society* (2nd edn), Oxford: Blackwell.

Castells, M. (2001) *The internet galaxy – reflections on the internet, business and society*, London: Oxford University Press.

Cha, D. (2001) *Internet communication structure in US congress: a network analysis*, paper prepared for the Annual American Political Science Association meeting, San Francisco.

Chandler, D. (1998) 'Personal home pages and the construction of identities on the web', available at http://www.aber.ac.uk/media/Documents/short/ webident.html.

Chartier, R. (ed.) (1995) 'Histoire de la lecture', *Un bilan des recherches*, Paris: IMEC, Editions de la MSH.

Cheta, R. (2002) 'Voicing disabled people', *movement through the online campaigning for access_@bility to ICTs*. Reflections from the GUIA/PASIG experience in Portugal.

Chroust, P. (2000) 'Neo-Nazis and Taliban on-line: anti-modern political movements and modern media', *Democratization* 7, 1: 102–119.

Chuck0 (2002) 'The sad decline of indymedia', http://amsterdam.nettime.org/ Lists-Archives/nettime-l-0212/msg00047.html, accessed 19 April 2003.

Cleaver, H. (1993) 'Theses on secular crisis in capitalism: the insurpassability of class antagonisms', http://www.eco.utexas.edu/facstaff/Cleaver/secularcrisis. html, accessed 24 December 2001.

Cleaver, H. (1997) 'Documents from the first intercontinental encounter: preface', http://www.geocities.com/CapitolHill/3849/italy_book.html, accessed 1 February 2002.

Cleaver, H. (1998) 'The Zapatistas and the international circulation of struggle: lessons suggested and problems raised', http://www.eco.utexas. edu/faculty/Cleaver/lessons.html, accessed 26 July 2001.

Cleaver, H. (1999) 'Computer-linked social movements and the global threat to capitalism', http://www.eco.utexas.edu/faculty/Cleaver/polnet.html, accessed 1 May 2001.

Cocco, G. and Lazzarato, M. (2002) 'An interview with Toni Negri', *Multitudes* 7, http://vancouver.indymedia.org/front.php3?article_id=9076 andgroup=webcast, accessed 1 March 2002.

Cockburn, C. (1997) 'Domestic technologies: Cinderella and the engineers', *Women's Studies International Forum* 20, 3: 361–371.

Cockburn, C. and Ormrod, S. (1993) *Gender and technology in the making*, London: Sage.

Cohen, J.L. (1985) 'Strategy or identity: new theoretical paradigms and contemporary social movements', *Social Research* 52, 4: 663–716.

Cohen, L. and Manion, L. (1989) *Research methods in education*, London: Routledge.

Cohen, R. and Rai, S. (eds) (2000) *Global social movements*, London: Athlone Press.

Cooper, M. (1999) 'The Australian disability rights movement lives', *Disability and Society* **14**, 2: 217–226.

Correll, S. (1995) 'The ethnography of an electronic bar: the lesbian café', *Journal of Contemporary Ethnography* **24**, 3: 270–298.

Cowell, A. (2000) 'Advocates gain ground in a globalized era', *The New York Times*, international business section, electronic edition of 18 December.

Cox, K.R. (1997) 'Spaces of dependence, spaces of engagement and the politics of scale, or: looking for local politics', *Political Geography* **17**, 1: 1–23.

Cox, L. (2001) 'Barbarian resistance and rebel alliances: social movements and empire', *Rethinking Marxism* **13**, 3/4: Fall/Winter.

Crook, S., Pakulski, J. and Waters, M. (1992) *Postmodernization – change in advanced societies*, London: Sage.

Crossley, N. (1996) *Intersubjectivity – the fabric of social becoming*, London: Sage.

Crossley, N. (2001) *Making sense of social movements*, Milton Keynes and Buckingham: Open University Press.

Dahlgren, P. (2000) 'L'espace public et l'internet. Structure, espace et communication', *Réseaux* **100**: 159–186.

Dalton, R.J. (1994) *The green rainbow. Environmental groups in Western Europe*. New Haven and London: Yale University Press.

Danitz, T. and Strobel, W.P. (1999) 'The internet's impact on activism: the case of Burma, *Studies in Conflict and Terrorism* **22**: 257–269.

Danziger, J.G., Dutton, W.H., Kling, R. and Kraemer, K.L. (1982) *Computers and politics. High technology in American local governments*, New York: Columbia University Press.

Davis, D. (1999) 'Media as public arena: reconceptualizing the role of media for a post-cold war and postmodern world', in Vincent, R., Nordenstreng, K. and Traber, M. (eds) *Towards equity in global communication*, Cresskill, NJ: Hampton Press.

Davis, K. (1996) *The disabled people's movement. Putting the power in empowerment*, paper presented at a seminar at the University of Sheffield, Department of Sociology, June, available at http://www.leeds.ac.uk/disability-studies/archiveuk/archframe/davisk1996.htm, accessed 11 November 2001.

Davis, R. (1999) *The web of politics: the internet's impact on the American political system*, New York: Oxford University Press.

Day, R. (1994) 'Animal songs: translation, community, the question of the "animal" information', http://www.lisp.wayne.edu/~ai2398/animal.htm, accessed 1 March 2002.

Day, R. (2001a) *The modern invention of information: discourse, history, and power*. Carbondale: Southern Illinois University Press.

Day, R. (2001b) 'Totality and representation. A history of knowledge management through European documentation, critical modernity, and postfordism', *Journal of the American Society for Information Science and Technology* 52, 9: June.

De Angelis, M. (1993) 'An interview with Harry Cleaver', http://www.geocities.com/CapitolHill/3843/cleaver.html, accessed 1 May 2000.

Debord, G. and Wolman, G. (1956) 'A user's guide to *détournement*', *Les Lèvres Nues*, no. 8 (May), http:/www.bopsecrets.org/SI/detourn.htm.

Deegan, D. (2001) *Managing activism: a guide to dealing with activists and pressure groups*, The Institute of Public Relations, London: Kegan Page.

Deibert, R.J. (2000) 'International plug 'n play? Citizen activism, the Internet, and global public policy', *International Studies Perspectives* 1: 255–272.

De Landtsheer, C., Krasnoboka, N. and Gomezllata, E. (2001a) *Userfriendliness of US presidential election websites*, paper prepared for the Conference 'Etmaal van de Communicatiewetenschap', Amsterdam, February.

De Landtsheer, C., Krasnoboka, N. and Neuner, C. (2001b) *Userfriendliness of political websites in Eastern and Western European countries*, paper prepared for the Conference of the International Communication Association in Washington, May.

Della Porta, D., Kriesi, H. and Rucht, D. (eds) (1999) *Social movements in a globalizing world*, London: Macmillan.

Depla, P.F.G. and Tops, P.W. (1995) 'Political parties in the digital era: the technological challenge?', in van de Donk, W.B.H.J., Snellen, I.Th.M. and Tops, P.W. (eds) *Orwell in Athens: a perspective on informatization and the future of democracy*, Amsterdam: IOS Press.

Diani, M. (1992) 'The concept of social movement', *The Sociological Review* 40, 1: 1–25.

Diani, M. (1995) *Green networks*, Edinburgh: Edinburgh University Press.

Diani, M. (1997) 'Social movements and social capital: a network perspective on movement outcomes', *Mobilization* 2: 129–147.

Diani, M. (2000) 'Social movement networks virtual and real', *Information, Communication and Society* 3: 3.

Diani, M. (2001) 'Social movement networks. Virtual and real', in Webster, F., *Culture and politics in the information age*, London: Routledge, pp. 117–127.

Diani, M. and Eyerman, R. (eds) (1992) *Studying collective action*, London: Sage.

Diggins, J.P. (1992) *The rise and fall of the American left* (originally published in 1973) New York and London: W.W. Norton.

Dijk, J.A.G.M. van (1996) 'The reality of virtual communities', *Trends in Communication* 1: 39–63.

Dodds, K.J. (2000) *Geopolitics in a changing world*, Harlow: Pearson Education.

Donk, W. van de and Foederer, B. (2001) 'E-movements or emotions? ICTs and social movements: some preliminary observations', in Prins, J. (ed.)

Ambitions and limits on the crossroads of technological innovation and institutional change, Cambridge, MA: Kluwer.

Donk, W.B.H.J. van de and Snellen, I.Th.M. (1998) 'Towards a theory of informatization of public administration', in Snellen, I.Th.M. and Donk, W.B.H.J. van de (ed.) *Public administration in an information age: a handbook*, Amsterdam: IOS Press.

Donk, W.B.H.J. van de, Snellen, I.Th.M. and Tops, P.W. (eds) (1995) *Orwell in Athens: a perspective on informatization and the future of democracy*, Amsterdam: IOS Press.

Donk, W.B.H.J. van de and Tops, P.W. (1992) 'Informatization and democracy: Orwell or Athens? A review of the literature, *Informatization and the Public Sector*, No. 2: 69–196.

Downing, J.D.H. (1989) 'Computers for political change: PeaceNet and public data access', *Journal of Communication* 39, 3: 154–162.

Downing, J. (2000) *Radical media: rebellious communication and social movements*. Thousand Oaks, CA: Sage.

Dupuy, G. (1998) 'Der Mai 1968 und das Projekt "Liberation"', in Gilcher-Holtey, I. (ed.) *1968. Vom Ereignis zum Gegenstand der Geschichtswissenschaft*, Göttingen: Vandenhoeck and Ruprecht.

Dutton, W. (1998) *Society on the line: information politics in the digital age*, Oxford: Oxford University Press.

Dutton W. (2000) *Networked citizens and e-democracy*, Presidência da República Portuguesa, Os Cidadãos e a Sociedade de Informação, Lisbon, INCM.

Duyvendak, J.W. (1995) *The power of politics: new social movements in France*, Boulder, CO: Westview Press.

Duyvendak, J.W. and Koopmans, R. (eds) (1992) *Tussen verbeelding en macht: 25 jaar nieuwe sociale bewegingen in Nederland*, Amsterdam: SUA.

Dyer-Witheford, N. (1999) *Cyber-Marx*, Champaign: University of Illinois Press.

Dyer-Witheford, N. (2001) 'Empire, immaterial labor, the new combinations, and the global worker', *Rethinking Marxism* 13, 3/4: Fall/Winter.

ECN (1992) 'ECN UK internal developments', http://www.etext.org/Politics/ECN/ecn.uk, accessed 12 August 2001.

Edwards, A.R. (2001) *De vrouwenbeweging online*, Rotterdam: Erasmus Universiteit Rotterdam, Faculteit Sociale Wetenschappen.

Edwards, M. and Hulme, D. (eds) (1992) *Making a difference: NGOs and development in a changing world*, London: Earthscan.

Esterberg, Kristin G. (1996) '"A certain swagger when I walk": performing lesbian identity', in Seidman, S. (ed.) *Queer theory/sociology*, Oxford: Blackwell.

ETAN, 'Santa Cruz massacre', available at http://etan.org/timor/Santa CRUZ.htm, accessed 28 February 2002.

Etzioni, A. and Etzioni, O. (1999) 'Face-to-face and computer-mediated communities, a comparative analysis', *The Information Society* 15: 241–248.

European Disability Forum (1999) *European manifesto on the information society and disabled people*, available at http://www.edf-feph.org/en/welcome.html, accessed 12 September 2001.

Fernback, J. (1997) 'The individual within the collective: virtual ideology and the realization of collective principles', in S.G. Jones (ed.) *Virtual Culture*, London: Sage.

Ferree, M.M., Gamson, W.A., Gerhards, J. and Rucht, D. (2002) *Shaping abortion discourse: democracy and the public sphere in Germany and the United States*, Cambridge and New York: Cambridge University Press.

Ferree, M.M. and Miller, F.D. (1985) 'Mobilization and meaning: some social–psychological contributions to the resource mobilization perspective on social movements', *Sociological Inquiry* 55: 38–61.

Fillieule, O. (1999) '"Plus ça change, moins ça change". Demonstrations in France during the Nineteen-Eighties', in Rucht, D., Koopmans, R. and Neidhardt, F. (eds) *Act of dissent: new developments in the study of protest*, Lanham, MD: Rowman & Littlefield.

Fincher, R. and Panelli, R. (2001) 'Making space: women's urban and rural activism and the Australian state', *Gender, Place and Culture* 8, 2: 129–148.

Fink, D. (1992) 'Farm wives and agrarianism in the United States', in M. Alston (ed.) *Key papers number 1: rural women*, Wagga Wagga: Centre for Rural Welfare Research.

Finkelstein, V. (1992) *Setting future agendas*, paper presented at the National Conference on *Researching Disability: Setting the Agenda for Change*, Sheffield, June.

Finkelstein, V. and Stuart, N. (1996) 'Developing new services', in Hales G. (ed.) *Beyond disability: towards an enabling society*, Milton Keynes and Buckingham: Open University.

Fiske, J. (1989) *Understanding popular culture*, Boston: Unwin Hyman.

Fitzgerald, J. (1997) 'Reclaiming the whole: self, spirit and society', *Disability and Rehabilitation*, 19: 407–413.

Flacks, R. (1998) 'Die philosophischen und politischen Ursprünge der amerikanischen New Left', in Gilcher-Holtey, I. (ed.) *1968. Vom Ereignis zum Gegenstand der Geschichtswissenschaft*, Göttingen: Vandenhoeck and Ruprecht.

Flieger, B. (1992) *Vom Alternativblatt zur linken Tageszeitung*, München: Ölschlager.

Ford, T. and Gil, G. (2000) 'Radical internet use', in Downing, J.D. (ed.) *Radical media – rebellious communication and social movements*, London: Sage.

Francissen, L. and Brants, K. (1998) 'Virtually going places: square-hopping in Amsterdam's Digital City', in Tsagarousianou, R., Tambini, D. and Bryan, C. (eds) *Cyberdemocracy, technology cities and civic networks*, London and New York: Routledge.

Frantzich, S.E. (1989) *Political parties in the technological age*, New York: Longman.

Fraser, N. (1997) 'Rethinking the public sphere: a contribution to the critique of actually existing democracy', in Calhoun, C. (ed.) *Habermas and the public sphere*, Cambridge, MA: MIT Press.

Fraser, R. (1988) *1968: a student generation in revolt*, New York: Pantheon.

Frederick, H. (1993) 'Computer networks and the emergence of global civil society', in Harasim, L.M. (ed.) *Global networks: computers and international communication*, Cambridge, MA: MIT Press.

Friedman, D. and McAdam, D. (1992) 'Collective identity and activism', in Aldon, D.M. and Mueller, C.M. (eds) *Frontiers in social movement theory*, New Haven, CT: Yale University Press.

Frissen, P.H.A. (1999) *Politics, governance and technology: a postmodern narrative on the virtual state*, Cheltenham: Edward Elgar.

Frissen, V. (1992) 'Trapped in electronic cages? Gender and new information technologies in the public and private domain: an overview of research', *Media, Culture and Society* **14**: 31–49.

Frissen, V. (1995) 'Gender is calling: some reflections on past, present and future uses of the telephone', in Grint, K. and Gill, R. (eds) *The gender-technology relation: contemporary theory and research*, London: Taylor & Francis.

Froehling, O. (1997) 'The cyberspace "war of ink and Internet"', *The Geographical Review* **87**, 2: 291–307.

Fuller, M. (2002) 'Behind the blip: software as culture', http://listserv.cddc. vt.edu/pipermail/softwareandculture/2002–January/000057.html, accessed 15 June 2002.

Gamson, J. (1996) 'Must identity movements self-destruct? A queer dilemma', in Seidman, S. (ed.) *Queer theory/sociology*, Oxford: Blackwell.

Gamson, W.A. (1992) 'The social psychology of collective action', in Morris, A.D. and Mueller, C.M. (eds) *Frontiers in social movement theory*, New Haven, CT: Yale University Press.

Gamson, W. (1996) 'Political discourse and the collective action', in McAdam, D., McCarthy, J. and Zald, M. (eds) *Opportunities, mobilizing, structures and frames: comparative applications of contemporary movement theory*, Cambridge: Cambridge University Press.

Gamson, W.A. (1998) 'Collective identity and the mass media', in Borgida, G. and Sullivan, J.L. (eds) *Minnesota symposium on political psychology*. New York: Cambridge University Press.

Gamson, W. (2001) 'Promoting political engagement', in Bennett W.L. and Entman, R.M. (eds) *Mediated politics: communication in the future of democracy*, New York: Cambridge University Press, 56–74.

Gamson, W. and Meyer, D. (1996) 'Framing political opportunity', in McAdam, D., McCarthy, J. and Zald, M. (eds) *Comparative perspectives on social movements*, Chicago: Cambridge University Press.

Gamson, W.A. and Modigliani, A. (1989) 'Media discourse and public opinion on nuclear power: a constructionist approach', *American Journal of Sociology* **95**, 1: S1–37.

Gamson, W.A. and Wolfsfeld, G. (1993) 'Movements and media as interacting systems', in Dalton, R.J (ed.) *Citizens, protest, and democracy*, The Annals of the American Academy of Political and Social Science, **529**: 114–125.

Garner, R. (1996) *Contemporary movements and ideologies*, New York: McGraw-Hill.

Gaxie, D. (1978) *Le Cens caché*, Paris: Seuil.

Geiecker, O. (1995) 'Social policy and the problems of handicapped persons: the concurrent influence of ethics and power', *Rehabilitation* **34**: 65–68.

George, S. (2000) 'Fixing or nixing the WTO', *Le Monde Diplomatique*, January.

George, S. (2001) *The global citizen's movement: a new actor for a new politics*, Conference on reshaping globalization, Central European University: Budapest, October, posted on the World Social Forum site www. portoalegre2002.org.

Gergen, K. (1995) *Social construction and the transformation of identity politics*, paper presented at a symposium at the New School of Social Research, April, available at http://www.swarthmore.edu/Soc.Sci/Kgergen1/text8.html, accessed 5 December 2001.

Gerhards, J. and Rucht, D. (1992) 'Mesomobilization: organizing and framing in two protest campaigns in West Germany', *American Journal of Sociology* **96**: 555–596.

Gerlach, L.P. (2001) 'The structure of social movements: environmental activism and its opponents', in Arquilla, J. and Ronfeldt, D. (eds) *Networks and netwars: the future of terror, crime, and militancy*, Santa Monica: Rand.

Gerlach, L.P. and Hine, V.H. (1970) *People, power, change: movements of social transformation*, Indianapolis: Bobbs-Merrill.

Gibbins, J. and Reimer, B. (1999) *The politics of postmodernity*, London: Sage.

Gibson, J. and Kelly, A. (2000) 'Become the media', *Arena Magazine* **49**: http://www.arena.org.au/archives/Mag_Archive/issue_49/against_the_current3_49.htm, accessed 3 January 2002.

Gibson, R.K., Nixon, P.G. and Ward, S. (2003) *Net gain? Political parties and the impact of new ICTs*, London: Routledge.

Giddens, A. (1991) *Modernity and self identity: self and society in the late modern age*, Cambridge: Polity Press.

Giddens, A. (1998) *As conseqüências da modernidade*, Oeiras: Celta.

Gilcher-Holtey, I. (1995) *Die Phantasie an die Macht. Mai 68 in Frankreich*, Frankfurt-on-Main: Suhrkamp.

Gilcher-Holtey, I. (2000) 'Der Transfer zwischen den Studentenbewegungen von 1968 und die Entstehung einer transnationalen Öffentlichkeit', *Berliner Journal für Soziologie* **10**, 4: 485–500.

Gilcher-Holtey, I. (2001) *Die 68er Bewegung. Deutschland, Westeuropa*, Munich: C.H. Beck.

Gitelman, I. and Pingree, G.B. (eds) (2003) *New media, 1740–1915*, Cambridge, MA: MIT Press.

Gitlin, T. (1980) *The whole world is watching: mass media in the making and unmaking of the new left*, Berkeley: University of California Press.

Gitlin, T. (1988) *The sixties: years of hope, days of rage*, Toronto: Bantam.

Graber, D.A., Bimber, B., Bennett, W., Davis, R. and Norris, P. (forthcoming) 'The internet and politics: emerging perspectives', in Price, M. and Nissenbaum, H. (eds) *The internet and the academy*, New York: Peter Lang.

Granjon, F. (2001) *L'Internet militant. Mouvement social et usage des réseaux télématiques*, Paris: Edition Apogée.

Green, E. and Adam, A. (1998) 'Online leisure: gender, and ICTs in the home', *Information, Communication and Society* 1, 3: 291–312.

Green, E., Hebron, S. and Woodward, D. (1990) *Women's leisure, what leisure?* London: Macmillan.

Green, E. and Keeble, L. (2001) 'The technological story of a women's centre: a feminist model of user-centred design', in Keeble, L. and Loader, B.D. (eds) *Community informatics: shaping computer-mediated social relations*, London: Routledge.

Greenberg, A. (1999) 'Reply to Pippa Norris' "who surfs?"', in Kamarck, E.C. and Nye, J.S. (eds) *Democracy.com. Governance in a networked world*, Hollis, NH: Hollis Publishing Company.

Greenhouse, S. (2002) 'Forum in New York: workers', *New York Times*, 1 February.

GUIA online, http://www.acessibilidade.net, accessed December 2001.

Gundelach, P. (1984) 'Social transformation and new forms of voluntary associations', *Social Science Information* 23: 1049–1081.

Gurak, L.J. (1999) 'The promise and the peril of social action in cyberspace', in Smith, M.A. and Kollock, P. (eds) *Communities in cyberspace*, London: Routledge.

Gurr, T.R. (1970) *Why men rebel*, Princeton, NJ: Princeton University Press.

Haas, P.M. (1992) 'Epistemic communities and international policy coordination', *International Organization* 49, 1: 1–35.

Habermas, J. (1981) 'New social movements', *Telos* 49: 33–37.

Habermas, J. (1987) *Theory of communicative action*, Cambridge: Polity Press.

Hague, B. and Loader, B. (eds) (1999) *Digital democracy: discourse and decision making in the information age*, London: Routledge.

Hajnal, P.I. (ed.) (2002) *Civil society in the information age*, Aldershot: Ashgate.

Halleck, D. (2002) *Gathering storm: the open cyber forum of indymedia*, paper presented at the 'Our media' pre-conference of the International Association for Media and Communication Research, Barcelona, 20 July, available at http://www.ourmedianet.org/om2002/papers2002/Halleck.IAMCR2002.pdf, accessed 28 April 2003.

Halloran, J., Elliott, P. and Murdock, G. (1970) *Demonstrations and communication: a case study*, Hammondsworth: Penguin.

Har, A. and Hutnyk, J. (1999) 'Languid, tropical, monsoonal time? Net-activism and hype in the context of South East Asian politics', *Saksi* **6**: July, http://www.saksi.com/jul99/huynyk.htm, accessed 26 December 2001.

Harasim, M. (ed.) *Global networks: computers and international communication*, Cambridge: Cambridge University Press.

Hardt, M. and Negri, A. (2000) *Empire*, Cambridge: Harvard University Press.

Heijden, H. van der (1997) 'Political opportunity structure and the institutionalisation of the environmental movement', *Environmental Politics* **6**, 4.

Hellmann, K.U. (1998) 'Paradigmen der bewegungsforschung', in Hellmann, K.U. and Koopmans, R. (eds) *Paradigmen der bewegungsforschung*, Opladen: Westdeutscher Verlag.

Hert, P. (1999) 'Quasi-oralité de l'écriture électronique et lien social: la construction du vraisemblable dans les communautés scientifiques', *Réseaux* **97**: 211–259.

Hilgartner, S. and Bosk, Ch.L. (1988) 'The rise and fall of social problems. A public arenas model', *American Journal of Sociology* **94**: 53–78.

Hill, K. and Hughes, J.E. (1998) *Cyberpolitics. Citizen activism in the age of the internet*, Lanham, MD: Rowman & Littlefield.

Hiltz, S. and Turoff, M. (1985) 'Structuring computer-mediated communications systems to avoid information overload', *Communications of the ACM*, **28**, 7, July: 680–689.

Hilwig, St. J. (1998) 'The revolt against the establishment: students versus the press in West Germany and Italy', in Fink, C., Gassert, P. and Junker, D. (eds) *1968: the world transformed*, Cambridge: Cambridge University Press.

Hocke, P. (1999) 'Determining the selection bias in local and national newspaper teports on protest events', in Rucht, D., Koopmans, R. and Neidhardt, F. (eds) *Act of dissent: new developments in the study of protest*, Lanham, MD: Rowman & Littlefield.

Hoff, J., Horrocks, I. and Tops, P. (eds) (2000) *Democratic governance and new technology: technologically mediated innovations in political practice in Western Europe*, London: Routledge.

Hübsch, H. (1980) *Alternative Öffentlichkeit. Freiräume der Information und Kommunikation*, Frankfurt-on-Main: Fischer.

Hudock, A.C. (1999) *NGOs and civil society. Democracy by proxy?* Cambridge: Polity Press.

Hughes, B. (1999) 'The constitution of impairment: modernity and the aesthetic of oppression', *Disability and Society* **14**, 2: 155–172.

Humphrey, J. (1999) 'Disabled people and the politics of difference', *Disability and Society* **14**, 2: 173–188.

Hutton, J. (1995) 'Technology and disability. Assessment needs and potential', *International Journal of Technology Assessment in Health Care*, **11**: 135–143.

Inglehart, R. (1997) *Modernization and post-modernization: cultural, economic and political change in 43 societies*, Princeton, NJ: Princeton University Press.

Ion, J. (1997) *La fin des militants?* Paris: Editions de l'Atelier.

Iozzi, D. (2002) 'Case materials and analysis of the North American fair trade coffee campaign', www.engagedcitizen.org (click on undergraduate research).

Jackson, M.H., Poole, M.S. and Kuhn, T. (2002) 'The social construction of technology in studies of the workplace', in Lievrouw, L.A. and Livingstone, S. (eds) *Handbook of new media: social shaping and consequences of ICTs*, London: Sage.

Jamison, A. and Eyerman, R. (1994) *Seeds of the sixties*, Berkeley and Los Angeles: University of California Press.

Jayassooria, D. (1999) 'Disabled people: active or passive citizens – reflections from the Malaysian experience', *Disability and Society* 14, 3: 341–352.

Jesover, L. (2001) *Stratégies d'utilisation des outils électroniques*, http://attac.org/temp/internet.pdf.

Johnson, K. (1998) 'Deinstitutionalisation: the management of the rights', *Disability and Society* 13, 3: 375–387.

Johnson, L. and Moxon, E. (1998) 'In whose service? Technology, care and disabled people: the case for a disability politics perspective', *Disability and Society* 13, 2: 241–258.

Johnson, T. and Kaye, B. (2000) 'Democracy's rebirth or demise? The influence of the internet on political attitudes', in Schultz, D. (ed.) *It's show time! Media, politics and popular culture*, New York: Peter Lang.

Johnston, H., Enrique, L. and Gusfield, J.R. (1994) 'Identities, grievances, and new social movements', in Laraña, E., Johnston, H. and Gusfield, J.R. (eds) *New social movements: from ideology to identity*, Philadelphia: Temple UP.

Jordan, J. and Whitney, J. (2002) 'Que Se Vayan Todos: Argentina's popular rebellion', http://www.chiapaslink.ukgateway.net/news/020501.html, accessed 1 February 2003.

Jordan, T. (1999) *Cyberpower. The culture and politics of cyberspace and the internet*, London: Routledge.

Jouët, J. (2000) 'Retour critique sur la sociologie des usages', *Réseaux* 100: 487–521.

Kaplan, Richard L. (2002) *Politics and the American press: the rise of objectivity, 1865–1920*, Cambridge: Cambridge University Press.

Katz, J.E. and Aspden, P. (1997) *Friendship formation in cyberspace, analysis of a national survey of users*, The Markle Foundation, available at http://www.iaginteractive.com/emfa/friendship.htm.

Keck, M.E. and Sikkink, K. (1998) *Activists beyond borders: advocacy networks in international politics*, Ithaca, NY: Cornell University Press.

Kerne, A. (1997) 'Re: equalizing the net and solving information overload', Web Foro Encounter 2, http://uts.cc.utexas.edu/cgi-bin/cgiwrap/nave/webforo.pl?read=27, accessed 25 October 2001.

Kidd, D. (2002) 'Which would you rather: Seattle or Porto Alegre?', paper presented at the 'Our media' pre-conference of the International Association for Media and Communication Research, Barcelona, 20 July, http://www.

ourmedianet.org/om2002/papers2002/Kidd.IAMCR2002.pdf, accessed 28 April 2003.

Kielbowicz, R.B. and Scherer, C. (1986) 'The role of the press in the dynamics of social movements', in Kriesberg L. (ed.) *Research in social movements, conflicts and change*, Greenwich, CT: JAI.

Kitschelt, H. (1986) 'Political opportunity structures and political protest: anti-nuclear movements in four democracies', *British Journal of Political Science*, 16: 57–85.

Klandermans, B. (1984) 'Mobilisation and participation: social–psychological expansions of resource mobilisation theory', *American Sociological Review* 49: 583–600.

Klandermans, B. and Oegema, D. (1987) 'Potentials, networks, motivation and barriers: steps towards participation in social movements', *American Sociological Review* 52: 519–531.

Klandermans, P.G. (1989) *Organizing for change: social movement to organizations in Europe and the USA*, Greenwich, CT: JAI.

Klein, H.K. and Kleinman, D.L. (2002) 'The social construction of technology: structural considerations', *Science, Technology, and Human Values* 27, 1: 28–52.

Klein, N. (2000) *No logo: taking aim at the brand bullies*, New York: Picador.

Kline, R. and Pinch, T. (1996) 'Users as agents of technological change: the social construction of the automobile in the rural United Sates', *Technology and Culture* 37, 4: 763–795.

Kline, R. and Pinch, T. (1999) 'The social construction of technology', in MacKenzie, D. and Wajcman, J. (eds) *The social shaping of technology*, 2nd edn, Buckingham: Open University Press.

Kollock, P. and Smith, M. (1996) 'Managing the virtual commons: co-operation and conflict in computer communities', in Herring, S.C. (ed.) *Computer-mediated communication: linguistic, social and cross-cultural perspectives*, Amsterdam: John Benjamins Publishing Company.

Kornhauser, W. (1962) *The politics of mass society*, Glencoe, IL: Free Press.

Kraushaar, W. (ed.) (1998) *Frankfurter Schule und Studentenbewegung. Von der Flaschenpost zum Molotowcocktail 1949–1995*, Vol. 1, Hamburg: Rogner and Bernhard.

Kriesi, H. (1996) 'The organizational structure of new social movements in a political context', in McAdam, D., McCarthy, D. and Zald, M.N. (eds) *Comparative perspectives on social movements*, Cambridge: Cambridge University Press.

Kriesi, H., Koopmans, R., Duyvendak, J.W. and Giugni, M. (1995) *New social movements in Western Europe. A comparative analysis*, Minneapolis: University of Minnesota Press.

Kurz, J. (2001) *Die Universität auf der Piazza. Entstehung und Zerfall der Studentenbewegung in Italien 1966–1968*, Cologne: SH-Verlag.

Kutner, L.A. (2000) 'Environmental activism and the internet', *Electronic Green Journal*, no. 12.

Lacey, A. (2001) *Networks of protest, communities of resistance: autonomous activism in contemporary Britain*, PhD thesis, Centre for European Studies, Monash University.

Lang, K. and Lang, G. (1961) *Collective dynamics*, New York: Crowell.

Lasn, K. (1999) *Culture jam: the uncooling of America*, New York: William Morrow.

Latour, B. (1987) *The pasteurization of French society, with irreductions*, Cambridge, MA: Harvard University Press.

Latté, S. (2000) 'Les usages sociaux d'une entreprise politique. Etude de deux comités ATTAC', Unpublished *Mémoire pour la maîtrise de Science politique*, Université Paris I.

Lawson, K. (1988) 'When linkage fails', in Lawson, K. and Merkl, P.H. (eds) *When parties fail*, Princeton, NJ: Princeton University Press.

Lax, S. (2000) 'The internet and democracy', in Gauntlett, D. (ed.) *Web.studies: rewiring media studies for the digital age*, London: Arnold.

Lee, E. (2000) 'What do [*sic*] want? A new chant! When do want it? Now!' http://www.antenna.nl/~waterman/inter-lee.html, accessed 20 February 2002.

Leizerov, S. (2000) 'Privacy advocacy groups versus Intel: a case study of how social movements are tactically using the internet to fight corporations', *Social Science Computer Review* **18**, 4: 461–483.

Lennie, J., Grace, M., Daws, L. and Simpson, L. (1999) 'Empowering online conversations: a pioneering Australian project to link rural and urban women', in Harcourt, W. (ed.) *Women @ internet: creating new cultures in cyberspace*, London: Zed Books.

Levi, M. and Olson, D. (2000) 'The battles in Seattle', *Politics & Society* **28**: 309–329.

Levitt, T. (1973) *The third sector: new tactics for a responsive society*, New York: Amacom.

Lichbach, M.I. and Almeida, P. (2001) *Global order and local resistance: the neoliberal institutional trilemma and the battle of Seattle*, unpublished manuscript, University of California: Riverside Center for Global Order and Resistance.

Liepins, R. (1994) '*We can do it': change for the invisible farmer*, paper presented at the Australian women's studies annual conference: women and the politics of change, Deakin University, 4–6 December.

Liepins, R. (1995) 'Women in agriculture: advocates for a gendered sustainable agriculture', *Australian Geographer* **26**: 118–126.

Liepins, R. (1996) 'Reading agricultural power: media as sites and processes in the construction of meaning', *New Zealand Geographer* **52**, 2: 3–10.

Limerick, B., Burgess-Limerick, T. and Grace, M. (1996) 'The politics of interviewing: power relations and accepting the gift', *Qualitative Studies in Education* **9**, 4: 449–460.

Little, J. (1987) 'Gender relations in rural areas: the importance of women's domestic role', *Journal of Rural Studies* **3**, 4: 335–342.

Little, J. (1997) 'Constructions of rural women's voluntary work', *Gender, Place and Culture* **4**, 2: 197–209.

Loader, B. (ed.) (1997) *The governance of cyberspace*, London: Routledge.

Loader, B. (ed.) (1998) *Cyberspace divide*, London: Routledge.

Löfgren, K. (2000) 'Danish political parties and new technology: interactive parties or new shop windows?', in Hoff, J., Horrocks, I. and Tops, P. (eds) *Democratic governance and new technology: technologically mediated innovations in political practice in Western Europe*, London: Routledge.

Lovink, G. (2002) *Dark fiber: tracking critical internet culture*. Cambridge, MA: MIT Press.

Lynch, C. (1998) 'Social movements and the problem of globalization', *Alternatives*, **23**: 149–174.

Macken, D. (2001) 'Chain reaction', *Australian Financial Review*, 21 April.

McAdam, D. (1982) *Political process and the development of black insurgency, 1930–1970*, Chicago and London: The University of Chicago Press.

McAdam, D. (1988) 'Micromobilisation contexts and the recruitment to activism', in Klandermans, B., Kriesi, H. and Tarrow, S. (eds) *From structure to action*, Greenwich, CT: JAI.

McAdam, D., McCarthy, J. and Zald, M. (eds) (1996a) *Comparative perspectives on social movements*, Chicago: Cambridge University Press.

McAdam, D., Tilly, C. and Tarrow, S. (1996b) 'To map contentious politics', *Mobilization* **1**: 17–34.

McAdam, D., Tarrow, S. and Tilly, C. (2001) *Dynamics of contention*, New York: Cambridge University Press.

McCarthy, J.D., McPhail, C. and Smith, J. (1996) 'Images of protest: dimensions of selection bias in media coverage of Washington demonstrations, 1982, 1991', *American Sociological Review* **61**: 478–499.

McCarthy, J. and Zald, M.N. (1977) 'Resource mobilization and social movements: a partial theory', *American Journal of Sociology* **82**, 6: 1212–1241.

McKay, Niall (1999) *Indonesia, Ireland in info war?*, http://www.wired.com/news/politics/0,1283,17562,00.html, accessed 27 January 1999.

MacKenzie, D. and Wajcman, J. (1999) *The social shaping of technology*, 2nd edn, Philadelphia and London: Open University Press and Taylor & Francis.

Mackenzie, F. (1994) 'Is where I sit, where I stand? The Ontario farm women's network, politics and difference', *Journal of Rural Studies* **10**, 2: 101–115.

McLaughlin, M.L., Osborne, K.K. and Smith, C.B. (1995) 'Standards of conduct on Usenet', in Jones, S.G. (ed.) *Cybersociety 2.0: revisiting computer-mediated communication and community*, Thousand Oaks, CA: Sage.

McLaughlin, M.L., Osborne, K.K. and Ellison, N.B. (1997) 'Virtual community in a telepresence environment', in Jones, S.G. (ed.) *Virtual culture: identity and communication in cybersociety*, London: Sage.

McQuail, D. (1998) *Mass communication theory*, London: Sage.

Maheu, L. (1993) 'Postmodernité et mouvements sociaux', in Audet, M. and Bouchikhi, H. (eds) *Structuration du social et modernité avancée – autour des travaux d'Anthony Giddens*, Saint-Foy: Les Presses de l'Université Laval.

Maheu, L. (ed.) (1995) *Social movements and social classes – the future of collective action*, London: Sage.

Manheim, J.B. (2001) *The death of a thousand cuts: corporate campaigns and the attack on the corporation*, Mahwah, NJ: Lawrence Erlbaum.

Margin, P. (1995) 'A summary of the recent debate within the ECN', *Italian Counterinfo* **12**: September, http://www.spunk.org/library/pubs/ci-it/sp001033.txt, accessed 12 August 2001.

Markham, A.N. (1998) *Life online: researching real experience in virtual space*, Walnut Creek, CA: AltaMira Press.

Marx, K. (1963) *The eighteenth brumaire of Louis Bonaparte*, New York: International Publishers.

Marx, K. (1973) *Grundrisse*. Harmondsworth: Penguin.

Mayer, M. (1991) 'Social movement research in the United States: a European perspective', *International Journal of Politics, Culture and Society* **4**, 4: 459–480.

Melucci, A. (1989) *Nomads of the present: social movements and individual needs in the contemporary society*, Philadelphia: Temple University Press.

Melucci, A. (1995a) 'Individualisation et globalisation: au-delà de la modernité?', in Dubet, F. and Wieviorka, M. (eds) *Penser le Sujet*, Paris: Fayard.

Melucci, A. (1995b) 'The new social movements revisited: reflections on a sociological misunderstanding', in Maheu, L. (ed.) *Social movements and social classes – the future of collective action*, London: Sage.

Melucci, A. (1995c) 'The process of collective identity', in Johnston, H. and Klandermans, B. (eds) *Social movements and culture*, London: UCL Press.

Melucci, A. (1996) *Challenging codes: collective action in the information age*, Cambridge: Cambridge University Press.

Meyer, D.S. and Tarrow, S. (1998) 'A movement society: contentious politics for a new century', in Meyer, D. and Tarrow, S. (eds) *The social movement society*, New York: Rowman & Littlefield.

Michailakis, D. (1997) 'When opportunity is the thing to be equalised', *Disability & Society* **12**, 1: 17–30.

Moglen, E. (1999) 'Anarchism triumphant: free software and the death of copyright', http://emoglen.law.columbia.edu/my_pubs/anarchism.html, accessed 3 February 2003.

Molotch, H. (1979) 'Media and movements', in Zald, M.N. and McCarthy, J.D. (eds) *The dynamics of social movements*, Cambridge, MA: Winthrop.

Molotch, H. and Lester, M. (1974) 'News as purposive behavior: on the strategic use of routine events, accidents, and scandals', *American Sociological Review* **39**: 101–112.

Morgan, E.P. (1991) *The 60s experience: hard lessons about modern America*, Philadelphia: Temple University Press.

Mouvements (1999) 'Y-a-t-il de nouveaux mouvements militants', Table Ronde, *Mouvements*, La Découverte 3: 32–45.

Mueller, C.M. (1992) 'Building social movement theory', in Morris, A.D. and Mueller, C.M. (eds) *Frontiers in social movement theory*, New Haven, CT: Yale University Press.

Münker, S. and Roesler, A. (eds) (1997) *Mythos Internet*, Frankfurt-on-Main: Suhrkamp.

Münker, S. and Roesler, A. (eds) (2000) *Praxis Internet. Kulturtechniken der vernetzten Welt*, Frankfurt-on-Main: Suhrkamp.

Myers, D. (1987) 'Anonymity is part of the magic: individual manipulation of computer-mediated communication contexts', *Qualitative Sociology* 10, 3: 251–266.

Myers, D.J. (1994) 'Communication technology and social movements: contributions of computer networks to activism', *Social Science Computer Review* 12, 2: 250–260.

Myers, D. (1998) 'Social activism through computer networks', American Sociological Association's Section on Collective Behavior and Social Movements, Working Paper Series 1 (3) http://www.nd.edu/~dmyers/cbsm/vol1/myers2.html, accessed 15 January 2002.

Naisbitt, J. (1982) *Megatrends*, New York: Warner Books.

National Forum (2001) 'How to lose money and influence people', in *Phi Kappa Phi Journal*, summer.

Naughton, J. (2001) 'Contested space: the internet and global civil society', in Anheier, H., Glasius, M. and Kaldor, M. (eds) *Global civil society 2001*, Oxford: Oxford University Press.

Negri, A. (1979) *Dall'operaio massa all'operaio sociale: intervista sull'operaismo*, Milan: Multhipla Edizioni.

Neidhardt, F. (1994) 'Öffentlichkeit, öffentliche Meinung, soziale Bewegungen', in Neidhardt, F. (ed.) *Öffentlichkeit, öffentliche Meinung, soziale Bewegungen*, Opladen: Westdeutscher Verlag.

Neidhardt, F. and Rucht, D. (1991) 'The state of the art and some perspectives for further research', in Rucht, D. (ed.) *Research on social movements: the state of the art in Western Europe and the USA*, Frankfurt-on-Main and Boulder, CO: Campus and Westview Press.

Neill, M. (1997a) 'Toward the new commons: working class strategies and the Zapatistas; IV. Localism, homogeneity, and networks', http://www.geocities.com/CapitolHill/3843/monty4.html, accessed 1 April 2000.

Neill, M. (1997b) 'Toward the new commons: working class strategies and the Zapatistas; V. Class composition and developing a new working class strategy', http://www.geocities.com/CapitolHill/3843/monty4.html, accessed 1 April 2000.

Neveu, E. (1996) *Sociologie des mouvements sociaux*, Paris: Éditions La Découverte.

Neveu, E. (1999) 'Médias, mouvement sociaux, espaces publique', *Reseaux* 98: 17–85.

Niels, H., Zadek, S. and Raynard, P. (eds) (2001) *Perspectives on the new economy of corporate citizenship*, Copenhagen: The Copenhagen Centre.

Nip, Y.M.J. (2001) *Methodological reflections from studying a message board on the World Wide Web*, paper presented at the Internet Political Economy Forum 2001: Internet and Development in Asia, Singapore, 14–15 September.

Nixon, P.G. and Johansson, H. (1999) 'Transparency through technology: a comparative analysis of the use of the internet by political parties', in Hague, B. and Loader, B.D. (eds) *Digital democracy: discourse and decision making in the information age*, London: Routledge.

Nordenstreng, K. and Traber, M. (eds) *Towards equity in global communication – MacBride update*, Cresskill, NJ: Hampton Press.

Norris, P. (2001) *Digital parties. Civic engagement and online democracy*, paper prepared for the ECPR Joint Sessions, Grenoble, 6–11 April.

Norris, P. (2002) *Democratic phoenix: political activism worldwide*, Cambridge: Cambridge University Press.

Nowé, K. (2001) 'Social movements and information management – an outline of a possible research project', http://www.hb.se/bhs/seminar/semdoc/nowe.htm, accessed 9 January 2002.

O'Brien, R., Goetz, A., Scholte, J. and Williams, M. (2000) *Contesting global governance. Multilateral economic institutions and global social movements*, Cambridge: Cambridge University Press.

Offe, C. (1985) 'New social movements: challenging the boundaries of institutional politics', *Social Research* 52, 4: 817–868.

Offerlé, M. (1994) *Sociologie des groupes d'intérêts*, Paris: Montchrestien.

Oliver, M. (1990) *Politics of disablement*, Basingstoke: Macmillan.

Oliver, M. (1993) *Disability, citizenship and empowerment*, Buckingham: Open University Press.

Oliver, M. (1999) 'Capitalism, disability and ideology: a materialist critique of the normalization principle', http://www.leeds.ac.uk/disability-studies/archiveuk/archframe/oliverm1999.htm, accessed 3 November 2001.

Oliver, M. and Barnes, C. (1998) *Disabled people and social policy: from exclusion to inclusion*, London: Longman.

Oliveri, A. (2003) 'Stop that train!', http://www.zmag.org/content/showarticle.cfm?SectionID=1andItemID=3165, accessed 25 April 2003.

Ollitrault, S. (1999) 'De la caméra à la pétition-web: le répertoire médiatique des écologistes', *Réseaux* 98: 156–186.

Ollitrault, S. (2001) 'Les écologistes français. Des experts en action', *Revue Française de Science Politique*, 51, 1–2: 105–130.

Olson, M. (1965) *The logic of collective action; public goods and the theory of groups*, Cambridge, MA: Harvard University Press.

Olson, M. (1978) *Logiques de l'action collective*, Paris: Presses Universitaires de France.

Outshoorn, J. (2000) 'Op zoek naar de vrouwenbeweging in de jaren negentig', in Sunier, T., Duyvendak J.W., Saharso, S. and Steijlen, F. (eds) *Emancipatie en subcultuur: sociale bewegingen in België en Nederland*, Amsterdam: Instituut voor Publiek en Politiek.

Oy, G. (2001) *Die Gemeinschaft der Lüge. Medien- und Öffentlichkeitskritik sozialer Bewegungen in der Bundesrepublik*, Münster: Westfälisches Dampfboot.

Pakulski, J. (1995) 'Social movements and class, the decline of the Marxist paradigm', in Maheu, L. (ed.) *Social movements and social classes – the future of collective action*, London: Sage.

Parks, M.R. and Floyd, K. (1996) 'Making friends in cyberspace', *Joint Issue of Journal of Communication* 46, 1 *and Journal of Computer-Mediated Communication* 1, 4, available at http://www.ascusc.org/jcmc/vol1/issue4/parks.html.

Patou, C. (2000) 'Usages militants de la formation et de l'information. Les exemples d'AC! et d'Attac', *Cahiers Politiques*, Université Paris-Dauphine, 4: 76–91.

Peck, A. (1985) *Uncovering the sixties: the life and times of the underground press*, New York: Pantheon.

Pellow, D.N. (1999) 'Framing emerging environmental movement tactics: mobilizing consensus, demobilizing conflict, *Sociological Forum* 14, 4: 659–683.

Peretti, J. (2003) 'Culture jamming, memes, social networks, and the emerging media ecology: the Nike sweatshop e-mail as object to think with', in Micheletti, M., Follesdal, A. and Dietlind, S. (eds) *The politics behind products*, New Brunswick, NJ: Transaction Books.

Perrolle, J.A. (1993) 'Comments from the special issue editor: the emerging dialogue on environmental justice', *Social Problems: Official Journal of the Society or the Study of Social Problems* 40, 1: 1–4.

Pew Internet and American Life Project (2000) *Tracking online life: how women use the internet to cultivate relationships with family and friends*, Washington, DC: Pew Internet and American Life Project: online, http://www.pewinternet.org/reports/toc.asp?Report=11, accessed 10 December 2002.

Phelan, S. (1993) '(Be)Coming out: Lesbian identity and politics', *Signs: Journal of Women in Culture and Society* 18: 765–790.

Pickerill, J. (2001) 'Weaving a green web. Environmental protest and computer-mediated communication in Britain', in Webster, F. (ed.) *Culture and politics in the information age*, London: Routledge.

Pilgrim, D., Todhunter, C. and Pearson, M. (1997) 'Accounting for disability: customer feedback or citizen complaints?', *Disability & Society* 12, 1: 3–15.

Pinch, T. and Bijker, W. (1984) 'The social construction of facts and artifacts', *Social Studies of Science* 14: 399–441.

Piven, F.F. and Cloward, R.A. (1977) *Poor people's movements: why they succeed, how they fail*, New York: Pantheon.

Piven, F.F. and Cloward, R.A. (1991) 'Collective protest: a critique of resource mobilization theory, *International Journal of Politics, Culture and Society* 4, 4: 435–458.

Pizzorno, A. (1978) 'Political science and collective identity in industrial conflict', in Crouch, C. and Pizzorno, A. (eds) *The resurgence of class conflict in Western Europe since 1968*, London: Macmillan.

Pizzorno, A. (1985) 'On the rationality of democratic choice', *Telos* 63, spring: 41–69.

Portugal Telecom (1999) *Timor: para que os Portugueses façam ouvir a sua voz*, available at http://www.telecom.pt/quemsomos/noticias/artigo.asp? Id_artigo=476, accessed 28 February 2002.

Price, R. (1998) 'Reversing the gun sights: transnational civil society targets land mines', *International Organization* 52, 3: 613–644.

Proença, L. (2000) *A Rádio Porta Estandarte: A TSF e o Pós-Referendo em Timor Leste*, post-degree dissertation on journalism, Lisbon: ISCTE/ESCS.

Prümm, P.D. (1996) *Politische Öffentlichkeitsarbeit bundesdeutscher Organizationen im World Wide Web,*. unpublished MA dissertation. Free University of Berlin, Department of Political Science.

Qualitative Solutions and Research. (1999) NUD*IST VIVO for qualitative research, Melbourne: La Trobe.

Raschke, J. (1985) *Soziale Bewegungen. Ein historisch-systematischer Grundriß*, Frankfurt-on-Main: Campus.

Reeder, H.M. (1996) 'A critical look at gender difference in communication research', *Communication Studies* 47, winter: 318–330.

Reinicke, W.H. (1998) *Global public policy. Governing without government?*, Washington, DC: Brookings Institution Press.

Rheingold, H. (1993) *The virtual community: homesteading on the electronic frontier*, available at http://www.rheingold.com/vc/book/.

Rheingold, H. (1996) 'A slice of my life in my virtual community', in Ludlow, P. (ed.) *High noon on the electronic frontier*, Cambridge, MA: MIT Press.

Rheingold, H. (1999) 'Community development in the cybersociety of the future', speech given in a live chat online, BBC, 4 October 1999, available at http://www.partnerships.org.uk/bol/howard.htm.

Rheingold, H. (2002) *Smart mobs: the next social revolution*, New York: Perseus.

RICA (1996) 'RICA: proposal for communication network/Propuesta para Red de Comunicacion', http://lists.village.virginia.edu/cgi-in/spoons/archive_ msgpl?file = aut-op-sy.archive/aut-op-sy_1996/96–09–24.223andmsgnum = 33andstart=4005andend=4460', accessed 1 May 2000.

Richardson, J. (1995) 'The market for political activism: interest groups as a challenge to political parties', *West European Politics* 18, 1: 116–139.

Richardson, J. (2001) 'Free software and GPL society: Stefan Merten of Oekonux interviewed by Joanne Richardson', http://subsol.c3.hu/subsol_2/ contributors0/mertentext.html, accessed 3 February 2003.

Rink, D. (2000) 'Soziale Bewegungen im 21. Jahrhundert', *Forschungsjournal Neue Soziale Bewegungen* 13, 1: 26–31.

Rocher, G. (1977–1979) *Sociologia Geral*, trans. Ana Ravara, Lisbon: Editorial Presença.

Roe, P. (1991) 'Telecommunications for all', in Von Tetzchner, S. (ed.) *Issues in telecommunications and disability*, Strasbourg: Commission of European Communities.

Rojecki, A. (2002) 'Modernism, state sovereignty and dissent: media and the new post-Cold War movements', *Critical Studies in Media Communication* 19: 152–171.

Rosati, P. and Prieur, L. (2000) 'La production de sens contre les portails de la "New Economy"', *Multitudes* 2 May.

Rosenberg, A. (1995) 'Equality, sufficiency and opportunity in a just society', *Social Philosophy & Policy* 2: 54–71.

RTS (eds) (1999) *Reflections on J18*, http://www.infoshop.org/octo/j18_reflections.html, accessed 9 June 2002.

Rucht, D. (1988) 'Themes, logics and arenas of social movements: a structural approach', in Klandermans, B., Kriesi, H. and Tarrow S. (eds) *From structure to action: comparing social movement research across cultures*, Greenwich, CT: JAI Press.

Rucht, D. (1989) 'Environmental movement organizations in West Germany and France – structure and interorganizational relations', in Klandermans, B. (ed.) *Organizing for change: social movement organizations across cultures*, Greenwich, CT: JAI Press.

Rucht, D. (1990) 'The strategies and action repertoires of new movements', in Dalton, R.J. and Kuechler, M. (eds) *Challenging the political order. New social and political movements in Western democracies*, Cambridge: Polity Press.

Rucht, D. (1994) *Modernisierung und neue soziale Bewegungen. Deutschland, Frankreich und USA im Vergleich*, Frankfurt/New York: Campus.

Rucht, D. (1996) 'The impact of national contexts on social movement structures: a cross-movement and cross-national comparison', in McAdam, D., McCarthy, J.M. and Zald, M. (eds) *Opportunities, mobilizing structures, and framing: comparative applications of contemporary movement theory*, Cambridge: Cambridge University Press.

Rucht, D. (1999) 'The transnationalization of social movements: trends, causes, problems', in Porta, D., Kriesi, H. and Rucht, D. (eds) *Social movements in a globalizing world*, London: Macmillan.

Rucht, D. (2001) 'Antikapitalistischer und ökologischer Protest als Medienereignis: Zur Resonanz der Proteste am 1. Mai 2000 in London', in Brunnengräber A., Klein A. and Walk, H. (eds) *Legitimationsressource NGOs. Zivilgesellschaftliche Partizipationsformen im Globalizierungsprozeß*, Opladen: Leske + Budrich.

Rucht, D. (2003) 'Interactions between social movements and states in comparative perspective', in Banaszak, L.A., Beckwith, K. and Rucht, D. (eds) *Women's movements facing the reconfigured state*, Cambridge: Cambridge University Press, pp. 242–274.

Rucht, D. and Roose, J. (2001) 'Neither decline nor sclerosis: the organisational structure of the German environmental movement', *West European Politics* 24, 4: 55–81.

Rucht, D., Blattert, B. and Rink, D. (1997) Von der Bewegung zur Institution? Alternative Gruppen in beiden Teilen Deutschlands, Frankfurt-on-Main: Campus.

Rucht, D. and Neidhardt, D. (2002) 'Towards a "movement society"? On the possibilities of institutionalizing social movements', *Social Movement Studies* 1, 1: 7–30.

Russell, S. (1986) 'The social construction of artifacts: a response to Pinch and Bijker', *Social Studies of Science* 16: 331–346.

Ryan, C. (1991) *Prime time activism: media strategies for grassroots organizing*, Boston, MA: South End Press.

Sachs, C. (1983) *The invisible farmers: women in agricultural production*, Totawa, NJ: Rowan and Allanheld.

Sachs, C. (1996) *Gendered fields: rural women, agriculture, and environment*, Boulder, CO: Westview Press.

Sack, F. (1984) 'Die Reaktion von Gesellschaft, Politik und Staat auf die Studentenbewegung', in Sack, F. and Steinert, H. (eds) *Protest und Reaktion. Analysen zum Terrorismus*, Opladen: Westdeutscher Verlag.

Sapey, B. (2000) 'Disablement in the informational age', *Disability & Society* 15, 4: 619–636.

Sarantakos, S. (1993) *Social research*, Melbourne: Macmillan Education.

Schulz, M. (1998) 'Collective action across borders: opportunity structures, network capacities, and communicative praxis in the age of advanced globalization', *Sociological Perspectives* 41, 3: 587–616.

Schulz, W. (1976) *Die Konstruktion von Realität in den Nachrichtenmedien. Analyse der aktuellen Berichterstattung*, Freiburg and Munich: Karl Alber.

Scott, A. (1990) *Ideology and the new social movements*, London: Unwin Hyman.

Scott, A. (2001) '(In)forming politics: processes of feminist activism in the information age', *Women's Studies International Forum* 24: 409–421.

Scott, A., Semmens, L. and Willoughby, L. (1999) 'Women and the internet: the natural history of a research project, *Information, Communication and Society* 2, 4: 541–565.

Scott, A. and Steer, J. (2001) 'From media politics to e-protest? The use of popular culture and new media in parties and social movements internet', in Webster, F. (ed.) *Culture and politics in the information age*, London: Routledge.

Sedgwick, E.K. (1994) *Tendencies*, London: Routledge.

Shah, H. (1999) 'Emancipation from modernization: development journalism and new social movements', in Nordenstreng, K., Traber, M. and Vincent, R. (eds) *Towards equity in global communication – MacBride update*, Cresskill, NJ: Hampton Press.

Shakespeare, T. (1993) 'Disabled people's self-organization: a new social movement?' *Disability & Society* **8**, 3: 249–264.

Shapiro, A.L. (1999) *The control revolution*, New York: Century Foundation.

Shenk, D. (1997) *Data smog: surviving the information glut*, New York: Harper Edge.

Shortall, S. (1994) 'Farm women's groups: feminist or farming or community groups, or new social movements?', *Industrial and Labor Relations Review* **28**, 1: 279–291.

Shriver, T.E., Cable, S., Norris, L. and Hastings, D.W. (2000) 'The role of collective identity in inhibiting mobilization: solidarity and suppression in Oak Ridge', *Sociological Spectrum* **20**: 41–64.

Shumway, C. (2001) 'Participatory media networks: a new model for producing and disseminating progressive news and information', http://chris.shumway.tripod.com/pmn.htm, accessed 1 August 2001.

Silva, R. (2000) *Guia do Activismo Online*, http://members.tripod.com/~Protesto_MC/timor.html, accessed 28 February 2002.

Silverstone, R. (1999) 'What's new about new media?', *New Media and Society* **1**: 10–12.

Simpson, L., Wood, L., Daws, L. and Seinen, A. (2001) *Creating rural connections book 1: project overview*, Brisbane: The Communication Centre, Queensland University of Technology.

Slocombe, M. (2003) 'Beware of the Troll', http://www.urban75.cim/Mag/trolling.html.

Smelser, N.J. (1962) *Theory of collective behaviour*, London: Routledge & Kegan Paul.

Smelser, N. (ed.) (1988, 1989) *Handbook of sociology*, Newbury Park, CA: Sage.

Smith, C. (1998) 'Political parties in the information age: from "mass party" to leadership organization?', in Snellen, I.Th.M. and. van de Donk, W.B.H.J. (eds) *Public administration in an information age; a handbook*, Amsterdam: IOS Press.

Smith, C. (2000) 'British political parties: continuity and change in the information age', in Hoff, J., Horrocks, I. and Tops, P.W. (eds) *Democratic governance and new technology: technologically mediated innovations in political practice in Western Europe*, London: Routledge.

Smith, J., Chatfield C. and Pagnucco, R. (eds) (1997) *Transnational social movements and global politics: solidarity beyond the state*, New York: Syracuse University Press.

Smith, J. (2001a) 'Cyber Subversion in the information economy', *Dissent* **48**, 2: http://www.dissentmagazine.org/archive/sp01/sp01.html.

Smith, J. (2001b) 'Behind the anti-globalization label', *Dissent*, fall, 14–18.

Smith, J. (2001c) Globalizing resistance: the battle of Seattle and the future of social movements, *Mobilization* **6**: 1–19.

Smith, P.J. and Smythe, E. (2000) *Sleepless in Seattle: challenging the WTO in a globalizing world*, paper presented at the meeting of the International Political Science Association, Quebec City, 1 August.

Smith, P.J. and Smythe, E. (2001) 'Globalization, citizenship and technology. The Multilateral Agreement on Investment meets the internet', in Webster, F., *Culture and politics in the information age*, London: Routledge.

Snellen, I.Th.M. (1994) 'ICT. A revolutionising force in public administration?', *Information and the Public Sector* 3/4: 283–304.

Snow, D. and Benford, R. (1988) 'Ideology, frame resonance, and participant mobilization', in Klandermans, B., Kriesi, H. and Tarrow, S. (eds) *From structure to action: comparing social movement research across cultures*, International Social Movement Research 1, Greenwich, CT: JAI Press.

Snow, D.A. and Benford, R. (1992) 'Master frames and cycles of protest', in Morris, A. and Mueller, C.M. (eds) *Frontiers in social movement theory*, New Haven, CT:Yale University Press.

Snow, D.A., Benford, R.D., Rochford, E.B. and Worden, S.K. (1986) 'Frame alignment processes, micromobilization and movement participation', *American Sociological Review* 51: 464–481.

Snow, D.A. and McAdam, D. (2000) 'Identity work process in the context of social movements: clarifying the identify/movement nexus', in Stryker, S., Owens, T.J. and White, R.W. (eds) *Self, identity and social movements*, London: University of Minnesota Press.

Sociaal en Cultureel Planbureau (1998) *Sociaal en Cultureel Rapport*, Rijswijk: SCP.

Sommier, I. (2001) *Les nouveaux mouvements contestataires à l'heure de la mondialisation*, Paris: Flammarion.

Sørensen, M. (2002) *Den politiske forbruger: en analyse af ideen og fænomenet*, Aarhus Universitet: Institut for Idéhistorie, Det Humanistiske Fakultet.

Staab, J.F. (1990) *Nachrichtenwert-Theorie. Formale Struktur und empirischer Gehalt*, Freiburg and Munich: Alber.

Stamm, K.H. (1988) *Alternative Öffentlichkeit. Die Erfahrungsproduktion neuer sozialer Bewegungen*, Frankfurt-on-Main and New York: Campus.

Star, S.L. (1991) 'Power, technology and the phenomenology of conventions: on being allergic to onions', in Law, J. (ed.) *A sociology of monsters: essays on power, technology and domination*, London and New York: Routledge.

Starr, A. (2000) *Naming the enemy: anti-corporate movements confront globalization*, London: Zed Books.

Stein, A. (1997) *Sex and sensibility: stories of a lesbian generation*, Berkeley, CA: University of California Press.

Stoecker, R. (2000) 'Cyberspace vs. face to face: community organizing in the new millennium', http://comm-org.utoledo.edu/papers2000/cyberorganize.htm, accessed 5 July 2001.

Sungu (1997) 'Re: equalizing the net and solving information overload', Web Foro Encounter 2, http://uts.cc.utexas.edu/cgi-bin/cgiwrap/nave/webforo.pl?read=32, accessed 25 October 2001.

Tanner, E. (2001) 'Chilean conversations: internet forum participants debate Augusto Pinochet's detention', *Journal of Communication* 51, 2, June: 383–403.

Tarrow, S. (1989) *Democracy and disorder: protest and politics in Italy, 1965–1975*, Oxford: Clarendon Press.

Tarrow, S. (1998) *Power in movement – social movements and contentious politics*, Cambridge: Cambridge University Press.

Tarrow, S. (1999) *Mad cows and activists: contentious politics in the trilateral democracies*, San Giacomo Working Papers 99.1, Institute for European Studies, Cornell University.

Tarrow, S. (2001) 'Transnational politics: contention and institutions in international politics', *Annual Review of Political Science* 4: 1–20.

Tarrow, S. (2002a) *The new transnational contention: organizations, coalitions, mechanisms*, paper prepared for delivery at the 2002 annual meeting of the American Political Science Association, 29 August–1 September, Boston.

Tarrow, S. (2002b) *Rooted cosmopolitans: transnational activists in a world of states*, unpublished manuscript.

Taylor, V. and Whittier, N.E. (1992) 'Collective identity in social movement communities: lesbian feminist mobilization', in Aldon, D.M. and Mueller, C.M. (eds) *Frontiers in social movement theory*, New Haven, CT: Yale University Press.

Thornton, P. (1993) 'Communications technology – empowerment or disempowerment?' *Disability, Handicap and Society* 8: 339–349.

Tilly, C. (1978) *From mobilization to revolution*, Reading, MA: Addison-Wesley.

Tilly, C. (1984) 'Social movements and national politics', in Bright, C. and Harding, S. (eds) *Statemaking and social movements. Essays in history and theory*, Ann Arbor: University of Michigan Press.

Tilly, C. (1986) *The contentious French*, Cambridge, MA and London: Belknap Press of Harvard University Press.

Touraine, A. (1981a) *O pós-socialismo*, trans. António M. Rollo Lucas, Oporto: Edições Afrontamento.

Touraine, A. (1981b) *The voice and the eye*, Cambridge: Cambridge University Press.

Trautmann, F. (2001) 'Internet au service de la démocratie? Le cas d'Attac', *Les Cahiers du Cevipof*, Paris: Sciences Po.

Tsang, D. (2000) 'Notes on queer 'n Asian virtual sex', in Bell, D. and Kennedy, B.M. (eds) *The cybercultures reader*, London: Routledge.

Tuchman, G. (1972) 'Objectivity as a strategic ritual', *American Journal of Sociology* 77: 660–679.

Turkle, S. (1995) *Life on the screen: identity in the age of the Internet*, New York: Touchstone.

Turner, R.H. (1969) 'The public perception of protest', *American Sociological Review* 34, 6: 815–831.

Valovic, T. (2000) *Digital mythologies: the hidden complexities of the internet*, New Brunswick: Rutgers University Press.

Vedel, T. (2000) 'Une nouvelle société de l'information, l'internet et la démocratie', *Cahiers français* 295: 25–30.

Viegas, H. (1999) 'Pressionar os Grandes através da internet', *O Público*, 7 September.

Viegas, H. and Gomes, S. (1999) 'BBC: duas mil mensagens', *O Público*, 9 September.

Viegas, J. and Costa, A. (eds) (1998) *Portugal, Que Modernidade?*, Oeiras: Celta.

Viegas, J.L. and Costa, A.F. (2000) '*Crossroads to modernity', contemporary Portuguese society*, Oeiras: Celta.

Virno, P. and Hardt, M. (eds) (1996) *Radical thought in Italy: a potential politics*, Minneapolis: University of Minnesota Press.

Voltmer, K. (2000) *Structures of diversity of press and broadcasting systems: the institutional context of political communication in Western democracies*, discussion paper FS III 00–201, Berlin: Wissenschaftszentrum Berlin für Sozialforschung.

Wajcman, J. (1991) *Feminism confronts technology*, Cambridge: Polity Press.

Wajcman, J. (2000) 'Reflections on gender and technology studies: in what state is the art?' *Social Studies of Science* 30, 3: 447–464.

Wakeford, N. (2000) 'New media, new methodologies: studying the web', in Gauntlett, D. (ed.) *Web.studies: rewiring media studies for the digital age*, London: Arnold.

Walch, J. (1999) *In the net: an internet guide for activists*, London: Zed Books.

Walgrave, S. and Manssens, J. (2000) 'The making of the white march: the mass media as a mobilizing alternative to movement organizations', *Mobilization* 5, 2: 217–246.

Wallerstein, I. (2001) 'America and the World: the twin towers as metaphor', http://fbc.binghamton.edu/iwbkln02.htm, accessed 19 October 2002.

Warkentin, C. (2001) *Reshaping world politics. NGOs, the internet and global civil society*, Lanham, MD: Rowman & Littlefield.

Waterman, P. (1992) *International labour communication by computer: the fifth international?*, The Hague: Institute of Social Studies.

Wearing, B. (1998) *Leisure and feminist theory*, London: Sage.

Webster, F. (ed.) (2001) *Culture and politics in the Information Age: a new politics?*, London: Routledge.

Weingartner, J. (2001) 'Interview on 2 year anniversary imc – DeeDee Halleck', http://news.openflows.org/telecom/01/12/03/1410214.shtml, accessed 1 January 2002.

Wellman, B. (2000) 'Changing connectivity: a future history of Y2.03K', *Sociological Research Online* 4, http://www.socresonline.org.uk/4/4/wellman.html.

Wellman, B. and Gulia, M. (1999) 'Virtual communities as communities: net surfers don't ride alone', in Smith, M.A. and Kollock, P. (eds) *Communities in cyberspace*, London: Routledge.

Wellman, B., Salaff, J., Dimitrova, D., Garton, L., Gulia, M. and Haythornthwaite, C. (1996) 'Computer networks as social networks', *Annual Review of Sociology* 22: 213–238.

Whatmore, S. (1991). *Farming women: gender, work and family enterprise*. Basingstoke: Macmillan.

Wieviorka, M. (1995) 'Plaidoyer pour un concept', in Dubet, F. and Wieviorka, M. (eds) *Penser le sujet*, Paris: Fayard.

Wilde, R. de, Vermeulen, N. and Reithler, M. (2003) *Bezeten van Genen. Een essay over de innovatieoorlog rondom genetisch gemanipuleerd voedsel* (Obsessed by genes. An essay about the innovation war regarding the genetic modification of food), The Hague: Scientific Council for Government Policy.

Williams, R. and Edge, D. (1996) 'The social shaping of technology', *Research Policy* 25, 8: 65–99.

Wittig, M.A. and Schmitz, J. (1996) 'Electronic grassroots organizing', *Journal of Social Issues* 52, 1: 53–69.

Wolfsfeld, G. (1984) 'Symbiosis of press and protest: an exchange analysis', *Journalism Quarterly* 61, 3: 550–555.

Woods, M. (1997) 'Researching rural conflicts: hunting, local politics and actor-networks, *Journal of Rural Studies* 14, 3: 321–340.

World Health Organization (1980) *ICIDH. International classification of impairments, disabilities and handicaps*, Geneva: WHO.

World Health Organization (2000 pre-final draft) *ICIDH-2. International classification of functioning, disability and health*, Geneva: WHO.

Wray, S. (1997) 'Equalizing the net and solving information overload', Web Foro Encounter 2, http://uts.cc.utexas.edu/cgi-bin/cgiwrap/nave/webforo.pl?read=22, accessed 25 October 2001.

Wright, S. (2000) '"A love born of hate": autonomist rap in Italy', *Theory, Culture & Society* 17, 3, June: 117–135.

Wright, S. (2002) *Storming heaven: class composition and struggle in Italian autonomist Marxism*, London: Pluto Press.

Wright, S. (2004) 'A party of autonomy?', in Mustapha, A. and Murphy, T. (eds) *Negri beyond Negri*, London: Verso.

Yin, R.K. (1994) *Case study research, design and methods*, Thousand Oaks, CA: Sage.

Zald, M.N. and Ash, R. (1966) 'Social movement organizations: growth, decay and change', *Social Forces* 44: 327–341.

Zald, M.N. and McCarthy, J.D. (1980) 'Social movement industries: competition and cooperation among movement organizations', in Kriesberg, L. (ed.) *Research in Social Movement, Conflicts and Change*, vol. 3, Greenwich, CT: JAI Press.

Zald, M. and McCarthy, J. (1990) *Social movements in an organizational society: collected essays*, New Brunswick, NJ: Transaction Books.

Zaller, J. (1992) *The nature and orgins of mass opinion*, Cambridge: Cambridge University Press.

Zelwietro, J. (1998) 'The politicization of environmental organizations through the internet', *The Information Society* 14: 45–56.

Zoonen, L. van (1992) 'The women's movement and the media: constructing a public identity', *European Journal of Communication* 7: 453–476.

Zoonen, L. van (2000) *Virtuele vrouwen: constructies van gender online* (oratie), Universiteit Maastricht.

Zoonen, L. van (2001) 'Les écologistes français. Des experts en action', *Revue Française de Science Politique* 51, 1–2: 105–130.

Index